PUTTING EVIDENCE *INTO* PRACTICE

A POCKET GUIDE TO
Cancer Symptom Management

Edited by
Margaret Irwin, PhD, RN, MN,
and Lee Ann Johnson, PhD(c), RN

Oncology Nursing Society
Pittsburgh, Pennsylvania

ONS Publications Department

Executive Director, Professional Practice and Programs: Elizabeth Wertz Evans, PhD, RN, MPM, CPHQ, CPHIMS, FHIMSS, FACMPE
Publisher and Director of Publications: William A. Tony, BA, CQIA
Managing Editor: Lisa M. George, BA
Assistant Managing Editor: Amy Nicoletti, BA, JD
Copy Editor: Laura Pinchot, BA
Graphic Designer: Dany Sjoen
Editorial Assistant: Judy Holmes

Library of Congress Cataloging-in-Publication Data

Putting evidence into practice. A pocket guide to cancer symptom management / edited by Margaret Irwin and Lee Ann Johnson.

p. ; cm.

Pocket guide to cancer symptom management

Includes bibliographical references and index.

ISBN 978-1-935864-54-7

I. Irwin, Margaret, editor. II. Johnson, Lee Ann (Registered nurse), editor. III. Oncology Nursing Society, issuing body. IV. Title: Pocket guide to cancer symptom management.

[DNLM: 1. Neoplasms--nursing--Handbooks. 2. Evidence-Based Nursing--Handbooks. 3. Neoplasms--therapy--Handbooks. WY 49]

RC266

616.99'40231--dc23

2014023452

Publisher's Note

This book is published by the Oncology Nursing Society (ONS). ONS neither represents nor guarantees that the practices described herein will, if followed, ensure safe and effective patient care. The recommendations contained in this book reflect ONS's judgment regarding the state of general knowledge and practice in the field as of the date of publication. The recommendations may not be appropriate for use in all circumstances. Those who use this book should make their own determinations regarding specific safe and appropriate patient care practices, taking into account the personnel, equipment, and practices available at the hospital or other facility at which they are located. The editors and publisher cannot be held responsible for any liability incurred as a consequence from the use or application of any of the contents of this book. Figures and tables are used as examples only. They are not meant to be all-inclusive, nor do they represent endorsement of any particular institution by ONS. Mention of specific products and opinions related to those products do not indicate or imply endorsement by ONS. Websites mentioned are provided for information only; the hosts are responsible for their own content and availability. Unless otherwise indicated, dollar amounts reflect U.S. dollars.

ONS publications are originally published in English. Publishers wishing to translate ONS publications must contact ONS about licensing arrangements. ONS publications cannot be translated without obtaining written permission from ONS. (Individual tables and figures that are reprinted or adapted require additional permission from the original source.) Because translations from English may not always be accurate or precise, ONS disclaims any responsibility for inaccuracies in words or meaning that may occur as a result of the translation. Readers relying on precise information should check the original English version.

Printed in the United States of America

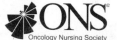

Integrity • Innovation • Stewardship • Advocacy • Excellence • Inclusiveness

Contributors

Editors

Margaret Irwin, PhD, RN, MN
Research Associate
Oncology Nursing Society
Pittsburgh, Pennsylvania
Chapter 1. PEP Up Your Practice: A Portable Evidence Guide for Clinicians; Chapter 2. Anorexia; Chapter 3. Anxiety; Chapter 4. Caregiver Strain and Burden; Chapter 7. Constipation; Chapter 9. Diarrhea; Chapter 11. Fatigue; Chapter 15. Pain; Chapter 16. Peripheral Neuropathy; Chapter 18. Radiodermatitis

Lee Ann Johnson, PhD(c), RN
Research Associate
Oncology Nursing Society
Pittsburgh, Pennsylvania
Chapter 6. Cognitive Impairment; Chapter 7. Constipation; Chapter 9. Diarrhea; Chapter 10. Dyspnea; Chapter 12. Hot Flashes; Chapter 13. Lymphedema; Chapter 14. Mucositis; Chapter 19. Skin Effects

Authors

Angela Adames, RN, BSN, OCN®
Memorial Sloan-Kettering Cancer Center
New York, New York
Chapter 10. Dyspnea

Deborah H. Allen, PhD, RN, AOCNP®
Duke University Hospital
Durham, North Carolina
Chapter 6. Cognitive Impairment

Marcia Beck, RN, ACNS-BC, CLT-LANA
Truman Medical Centers
Kansas City, Missouri
Chapter 13. Lymphedema

Ann M. Berger, PhD, APRN, AOCNS®, FAAN
College of Nursing
University of Nebraska Medical Center
Omaha, Nebraska
Chapter 20. Sleep-Wake Disturbances

Jeannine M. Brant, PhD, APRN, AOCN®
Billings Clinic Cancer Center
Billings, Montana
Chapter 15. Pain

Catherine Cherwin, MS, RN
School of Nursing
University of Wisconsin at Madison
Madison, Wisconsin
Chapter 5. Chemotherapy-Induced Nausea and Vomiting

Jie Deng, PhD, RN, OCN®
School of Nursing
Vanderbilt University
Nashville, Tennessee
Chapter 13. Lymphedema

Genevieve Desaulniers, MS, CPNP-PC, RN
WellStar Health System
Kennesaw, Georgia
Chapter 20. Sleep-Wake Disturbances

Colleen H. Erb, MSN, ACNP-BC, AOCNP®
Hospital of the University of Pennsylvania
Philadelphia, Pennsylvania
Chapter 17. Prevention of Infection

Maria Paz Fernandez-Ortega, PhD(c), RN
Catalan Institute of Oncology
Durán i Reynals Hospital
Barcelona, Spain
Chapter 12. Hot Flashes

Caryl D. Fulcher, MSN, RN, CNS-BC
Duke University Hospital
Durham, North Carolina
Chapter 8. Depression

Tracy K. Gosselin, PhD, RN, MSN, AOCN®
Duke Cancer Institute
Durham, North Carolina
Chapter 18. Radiodermatitis

Dale Grimmer, RN, MS, AOCN®, CCRC
Fox Valley Hematology and Oncology
Appleton, Wisconsin
Chapter 12. Hot Flashes

Marilyn J. Hammer, PhD, DC, RN
College of Nursing
New York University
New York, New York
Chapter 17. Prevention of Infection

Karen S. Henry, ARNP, FNP-BC, MSN, AOCNP®
Sylvester Comprehensive Cancer Center
University of Miami Health System
Miami, Florida
Chapter 14. Mucositis

Ahlam Jadalla, PhD, RN
California State University, Long Beach
Long Beach, California
Chapter 4. Caregiver Strain and Burden

Catherine E. Jansen, PhD, RN, AOCNS®
Kaiser Permanente Medical Center
San Francisco, California
Chapter 6. Cognitive Impairment

Heeju Kim, PhD, RN, OCN®
College of Nursing
Catholic University of Korea
Seoul, South Korea
Chapter 8. Depression

Colleen Lewis, MSN, ANP-BC, AOCNP®
Emory Healthcare
Atlanta, Georgia
Chapter 5. Chemotherapy-Induced Nausea and Vomiting

Ellyn E. Matthews, PhD, RN, AOCN®, CBSM
College of Nursing
University of Colorado
Aurora, Colorado
Chapter 20. Sleep-Wake Disturbances

Sandra A. Mitchell, PhD, CRNP, AOCN®
National Cancer Institute
Rockville, Maryland
Chapter 11. Fatigue

Marilyn Omabegho, RN, MSN, OCN®, NE-BC
Robert Wood Johnson Hospital
New Brunswick, New Jersey
Chapter 18. Radiodermatitis

Julie L. Otte, PhD, RN, OCN®
School of Nursing
Indiana University
Indianapolis, Indiana
Chapter 20. Sleep-Wake Disturbances

Margaretta S. Page, MS, RN
University of California,
   San Francisco
San Francisco, California
Chapter 20. Sleep-Wake Disturbances

Mary E. Peterson, MS, RN,
ANP-BC, AOCNP®
Banner MD Anderson Cancer
   Center
Gilbert, Arizona
Chapter 17. Prevention of Infection

Patricia Poirier, PhD, RN, AOCN®
University of Maine
Orono, Maine
Chapter 11. Fatigue

Barbara B. Rogers, CRNP, MN,
AOCN®, ANP-BC
Fox Chase Cancer Center
Philadelphia, Pennsylvania
Chapter 2. Anorexia

Hanan Saca-Hazboun, PhD(c), RN
Bethlehem University
Bethlehem, Palestine
Chapter 14. Mucositis

Celestine Samuel-Blalock, MSNL-
HCS, PHN, RN-BC
St. Francis Medical Center
Lynnwood, California
Chapter 14. Mucositis

Deborah L. Selm-Orr, RN, MS,
DNP(c), CRNP, AOCN®
Cancer Treatment Centers of
   America
Philadelphia, Pennsylvania
*Chapter 5. Chemotherapy-
Induced Nausea and Vomiting*

Bethany Sterling, MSN, CRNP,
ANP-BC, OCN®, CHPN
Abramson Cancer Center
University of Pennsylvania
Philadelphia, Pennsylvania
Chapter 15. Pain

Cindy Tofthagen, PhD, ARNP,
AOCNP®, FAANP
University of South Florida
Tampa, Florida
Chapter 16. Peripheral Neuropathy

Karen L. Visich, MSN, ANP-BC,
AOCNP®
Virtua Memorial Hospital
Mount Holly, New Jersey
Chapter 15. Pain

Diane Von Ah, PhD, RN
Science of Nursing Care
   Department
Indiana University
Indianapolis, Indiana
Chapter 6. Cognitive Impairment

Deborah K. Walker, DNP, FNP-BC,
AOCN®
School of Nursing
University of Alabama at
   Birmingham
Birmingham, Alabama
Chapter 3. Anxiety

Dwanna M. Ward-Boahen, RN,
BSN, MSN, AOCNP®
St. Vincent's Medical Center
Bridgeport, Connecticut
*Chapter 5. Chemotherapy-
Induced Nausea and Vomiting*

Stacy Whiteside, RN, MS,
CPNP-AC/PC, CPON®
Hematology/Oncology Depart-
   ment
Nationwide Children's Hospital
Columbus, Ohio
*Chapter 5. Chemotherapy-
Induced Nausea and Vomiting*

Barbara J. Wilson, MS, RN,
ACNS-BC, AOCN®
WellStar Regional Medical Center
Marietta, Georgia
Chapter 17. Prevention of Infection

Laura J. Zitella, MS, RN,
ACNP-BC, AOCN®
Stanford University Medical Center
Stanford, California
Chapter 17. Prevention of Infection

Oncology Nursing Society Staff

Christine Maloney, BA
Associate Archivist

Mark Vrabel, MLS, AHIP, ELS
Information Resources Supervisor

Kerri Moriarty, MLS
Research Specialist

Disclosure

Editors and authors of books and guidelines provided by the Oncology Nursing Society are expected to disclose to the readers any significant financial interest or other relationships with the manufacturer(s) of any commercial products.

A vested interest may be considered to exist if a contributor is affiliated with or has a financial interest in commercial organizations that may have a direct or indirect interest in the subject matter. A "financial interest" may include, but is not limited to, being a shareholder in the organization; being an employee of the commercial organization; serving on an organization's speakers bureau; or receiving research from the organization. An "affiliation" may be holding a position on an advisory board or some other role of benefit to the commercial organization. Vested interest statements appear in the front matter for each publication.

Contributors are expected to disclose any unlabeled or investigational use of products discussed in their content. This information is acknowledged solely for the information of the readers.

The contributors provided the following disclosure and vested interest information:

Margaret Irwin, PhD, RN, MN: Boehringer Ingelheim, consultant or advisory role

Lee Ann Johnson, PhD(c), RN: American Cancer Society, research funding

Jeannine M. Brant, PhD, APRN, AOCN®: American Society of Clinical Oncology, Palliative Care Symposium Committee; *Journal of the Advanced Practitioner in Oncology*, associate editor, leadership positions; American Society of Clinical Oncology, Genentech Oncology, honoraria

Maria Paz Fernandez-Ortega, PhD(c), RN: Regional Conference on Chemical Engineering, Enfermeria Clinica, reviewer; Scientific Committee European Congress, expert testimony

Tracy K. Gosselin, PhD, RN, MSN, AOCN®: Oncology Nursing Society, honoraria; The DAISY Foundation, research funding

Julie L. Otte, PhD, RN, OCN®: On Q Health, honoraria

Deborah L. Selm-Orr, RN, MS, DNP(c), CRNP, AOCN®: Bayer, Amgen, honoraria

Cindy Tofthagen, PhD, ARNP, AOCNP®, FAANP: Oncology Nursing Society, Medscape Oncology, honoraria; American Cancer Society, ONS Foundation, research funding

Deborah K. Walker, DNP, FNP-BC, AOCN®: Hematology/Oncology Associates of Alabama, inPractice Oncology, STV Health System, Regional Medical Center, honoraria; Women's Breast Health Fund, research funding

Barbara J. Wilson, MS, RN, ACNS-BC, AOCN®: Amgen, honoraria

Laura J. Zitella, MS, RN, ACNP-BC, AOCN®: Teva Oncology, On Q Health, Gilead, consultant or advisory role

Acknowledgments

Special thanks to the following individuals for their contributions to previous versions of the PEP resources:

Anorexia
Lynn A. Adams, RN, MS, ANP, AOCN®, Rose Ann Caruso, RN, OCN®, Regina S. Cunningham, PhD, RN, AOCN®, Martha J. Norling, RN, OCN®, and Nancy Shepard, RN, MS, AOCN®

Anxiety
Terry A. Badger, PhD, RN, CS, FAAN, Amy H. Dolce, RN, APN, MS, AOCN®, CHPN, Kathy Marsh, RN, Lisa Kennedy Sheldon, PhD, APRN-BC, AOCNP®, Julie A. Summers, RN, BSN, and Susan A. Swanson, RN, MS, AOCN®

Caregiver Strain and Burden
Ruth Ann Brintnall, PhD, RN, CHPN, Deirdre B. Colao, RN, OCN®, Barbara A. Given, PhD, RN, FAAN, Norissa J. Honea, PhD(c), MSN, RN, AOCN®, CCRP, Laurel L. Northouse, PhD, RN, FAAN, Paula R. Sherwood, PhD, RN, CNRN, and Susan Claire Somers, RN, BSN, OCN®

Chemotherapy-Induced Nausea and Vomiting
Laurel A. Barbour, MSN, RN, AOCN®, Patricia J. Friend, PhD, APRN, AOCN®, Mary Pat Johnston, RN, MS, AOCN®, Marilyn K. Kayne, BSN, RN, OCN®, Roxanne W. McDaniel, PhD, RN, Marita L. Ripple, RN, and Janelle M. Tipton, MSN, RN, AOCN®

Cognitive Impairment
Rachel Behrendt, DNP, MSN, APN-C, AOCNS®, Phyllis Gagnon, RN, BSN, OCN®, and Rosalina M. Schiavone, RN, BSN, OCN®

Constipation
Annette Kay Bisanz, RN, BSN, MPH, Stephanie Fulton, MSIS, Lindsay Gaido, MSN, RN, Hannah F. Lyons, MSN, RN, BC, AOCN®, Myra J. Woolery, MN, RN, CPON®, and Mary Yenulevich, BSN, RN, OCN®

Depression
Terry A. Badger, PhD, RN, CS, FAAN, Ashley K. Gunter, RN, BSN, OCN®, Joyce A. Marrs, MS, APRN-BC, AOCNP®, and Jill M. Reese, RN, BSN, OCN®

Diarrhea
Rachel Christine Drabot, MPH, CNSD, RD, Elizabeth S. Kiker, RN, OCN®, Paula Muehlbauer, RN, MSN, OCN®, ACHPN, and Barbara L. Rawlings, RN, BSN

Dyspnea
Ann E. Culkin, RN, OCN®, Wendye M. DiSalvo, RN, ARNP, MS, AOCN®, Kathleen Mackay, RN, BSN, OCN®, and Leslie B. Tyson, MS, APRN-BC, OCN®

Fatigue
Susan L. Beck, PhD, APRN, AOCN®, Linda Edwards Hood, MSN, RN, AOCN®, Katen Moore, MSN, APRN, AOCN®, and Ellen R. Tanner, RN, BSN, OCN®

Hot Flashes
Diane Cope, RN, PhD, ARNP-BC, AOCNP®, Stacey Hill, RN, BSN, Marcie Jacobson, RN, BSN, OCN®, Elizabeth Keating, RN, MS, NP, CBCN®, and Suzanne Mahon, RN, DNSc, AOCN®, APNG

Lymphedema
Ellen G. Poage, MSN, FNP-C, MPH, CLT-LANA, Melanie D. Poundall, RN, M. Jeanne Shellabarger, RN, BSN, and Marybeth Singer, MS, APRN-BC, AOCN®, ACHPN

Mucositis
Jane M. Armer, RN, PhD, Barbara J. Cashavelly, MSN, RN, AOCN®, and Amber Harriman, RN

Pain
Lisa B. Aiello-Laws, RN, MSN, APNG, AOCNS®, Suzanne W. Ameringer, PhD, RN, Marie A. Bakitas, RN, DNSc, ARNP, AOCN®, FAAN, Nancy A. Delzer, MSN, RN, AOCN®, BC-PCM, Mary E. Peterson, RN, OCN®, and Janice K. Reynolds, RN, BSN, OCN®

Peripheral Neuropathy
Linda I. Abbott, RN, MSN, AOCN®, CWON, Julie A. Aschenbrenner, RN, OCN®, and Connie Hart, RN, BSN, OCN®

Prevention of Infection
Felicia Andrews, RN, BSN, Christopher R. Friese, PhD, MS, RN, AOCN®, Barbara Holmes Gobel, MS, RN, AOCN®, Jody Hauser, RN, MS, NP, Colleen O'Leary, MSN, RN, AOCNS®, and Myra Woolery, RN, MN

Radiodermatitis
Tara Baney, RN, MS, ANP-BC, AOCN®, Kathleen Bell, RN, MSN, OCN®, Susan Bruce, RN, MSN, OCN®, Marilyn Haas, PhD, RN, CNS, ANP-C, and Linda Weis-Smith, RN, OCN®

Skin Effects
Therese Carpizo, MSN, RN, AOCN®, and Denise Portz, BSN, RN, OCN®

Sleep-Wake Disturbances
Lauran B. Johnson, RN, MSN

Contents

PEP UP YOUR PRACTICE: A Portable Evidence Guide for Clinicians

Margaret Irwin, PhD, RN, MN

Introduction

The importance of using evidence in clinical practice to provide high-quality patient care is well recognized. Evidence-based practice necessitates availability of evidence that is systematically appraised and synthesized. Since 2006, the Oncology Nursing Society (ONS) Putting Evidence Into Practice (PEP) program has provided clinicians with resources to meet this need in caring for patients with cancer and their caregivers.

The ONS PEP program began with four teams that synthesized evidence for interventions in four topic areas. Since that time, the PEP program has expanded to 20 topics with synthesis of evidence from more than 1,700 publications. Currently, more than 150 ONS members from across the United States and several other countries contribute to this work. PEP resources are currently provided in multiple formats including books, articles, monographs, and open-access web-based materials that are available on the ONS website at www.ons.org/practice-resources/pep. Several publications are also currently available through the National Guideline Clearinghouse (www.guidelines.gov).

In 2012, an ONS project team was formed to review the PEP program and make recommendations for future directions. This book was created to meet one of those recommendations—provision of a practical and abbreviated version of PEP evidence syntheses in a format that can be used as a reference in clinical practice. This book updates evidence in 19 of the PEP topics for which substantial new evidence was found; Prevention of Bleeding is not included here due to minimal additional evidence. Specific information for application to practice is included for each topic to assist clinicians with applying the evidence.

The PEP Process

Search Strategy

In 2010, literature searching was centralized at ONS and specific inclusion and exclusion criteria were established. The standard databases used are Medline, CINAHL® (Cumulative Index to Nursing and Allied Health Literature), and the Cochrane Collaboration. For all topics, inclusion criteria are (a) the sample must include patients with cancer, (b) research articles must report results in the specific outcome/topic of interest, (c) the articles must be in English, (d) research studies, systematic reviews, professional consensus, and evidence-based guidelines are included, and (e) the reference addresses interventions. Exclusion criteria are (a) gray literature, (b) studies that are only descriptive in nature, and (c) studies that use only qualitative methods. Some topic teams have identified additional topic-specific inclusion and exclusion criteria. A full description of search terms and criteria for each topic can be found on the ONS website. Evidence that was obtained prior to establishing these criteria in 2010 has been retained in the resources, although some of this is not specific to the care of patients with cancer.

It should be noted that the publication and retrieval of evidence is a dynamic process with ongoing additions to the full body of knowledge about interventions. In each chapter of this book, the time frame in which the evidence was retrieved is identified. Evidence retrieved after these dates will be included in future PEP updates.

Evidence Summary and Synthesis

An ONS staff member reviews published abstracts that were retrieved against the inclusion and exclusion criteria. Another

ONS staff member then reviews the full article and, if criteria are met, assigns the summary and appraisal to a PEP topic team member. Topic team members then confirm full articles meet the criteria. Team members appraise the evidence and complete a summary for the evidence on a standardized form. Another team member peer-reviews the summary. The topic team reviews the results of all summaries via web and phone conferences, and the summaries are categorized according to the PEP classification schema shown in Figure 1. Complete details of the criteria for each PEP classification level can be found at www.ons.org/ons-pep-weight-evidence-classification-schema. PEP topic teams include nurse scientists, advanced practice nurses, and staff nurses who have expertise and interest in the topic.

How to Use This Book

This book is intended to identify the strength of the evidence to answer, "What interventions are effective?" This book is not intended to provide a detailed analysis of literature included. Further detail in summaries for each reference can be accessed on the ONS website. These summaries provide description of the sample, the intervention, research design, findings, limitations, and implications for nursing. Web-based resources can be viewed via computer or mobile devices, and print capability is provided.

Each chapter in this book outlines the nature, incidence, and impact of the symptom for patients with cancer, factors that create the highest risk, key aspects of assessment and identification of some assessment tools, intervention evidence, and suggestions for application to practice. Risk factors can be used to prioritize those patients who are most likely to experience the problem and need further assessment and intervention for prevention or symptom management. Classification of each intervention identifies those with the strongest supportive evidence of effectiveness. This information can be used to select interventions that are feasible and acceptable to and appropriate for the patient and have the strongest supportive evidence for application in patient care.

Through personal feedback and surveys, nurses have indicated that they apply and use PEP resources in the following ways.

- Inclusion of interventions with strong evidence into nursing care plans
- Inclusion of interventions with strong evidence into standing physician orders and order sets
- Patient teaching and development of patient teaching aids
- Provision of summaries in interdisciplinary discussions and meetings. Nurses have told us that sharing PEP evidence summaries establishes credibility with other professional groups.
- Education of nursing and other professional staff
- Identification of the evidence in nursing policies and procedures
- Provision of the ONS PEP web address on the organization's intranet or library site to facilitate access
- Identification of areas for research, quality improvement, and evidence-based practice implementation projects

Figure 1. ONS PEP Classification Schema

Recommended for Practice—Interventions for which effectiveness has been demonstrated by strong evidence from rigorously designed studies, meta-analyses, or systematic reviews and for which expectation of harms is small compared with the benefits

Likely to Be Effective—Interventions for which the evidence is less well-established than for those listed under Recommended for Practice

Benefits Balanced With Harms—Interventions for which clinicians and patients should weigh the beneficial and harmful effects according to individual circumstances and priorities

Effectiveness Not Established—Interventions for which there are currently insufficient data or data of inadequate quality

Effectiveness Unlikely—Interventions for which lack of effectiveness is less well-established than for those listed under Not Recommended for Practice

Not Recommended for Practice—Interventions for which ineffectiveness or harmfulness has been demonstrated by clear evidence, or the cost or burden necessary for the intervention exceeds anticipated benefit

Expert Opinion—Interventions that are low risk, recommended by an expert in the field, and consistent with sound clinical practice

Specific criteria for each of these categories are applied. A full listing of all classification criteria can be found at www.ons.org/ons-pep-weight-evidence-classification -schema.

Note. From "ONS PEP Weight-of-Evidence Classification Schema: Decision Rules for Summative Evaluation of a Body of Evidence," by S.A. Mitchell and C.R. Friese, n.d. Retrieved from https://www.ons.org/ons-pep-weight-evidence-classification -schema. Copyright by the Oncology Nursing Society. Adapted with permission.

2

Anorexia

*Margaret Irwin, PhD, RN, MN,
and Barbara B. Rogers, CRNP, MN, AOCN®, ANP-BC*

Problem and Incidence

Anorexia is a common symptom in people with cancer and a component of the anorexia-cachexia syndrome. It is the lack or loss of appetite or desire to eat. Anorexia leads to reduced intake; however, anorexia alone does not account for the complex alterations that characterize the anorexia-cachexia syndrome.[1] Anorexia is associated with metabolic derangements, including release of pro-inflammatory cytokines such as interleukin (IL)-1, IL-6, and tumor necrosis factor-alpha produced by the immune system and tumor cells.[1,2] Anorexia is the most common cause of decreased nutrient intake that triggers malnutrition and muscle wasting.[3] The prevalence of anorexia in individuals with cancer is highly variable but has been reported to be 40% at diagnosis and 70% in advanced disease.[3]

Risk Factors and Assessment

Risk factors for anorexia include
- Advanced disease
- Symptoms such as depression and pain that affect appetite
- Treatment side effects such as nausea and vomiting
- Location of tumor that interferes with ability to eat (e.g., head and neck, gastrointestinal).

Assessment related to anorexia should include
- Measurement of body weight and lean body mass
- Identification of any unplanned weight loss
- Assessment of appetite and changes in appetite.

Assessment tools include
- Functional Assessment of Anorexia/Cachexia Therapy Questionnaire
- Numeric or visual analog scale for patient self-report of appetite.

What interventions are effective in managing anorexia in people with cancer?

Evidence retrieved through December 31, 2013

Recommended for Practice

Corticosteroids have been recommended in professional guidelines[4] and were associated with some improvement in appetite.[5,6]

Progestins (megestrol/megestrol acetate) improved appetite in patients at various phases of care in multiple research studies and systematic reviews.[4,7-12]

Likely to Be Effective

Dietary counseling with and without use of oral nutritional supplements improved energy intake and appetite.[13-15]

Effectiveness Not Established

Several interventions have shown mixed results in studies or were examined in small groups of patients with inconclusive findings. These include
- **Astragali Radix**, an herbal mixture[16]
- **Cyproheptadine**, an antihistamine[4]
- **Ghrelin**, a hormone that acts on the hypothalamus[17-19]

- **Melatonin,**[20] which was not found to be effective in a systematic review[6]
- **Mirtazapine**[21]
- **OHR-118,** a peptide nucleic acid[22]
- **Omega-3 fatty acid supplementation** alone or in combination with megestrol[23,24]—A systematic review showed no difference in appetite with this intervention.[6]
- **Oral branched-chain amino acids**[25]
- **Pentoxifylline**[4]
- **Rikkunshito,** a traditional Japanese medicine[26]
- **Thalidomide,** which had mixed results for tolerability and effectiveness.[12,27-32]

Effectiveness Unlikely

Carnitine/L-carnitine did not improve appetite in patients with cancer in several research studies.[30,33,34]

Not Recommended for Practice

Cannabis/cannabinoids did not improve anorexia in a large multicenter trial[35] or in a systematic review.[6]

Application to Practice

Patients at risk for anorexia should be assessed for appetite level, appetite changes, and weight loss during cancer treatment.

Interventions for which there is strong evidence of effectiveness, including administration of progestins and corticosteroids, should be considered for management.

Nurses can counsel patients regarding nutritional needs and teach patients about the use of nutritional supplements that are likely to be effective.

Patients with severe anorexia, weight loss, or comorbid conditions that necessitate dietary restrictions or specific dietary interventions should be referred to a registered dietitian for in-depth counseling and education.

Anorexia Resource Contributors

Paula Caron, MS, ARNP, ACHPN, Barbara B. Rogers, CRNP, MN, AOCN®, ANP-BC, and Meghan L. Underhill, PhD, RN, AOCNS®

References

1. Mantovani, G., Madeddu, C., & Maccio, A. (2013). Drugs in development for treatment of patients with cancer-related anorexia and cachexia syndrome. *Drug Design, Development and Therapy, 7,* 645–656. doi:10.2147/DDDT.S39771

2. Argilés, J.M., Busquets, S., Toledo, M., & López-Soriano, F.J. (2009). The role of cytokines in cancer cachexia. *Current Opinion in Supportive and Palliative Care, 3,* 263–268. doi:10.1097/SPC.0b013e3283311d09

3. Ribaudo, J.M., Cella, D., Hahn, E.A., Lloyd, S.R., Tchekmedyian, N.S., Von Roenn, J., & Leslie, W.T. (2001). Re-validation and shortening of the Functional Assessment of Anorexia/Cachexia Therapy (FAACT) Questionnaire. *Quality of Life Research, 9,* 1137–1146. doi:10.1023/A:1016670403148

4. Desport, J.C., Gory-Delabaere, G., Blanc-Vincent, M.P., Bachmann, P., Béal, J., Benamouzig, R., ... Senesse, P. (2003). Standards, options and recommendations for the use of appetite stimulants in oncology (2000). *British Journal of Cancer, 89*(Suppl. 1), S98–S100. doi:10.1038/sj.bjc.6601090

5. Bruera, E., Roca, E., Cedaro, L., Carraro, S., & Chacon, R. (1985). Action of oral methylprednisolone in terminal cancer patients: A prospective randomized double-blind study. *Cancer Treatment Reports, 69,* 751–754.

6. Yavuzsen, T., Davis, M.P., Walsh, D., LeGrand, S., & Lagman, R. (2005). Systematic review of the treatment of cancer-associated anorexia and weight loss. *Journal of Clinical Oncology, 23,* 8500–8511. doi:10.1200/JCO.2005.01.8010

7. Berenstein, E.G., & Ortiz, Z. (2005). Megestrol acetate for the treatment of anorexia-cachexia syndrome. *Cochrane Database of Systematic Reviews, 2005*(2). doi:10.1002/14651858.CD004310.pub2

8. Jatoi, A., Windschitl, H.E., Loprinzi, C.L., Sloan, J.A., Dakhil, S.R., Mailliard, J.A., ... Christensen, B. (2002). Dronabinol versus megestrol acetate versus combination therapy for cancer-associated anorexia: A North Central Cancer Treatment Group study. *Journal of Clinical Oncology, 20,* 567–573. doi:10.1200/JCO.20.2.567

9. Lesniak, W., Bala, M., Jaeschke, R., & Krzakowski, M. (2008). Effects of megestrol acetate in patients with cancer anorexia-cachexia syndrome—A systematic review and meta-analysis. *Polskie Archiwum Medycyny Wewnętrznej, 118,* 636–644.

10. Ruiz Garcia, V., López-Briz, E., Carbonell Sanchis, R., Gonzalvez Perales, J.L., & Bort-Marti, S. (2013). Megestrol acetate for treatment of anorexia-cachexia syndrome. *Cochrane Database of Systematic Reviews, 2013*(3). doi:10.1002/14651858.CD004310.pub3

11. Tomiska, M., Tomiskova, M., Salajka, F., Adam, Z., & Vorlicek, J. (2003). Palliative treatment of cancer anorexia with oral suspension of megestrol acetate. *Neoplasma, 50,* 227–233.

12. Wen, H.-S., Li, X., Cao, Y.-Z., Zhang, C.-C., Yang, F., Shi, Y.-M., & Peng, L.-M. (2012). Clinical studies on the treatment of cancer cachexia with megestrol acetate plus thalidomide. *Chemotherapy, 58,* 461–467. doi:10.1159/000346446

13. Baldwin, C., Spiro, A., Ahern, R., & Emery, P.W. (2012). Oral nutritional interventions in malnourished patients with cancer: A systematic review and meta-analysis. *Journal of the National Cancer Institute, 104,* 371–385. doi:10.1093/jnci/djr556

14. Brown, J.K. (2002). A systematic review of the evidence on symptom management of cancer-related anorexia and cachexia. *Oncology Nursing Forum, 29,* 517–530. doi:10.1188/02.ONF.517-532

15. Ravasco, P., Monteiro-Grillo, I., Vidal, P.M., & Camilo, M. (2005). Dietary counseling improves patient outcomes: A prospective, randomized, controlled trial in colorectal cancer patients undergoing radiotherapy. *Journal of Clinical Oncology, 23,* 1431–1438. doi:10.1200/JCO.2005.02.054

16. Lee, J.J., & Lee, J.J. (2010). A phase II study of an herbal decoction that includes Astragali Radix for cancer-associated anorexia in patients with advanced cancer. *Integrative Cancer Therapies, 9,* 24–31. doi:10.1177/1534735409359180

17. Garcia, J.M., Friend, J., & Allen, S. (2013). Therapeutic potential of anamorelin, a novel, oral ghrelin mimetic, in patients with cancer-related cachexia: A multicenter, randomized, double-blind, crossover, pilot study. *Supportive Care in Cancer, 21,* 129–137. doi:10.1007/s00520-012-1500-1

18. Hiura, Y., Takiguchi, S., Yamamoto, K., Takahashi, T., Kurokawa, Y., Yamasaki, M., ... Doki, Y. (2012). Effects of ghrelin administration during chemotherapy with advanced esophageal cancer patients: A prospective, randomized, placebo-controlled phase 2 study. *Cancer, 118,* 4785–4794. doi:10.1002/cncr.27430

19. Neary, N.M., Small, C.J., Wren, A.M., Lee, J.L., Druce, M.R., Palmieri, C., ... Bloom, S.R. (2004). Ghrelin increases energy intake in cancer patients with impaired appetite: Acute, randomized, placebo-controlled trial. *Journal of Clinical Endocrinology and Metabolism, 89,* 2832–2836. doi:10.1210/jc.2003-031768

20. Del Fabbro, E., Dev, R., Hui, D., Palmer, L., & Bruera, E. (2013). Effects of melatonin on appetite and other symptoms in patients with advanced cancer and cachexia: A double-blind placebo-controlled trial. *Journal of Clinical Oncology, 31,* 1271–1276. doi:10.1200/JCO.2012.43.6766

21. Riechelmann, R.P., Burman, D., Tannock, I.F., Rodin, G., & Zimmermann, C. (2010). Phase II trial of mirtazapine for cancer-related cachexia and anorexia. *American Journal of Hospice and Palliative Care, 27,* 106–110. doi:10.1177/1049909109345685

22. Chasen, M., Hirschman, S.Z., & Bhargava, R. (2011). Phase II study of the novel peptide-nucleic acid OHR118 in the management of cancer-related anorexia/cachexia. *Journal of the American Medical Directors Association, 12,* 62–67. doi:10.1016/j.jamda.2010.02.012

23. Bruera, E., Strasser, F., Palmer, J.L., Willey, J., Calder, K., Amyotte, G., & Baracos, V. (2003). Effect of fish oil on appetite and other symptoms in patients with advanced cancer and anorexia/cachexia: A double-blind, placebo-controlled study. *Journal of Clinical Oncology, 21,* 129–134. doi:10.1200/JCO.2003.01.101

24. Jatoi, A., Rowland, K., Loprinzi, C.L., Sloan, J.A., Dakhil, S.R., MacDonald, N., ... Christensen, B. (2004). An eicosapentaenoic acid supplement versus megestrol acetate versus both for patients with cancer-associated wasting: A North Central Cancer Treatment Group and National Cancer Institute of Canada collaborative effort. *Journal of Clinical Oncology, 22,* 2469–2476. doi:10.1200/JCO.2004.06.024

25. Cangiano, C., Laviano, A., Meguid, M.M., Mulieri, M., Conversano, L., Preziosa, I., & Rossi-Fanelli, F. (1996). Effects of administration of oral branched-chain amino acids on anorexia and caloric intake in cancer patients. *Journal of the National Cancer Institute, 88,* 550–552. doi:10.1093/jnci/88.8.550

26. Ohno, T., Yanai, M., Ando, H., Toyomasu, Y., Ogawa, A., Morita, H., ... Kuwano, H. (2011). Rikkunshito, a traditional Japanese medicine, suppresses cisplatin-induced anorexia in humans. *Clinical and Experimental Gastroenterology, 4,* 291–296. doi:10.2147/CEG.S26297

27. Bruera, E., Neumann, C.M., Pituskin, E., Calder, K., Ball, G., & Hanson, J. (1999). Thalidomide in patients with cachexia due to terminal cancer: Preliminary report. *Annals of Oncology, 10,* 857–859. doi:10.1023/A:1008329821941

28. Davis, M., Lasheen, W., Walsh, D., Mahmoud, F., Bicanovsky, L., & Lagman, R. (2012). A phase II dose titration study of thalidomide for cancer-associated anorexia. *Journal of Pain and Symptom Management, 43,* 78–86. doi:10.1016/j.jpainsymman.2011.03.007

29. Gordon, J.N., Trebble, T.M., Ellis, R.D., Duncan, H.D., Johns, T., & Goggin, P.M. (2005). Thalidomide in the treatment of cancer cachexia: A randomised placebo controlled trial. *Gut, 54,* 540–545. doi:10.1136/gut.2004.047563

30. Mantovani, G., Maccio, A., Madeddu, C., Serpe, R., Massa, E., Dessi, M., ... Contu, P. (2010). Randomized phase III clinical trial of five different arms of treatment in 332 patients with cancer cachexia. *Oncologist, 15,* 200–211. doi:10.1634/theoncologist.2009-0153

31. Wilkes, E.A., Selby, A.L., Cole, A.T., Freeman, J.G., Rennie, M.J., & Khan, Z.H. (2011). Poor tolerability of thalidomide in end-stage oesophageal cancer. *European Journal of Cancer Care, 20,* 593–600. doi:10.1111/j.1365-2354.2011.01255.x

32. Yennurajalingam, S., Willey, J.S., Palmer, J.L., Allo, J., Del Fabbro, E., Cohen, E.N., ... Bruera, E. (2012). The role of thalidomide and placebo for the treatment of cancer-related anorexia-cachexia symptoms: Results of a double-blind placebo-controlled randomized study. *Journal of Palliative Medicine, 15,* 1059–1064. doi:10.1089/jpm.2012.0146

33. Maccio, A., Madeddu, C., Gramignano, G., Mulas, C., Floris, C., Sanna, E., ... Mantovani, G. (2012). A randomized phase III clinical trial of a combined treatment for cachexia in patients with gynecological cancers: Evaluating the impact on metabolic and inflammatory profiles and quality of life. *Gynecologic Oncology, 124,* 417–425. doi:10.1016/j.ygyno.2011.12.435

34. Madeddu, C., Dessi, M., Panzone, F., Serpe, R., Antoni, G., Cau, M.C., ... Mantovani, G. (2012). Randomized phase III clinical trial of a combined treatment with carnitine + celecoxib ± megestrol acetate for patients with cancer-related anorexia/cachexia syndrome. *Clinical Nutrition, 31,* 176–182. doi:10.1016/j.clnu.2011.10.005

35. Strasser, F., Luftner, D., Possinger, K., Ernst, G., Ruhstaller, T., Meissner, W., ... Cerny, T. (2006). Comparison of orally administered cannabis extract and delta-9-tetrahydrocannabinol in treating patients with cancer-related anorexia-cachexia syndrome: A multicenter, phase III, randomized, double-blind, placebo-controlled clinical trial from the Cannabis-In-Cachexia-Study-Group. *Journal of Clinical Oncology, 24,* 3394–3400. doi:10.1200/JCO.2005.05.1847

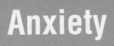

3

Anxiety

Margaret Irwin, PhD, RN, MN,
and Deborah K. Walker, DNP, FNP-BC, AOCN®

Problem and Incidence

Anxiety is an emotional and/or physical reaction to known or unknown causes.[1] Cancer is threatening, and patients may become anxious in response to that threat. In some circumstances, anxiety becomes maladaptive and persists, manifesting as panic attacks, physical symptoms, and disruption of ability to function.[2] Clinically diagnosed anxiety disorders meeting *Diagnostic and Statistical Manual of Mental Disorders* criteria have been reported in 1.3%–29% of patients with cancer.[2-5] Symptoms of anxiety may be episodic and associated with high-stress phases of cancer care.[6] Among cancer survivors, the prevalence of anxiety is significantly higher than in a health-matched control group.[7,8]

Risk Factors and Assessment

Patients may be at greater risk at certain points in the cancer trajectory, such as at diagnosis, during initial stages of treatment, before invasive procedures, and at follow-up because of concern about recurrence. Risk factors that have been identified include the following.[4,5,9]

- High risk
  - Younger age
  - Female gender
  - History of abuse
  - Social isolation
  - Home, work, and/or financial problems
  - Lower level of education
  - Inability to perform activities of daily living (ADLs)
  - History of anxiety and depression

- Uncontrolled pain or symptoms from treatment or disease
- Moderate risk
  - Drugs (e.g., corticosteroids)
  - Comorbidities (e.g., cardiac, central nervous system, endocrine, pulmonary)

Assessment for signs and symptoms of anxiety[9,10] should include the following.
- Changes in ability to perform ADLs
- Insomnia and difficulty getting to sleep because of worry
- Changes in thinking, such as apprehension, worry, feeling on edge or mentally tense, difficulty concentrating, or lack of interest
- Physical symptoms, such as muscle tension and fatigue
- Behaviors indicating irritability, restlessness, and reassurance seeking
- History of anxiety

Assessment tools include
- National Comprehensive Cancer Network Distress Thermometer Screening Tool (open access)[11]
- Generalized Anxiety Disorder-7 (GAD-7) (open access)[12]
- Hospital Anxiety and Depression Scale
- State-Trait Anxiety Inventory.

What interventions are effective in preventing and managing anxiety in people with cancer?

Evidence retrieved through June 30, 2013

Likely to Be Effective

Coaching using prompts to identify needs was examined in two studies. One small study showed no effect[13]; however, in one large randomized controlled trial, coaching reduced the prevalence of anxiety.[14]

Cognitive behavioral therapy (CBT) interventions were effective in individual[15-20] and group settings.[21-24] In one study, the intervention was provided via group videoconferencing for rural patients.[25] Two meta-analyses demonstrated significant improvements in anxiety with CBT interventions.[26,27]

Exercise showed mixed results in small studies.[28-36] One meta-analysis showed a significant effect of exercise.[37]

Massage/aromatherapy massage was examined in several studies.[20,38-47] Two systematic reviews demonstrated that massage reduced anxiety level.[48,49]

Mindfulness-based stress reduction interventions involving combinations of education and mindfulness practices such as meditation and yoga were effective in several studies.[50-55] A systematic review and meta-analysis showed a moderate to significant effect in reducing anxiety, but most studies were in women with breast cancer, study quality tended to be low, most did not include patients with clinically significant anxiety at baseline, and high heterogeneity existed among the studies, suggesting that results need to be viewed with caution.[56]

Music/music therapy was studied in adults and children.[57-66] A meta-analysis showed a positive effect of music on anxiety.[67]

Progressive muscle relaxation was associated with reduced anxiety.[68,69]

Psychoeducational interventions showed mixed results.[26,27,68-84] Four out of five meta-analyses showed small but significant reductions in anxiety. No strong support exists for any single type of psychoeducational intervention, and duration of effect is unclear.

Supportive care/support interventions had mixed results, but the bulk of evidence showed improvement in anxiety at several points in the cancer trajectory.[14,28,78,85-89] Support has been provided in person or via telephone.

Effectiveness Not Established

Numerous pharmacologic and nonpharmacologic interventions have been examined for effects on anxiety. Findings were generally mixed, and many studies were small and of nonrandomized designs.

- **Pharmacologic interventions**
  - **Antidepressants**[90-92]
  - **Anxiolytics**[93-95]
  - **Gabapentin** for women with hot flash symptoms[96]
  - **Methylphenidate**[97]
  - **Pregabalin** in patients with neuropathic pain[98]
  - **Psilocybin**, a psychotropic drug[99]
- **Communication and care coordination interventions**
  - **Computer-assisted communication** involving telephone interviews and automated feedback to caseworkers and physicians[100]
  - **Medical record access** provided proactively to patients rather than upon patient request[101]
  - **Navigation/care coordination**[102,103]
  - **Provider communication skill training**, to improve physician communication with patients newly diagnosed with cancer[104]
  - **Tailored information** including written materials, interactive computer software, and computer animation[105]
- **Complementary and alternative therapies**
  - **Acupuncture**[106,107]—A systematic review reported mixed results of acupuncture on anxiety.[108]
  - **Ama-Deus® energy healing**, a specific hand-mediated approach for energy healing[109]
  - **Art/art therapy**[110-113]
  - **Caregiver/partner interventions**[114,115]
  - **Expressive writing** to promote emotional disclosure[116,117]
  - **Homeopathy**[118]
  - **Hypnosis/hypnotherapy** before invasive procedures.[119,120] In one study, not all patients achieved induction, so effectiveness could not be determined.
  - **Meditation**[121-123]
  - **Progressive muscle relaxation and guided imagery**[26,124,125]—Although progressive muscle relaxation

has strong evidence, the addition of guided imagery did not provide additional benefit.

- **Qigong/mind-body-spirit therapy** exercises and activities based in Eastern philosophies[79]
- **Reflexology**[126-129]
- **Reiki**[130-132]
- **Relaxation therapy** involving only breathing exercises[133,134]
- **Relaxation/visual imagery** including breathing exercises and guided imagery[135]—A systematic review did not show supportive evidence.[26]
- **Structured rehabilitation services** provided by multidisciplinary teams[136-138]
- **Therapeutic touch**[43]
- **Virtual reality** during chemotherapy[139] and in children hospitalized for cancer treatment[140]
- **Yoga**[141-146]

Effectiveness Unlikely

Orientation and information provision, orienting patients to setting and processes, was examined in four studies[83, 147-149] and two systematic reviews.[27,150] No effects on anxiety were reported.

Application to Practice

Nurses can identify patients at risk for anxiety and use objective tools to assess patients for clinically relevant anxiety.

Interventions that evidence shows are likely to be effective in managing anxiety include the following.
- Listening to music during invasive procedures may benefit adults and children.
- Providing psychoeducational, cognitive behavioral, and supportive care can help reduce anxiety. It should be noted that simple provision of information and orientation to facilities and care navigation alone appear to be insufficient to reduce anxiety. Interventions that include two-way

communication, active listening, counseling, and support are supported by evidence, whether delivered in person, via telephone, or through computer applications.

- Patients may benefit from learning and practicing progressive muscle relaxation techniques. Training is often delivered in a practical way by providing patients with a CD and written guidance.
- Nurses can educate and encourage patients to get regular exercise and physical activity, which may help reduce anxiety.
- Referral to support groups can be helpful for interested patients.

For patients whose symptoms are severe or persistent, appropriate referrals for psychological care need to be made.

Anxiety Resource Contributors

*Topic leader: Caryl D. Fulcher, MSN, RN, CNS-BC
Angelia Berkowitz, MSN, APRN, FNP-BC, Diane G. Cope, RN,
PhD, ARNP-BC, AOCNP®, Patricia J. Friend, PhD, APRN, AOCN®,
Heeju Kim, PhD, RN, OCN®, Tammie L. Sherner, MSN, APRN-
CNS, Patsy Smith, RN, PhD, Thiruppavai Sundaramurthi, MSN,
RN, CCRN, Meghan L. Underhill, PhD, RN, AOCNS®, and
Deborah K. Walker, DNP, FNP-BC, AOCN®*

References

1. Eaton, L.H., & Tipton, J.M. (Eds.). (2009). *Putting evidence into practice: Improving oncology patient outcomes.* Pittsburgh, PA: Oncology Nursing Society.
2. Stark, D.P.H., & House, A. (2000). Anxiety in cancer patients. *British Journal of Cancer, 83,* 1261–1267. doi:10.1054/bjoc.2000.1405
3. Kadan-Lottick, N.S., Vanderwerker, L.C., Block, S.D., Zhang, B., & Prigerson, H.G. (2005). Psychiatric disorders and mental health service use in patients with advanced cancer. *Cancer, 104,* 2872–2881. doi:10.1002/cncr.21532
4. Strong, V., Waters, R., Hibberd, C., Rush, R., Cargill, A., Storey, D., ... Sharpe, M. (2007). Emotional distress in cancer patients: The Edinburgh Cancer Centre symptom study. *British Journal of Cancer, 96,* 868–874. doi:10.1038/sj.bjc.6603626
5. Vodermaier, A., Linden, W., MacKenzie, R., Greig, D., & Marshall, C. (2011). Disease stage predicts post-diagnosis anxiety and depression only in some types of cancer. *British Journal of Cancer, 105,* 1814–1817. doi:10.1038/bjc.2011.503
6. Meraner, V., Gamper, E.-M., Grahmann, A., Giesinger, J.M., Wiesbauer, P., Sztankay, M., ... Holzner, B. (2012). Monitoring physical and psychosocial symptom trajectories in ovarian cancer patients receiving chemotherapy. *BMC Cancer, 12,* 77. doi:10.1186/1471-2407-12-77

7. Greer, J.A., Solis, J.M., Temel, J.S., Lennes, I.T., Prigerson, H.G., & Maciejewski, P.K., & Pirl, W.F. (2011). Anxiety disorders in long-term survivors of adult cancers. *Psychosomatics, 52,* 417–423. doi:10.1016/j.psym.2011.01.014

8. Schumacher, J.R., Palta, M., LoConte, N.K., Trentham-Dietz, A., Witt, W.P., Heidrich, S.M., & Smith, M.A. (2013). Characterizing the psychological distress response before and after a cancer diagnosis. *Journal of Behavioral Medicine, 36,* 591–600. doi:10.1007/s10865-012-9453-x

9. National Cancer Institute. (2013, November 19). Adjustment to cancer: Anxiety and distress (PDQ®) [Health professional version]. Retrieved from http://www.cancer.gov/cancertopics/pdq/supportivecare/adjustment/HealthProfessional

10. National Comprehensive Cancer Network. (2013). *NCCN Clinical Practice Guidelines in Oncology: Survivorship* [v.1.2013]. Retrieved from http://www.nccn.org/professionals/physician_gls/pdf/survivorship.pdf

11. National Comprehensive Cancer Network. (2012). *NCCN Clinical Practice Guidelines in Oncology: Distress management* [v.2.2013]. Retrieved from http://www.nccn.org/professionals/physician_gls/pdf/distress.pdf

12. Spitzer, R.L., Kroenke, K., Williams, J., & Lowe, B. (2006). A brief measure for assessing generalized anxiety disorder: The GAD-7. *Archives of Internal Medicine, 166,* 1092–1097. doi:10.1001/archinte.166.10.1092

13. Shields, C.G., Ziner, K.W., Bourff, S.A., Schilling, K., Zhao, Q., Monahan, P., ... Champion, V. (2010). An intervention to improve communication between breast cancer survivors and their physicians. *Journal of Psychosocial Oncology, 28,* 610–629. doi:10.1080/07347332.2010.516811

14. White, V.M., Macvean, M.L., Grogan, S., D'Este, C., Akkerman, D., Ieropoli, S., ... Sanson-Fisher, R. (2012). Can a tailored telephone intervention delivered by volunteers reduce the supportive care needs, anxiety and depression of people with colorectal cancer? A randomised controlled trial. *Psycho-Oncology, 21,* 1053–1062. doi:10.1002/pon.2019

15. Arving, C., Sjoden, P.-O., Bergh, J., Hellbom, M., Johansson, B., Glimelius, B., & Brandberg, Y. (2007). Individual psychosocial support for breast cancer patients: A randomized study of nurse versus psychologist interventions and standard care. *Cancer Nursing, 30*(3), E10–E19. doi:10.1097/01.NCC.0000270709.64790.05

16. Greer, J.A., Traeger, L., Bemis, H., Solis, J., Hendriksen, E.S., Park, E.R., ... Safren, S.A. (2012). A pilot randomized controlled trial of brief cognitive-behavioral therapy for anxiety in patients with terminal cancer. *Oncologist, 17,* 1337–1345. doi:10.1634/theoncologist.2012-0041

17. Hopko, D.R., Armento, M.E., Robertson, S.M., Ryba, M.M., Carvalho, J.P., Colman, L.K., ... Lejuez, C.W. (2011). Brief behavioral activation and problem-solving therapy for depressed breast cancer patients: Randomized trial. *Journal of Consulting and Clinical Psychology, 79,* 834–849. doi:10.1037/a0025450

18. Kangas, M., Milross, C., Taylor, A., & Bryant, R.A. (2013). A pilot randomized controlled trial of a brief early intervention for reducing posttraumatic stress disorder, anxiety and depressive symptoms in newly diagnosed head and neck cancer patients. *Psycho-Oncology, 22,* 1665–1673. doi:10.1002/pon.3208

19. Pitceathly, C., Maguire, P., Fletcher, I., Parle, M., Tomenson, B., & Creed, F. (2009). Can a brief psychological intervention prevent anxiety or depressive disorders in cancer patients? A randomised controlled trial. *Annals of Oncology, 20,* 928–934. doi:10.1093/annonc/mdn708

20. Serfaty, M., Wilkinson, S., Freeman, C., Mannix, K., & King, M. (2012). The ToT study: Helping with Touch or Talk (ToT): A pilot randomised controlled trial to examine the clinical effectiveness of aromatherapy massage versus cognitive behaviour therapy for emotional distress in patients in cancer/palliative care. *Psycho-Oncology, 21,* 563–569. doi:10.1002/pon.1921

21. Ames, S.C., Tan, W.W., Ames, G.E., Stone, R.L., Rizzo, T.D., Jr., Crook, J.E., ... Rummans, T.A. (2011). A pilot investigation of a multidisciplinary quality of life intervention for men with biochemical recurrence of prostate cancer. *Psycho-Oncology, 20,* 435–440. doi:10.1002/pon.1769

22. Boesen, E.H., Karlsen, R., Christensen, J., Paaschburg, B., Nielsen, D., Bloch, I.S., ... Johansen, C. (2011). Psychosocial group intervention for patients with primary breast cancer: A randomised trial. *European Journal of Cancer, 47,* 1363–1372. doi:10.1016/j.ejca.2011.01.002

23. Dolbeault, S., Cayrou, S., Bredart, A., Viala, A.L., Desclaux, B., Saltel, P., ... Dickes, P. (2009). The effectiveness of a psycho-educational group after early-stage breast cancer treatment: Results of a randomized French study. *Psycho-Oncology, 18,* 647–656. doi:10.1002/pon.1440

24. Korstjens, I., Mesters, I., May, A.M., van Weert, E., van den Hout, J.H., Ros, W., ... van den Borne, B. (2011). Effects of cancer rehabilitation on problem-solving, anxiety and depression: A RCT comparing physical and cognitive-behavioural training versus physical training. *Psychology and Health, 26*(Suppl. 1), 63–82. doi:10.1080/08870441003611569

25. Shepherd, L., Goldstein, D., Whitford, H., Thewes, B., Brummell, V., & Hicks, M. (2006). The utility of videoconferencing to provide innovative delivery of psychological treatment for rural cancer patients: Results of a pilot study. *Journal of Pain and Symptom Management, 32,* 453–461. doi:10.1016/j.jpainsymman.2006.05.018

26. Naaman, S.C., Radwan, K., Fergusson, D., & Johnson, S. (2009). Status of psychological trials in breast cancer patients: A report of three meta-analyses. *Psychiatry, 72,* 50–69. doi:10.1521/psyc.2009.72.1.50

27. Osborn, R.L., Demoncada, A.C., & Feuerstein, M. (2006). Psychosocial interventions for depression, anxiety and quality of life in cancer survivors: Meta-analyses. *International Journal of Psychiatry in Medicine, 36,* 13–34. doi:10.2190/EUFN-RV1K-Y3TR-FK0L

28. Badger, T., Segrin, C., Dorros, S.M., Meek, P., & Lopez, A.M. (2007). Depression and anxiety in women with breast cancer and their partners. *Nursing Research, 56,* 44–53. doi:10.1097/00006199-200701000-00006

29. Blacklock, R., Rhodes, R., Blanchard, C., & Gaul, C. (2010). Effects of exercise intensity and self-efficacy on state anxiety with breast cancer survivors. *Oncology Nursing Forum, 37,* 206–212. doi:10.1188/10.ONF.206-212

30. Burnham, T.R., & Wilcox, A. (2002). Effects of exercise on physiological and psychological variables in cancer survivors. *Medicine and Science in Sports and Exercise, 34,* 1863–1867. doi:10.1097/00005768-200212000-00001

31. Courneya, K.S., Segal, R.J., Gelmon, K., Reid, R.D., Mackey, J.R., Friedenreich, C.M., ... McKenzie, D.C. (2007). Six-month follow-up of patient-rated outcomes in a randomized controlled trial of exercise training during breast cancer chemotherapy. *Cancer Epidemiology, Biomarkers and Prevention, 16,* 2572–2578. doi:10.1158/1055-9965.EPI-07-0413

32. Kolden, G.G., Strauman, T.J., Ward, A., Kuta, J., Woods, T.E., Schneider, K.L., ... Mullen, B. (2002). A pilot study of group exercise training (GET) for women with primary breast cancer: Feasibility and health benefits. *Psycho-Oncology, 11,* 447–456. doi:10.1002/pon.591

33. Mehnert, A., Veers, S., Howaldt, D., Braumann, K.-M., Koch, U., & Schulz, K.-H. (2011). Effects of a physical exercise rehabilitation group program on anxiety, depression, body image, and health-related quality of life among breast cancer patients. *Onkologie, 34,* 248–253. doi:10.1159/000327813

34. Midtgaard, J., Rørth, M., Stelter, R., Tveterås, A., Andersen, C., Quist, M., ... Adamsen, L. (2005). The impact of a multidimensional exercise program on self-reported anxiety and depression in cancer patients undergoing chemotherapy: A phase II study. *Palliative and Supportive Care, 3,* 197–208. doi:10.1017/S1478951505050327

35. Midtgaard, J., Stage, M., Møller, T., Andersen, C., Quist, M., Rörth, M., ... Adamsen, L. (2011). Exercise may reduce depression but not anxiety in self-referred cancer patients undergoing chemotherapy. Post-hoc analysis of data from the 'Body & Cancer' trial. *Acta Oncologica, 50,* 660–669. doi:10.3109/0284186X.2010.543145

36. Thorsen, L., Skovlund, E., Strømme, S.B., Hornslien, K., Dahl, A.A., & Fosså, S.D. (2005). Effectiveness of physical activity on cardiorespiratory fitness and health-related quality of life in young and middle-aged cancer

patients shortly after chemotherapy. *Journal of Clinical Oncology, 23,* 2378–2388. doi:10.1200/JCO.2005.04.106

37. Mishra, S.I., Scherer, R.W., Geigle, P.M., Berlanstein, D.R., Topaloglu, O., Gotay, C.C., & Snyder, C. (2012). Exercise interventions on health-related quality of life for cancer survivors. *Cochrane Database of Systematic Reviews, 2012*(8).doi:10.1002/14651858.CD007566.pub2

38. Campeau, M.P., Gaboriault, R., Drapeau, M., Van Nguyen, T., Roy, I., Fortin, B., … Nguyen-Tân, P.F. (2007). Impact of massage therapy on anxiety levels in patients undergoing radiation therapy: Randomized controlled trial. *Journal of the Society for Integrative Oncology, 5,* 133–138. doi:10.2310/7200.2007.018

39. Currin, J., & Meister, E.A. (2008). A hospital-based intervention using massage to reduce distress among oncology patients. *Cancer Nursing, 31,* 214–221. doi:10.1097/01.NCC.0000305725.65345.f3

40. Hernandez-Reif, M., Field, T., Ironson, G., Beutler, J., Vera, Y., Hurley, J., … Fraser, M. (2005). Natural killer cells and lymphocytes increase in women with breast cancer following massage therapy. *International Journal of Neuroscience, 115,* 495–510. doi:10.1080/00207450590523080

41. Jane, S.-W., Chen, S.-L., Wilkie, D.J., Lin, Y.-C., Foreman, S.W., Beaton, R.D., … Liao, M.-N. (2011). Effects of massage on pain, mood status, relaxation, and sleep in Taiwanese patients with metastatic bone pain: A randomized clinical trial. *Pain, 152,* 2432–2442. doi:10.1016/j.pain.2011.06.021

42. Kutner, J.S., Smith, M.C., Corbin, L., Hemphill, L., Benton, K., Mellis, B.K., … Fairclough, D.L. (2008). Massage therapy versus simple touch to improve pain and mood in patients with advanced cancer: A randomized trial. *Annals of Internal Medicine, 149,* 369–379. doi:10.7326/0003-4819 -149-6-200809160-00003

43. Post-White, J., Kinney, M.E., Savik, K., Gau, J.B., Wilcox, C., & Lerner, I. (2003). Therapeutic massage and healing touch improve symptoms in cancer. *Integrative Cancer Therapies, 2,* 332–344. doi: 10.1177/1534735403259064

44. Smith, M.C., Kemp, J., Hemphill, L., & Vojir, C.P. (2002). Outcomes of therapeutic massage for hospitalized cancer patients. *Journal of Nursing Scholarship, 34,* 257–262. doi:10.1111/j.1547-5069.2002.00257.x

45. Soden, K., Vincent, K., Craske, S., Lucas, C., & Ashley, S. (2004). A randomized controlled trial of aromatherapy massage in a hospice setting. *Palliative Medicine, 18,* 87–92. doi:10.1191/0269216304pm874oa

46. Sturgeon, M., Wetta-Hall, R., Hart, T., Good, M., & Dakhil, S. (2009). Effects of therapeutic massage on the quality of life among patients with breast cancer during treatment. *Journal of Alternative and Complementary Medicine, 15,* 373–380. doi:10.1089/acm.2008.0399

47. Wilkinson, S.M., Love, S.B., Westcombe, A.M., Gambles, M.A., Burgess, C.C., Cargill, A., … Ramirez, A.J. (2007). Effectiveness of aromatherapy massage in the management of anxiety and depression in patients with cancer: A multicentre randomized controlled trial. *Journal of Clinical Oncology, 25,* 532–539. doi:10.1200/JCO.2006.08.9987

48. Fellowes, D., Barnes, K., & Wilkinson, S. (2004). Aromatherapy and massage for symptom relief in patients with cancer. *Cochrane Database of Systematic Reviews, 2004*(3). doi:10.1002/14651858.CD002287.pub2

49. Wilkinson, S., Barnes, K., & Storey, L. (2008). Massage for symptom relief in patients with cancer: Systematic review. *Journal of Advanced Nursing, 63,* 430–439. doi:10.1111/j.1365-2648.2008.04712.x

50. Garland, S.N., Tamagawa, R., Todd, S.C., Speca, M., & Carlson, L.E. (2013). Increased mindfulness is related to improved stress and mood following participation in a mindfulness-based stress reduction program in individuals with cancer. *Integrative Cancer Therapies, 12,* 31–40. doi:10.1177/1534735412442370

51. Hoffman, C.J., Ersser, S.J., Hopkinson, J.B., Nicholls, P.G., Harrington, J.E., & Thomas, P.W. (2012). Effectiveness of mindfulness-based stress reduction in mood, breast- and endocrine-related quality of life, and well-being in stage

0 to III breast cancer: A randomized, controlled trial. *Journal of Clinical Oncology, 30,* 1335–1342. doi:10.1200/JCO.2010.34.0331

52. Lengacher, C.A., Reich, R.R., Post-White, J., Moscoso, M., Shelton, M.M., Barta, M., … Budhrani, P. (2012). Mindfulness based stress reduction in post-treatment breast cancer patients: An examination of symptoms and symptom clusters. *Journal of Behavioral Medicine, 35,* 86–94. doi:10.1007/s10865-011-9346-4

53. Monti, D.A., Kash, K.M., Kunkel, E.J.S., Brainard, G., Wintering, N., Moss, A.S., … Newberg, A.B. (2012). Changes in cerebral blood flow and anxiety associated with an 8-week mindfulness programme in women with breast cancer. *Stress and Health, 28,* 397–407. doi:10.1002/smi.2470

54. Sharplin, G.R., Jones, S.B., Hancock, B., Knott, V.E., Bowden, J.A., & Whitford, H.S. (2010). Mindfulness-based cognitive therapy: An efficacious community-based group intervention for depression and anxiety in a sample of cancer patients. *Medical Journal of Australia, 193*(Suppl. 5), S79–S82.

55. Würtzen, H., Dalton, S.O., Elsass, P., Sumbundu, A.D., Steding-Jensen, M., Karlsen, R.V., … Johansen, C. (2013). Mindfulness significantly reduces self-reported levels of anxiety and depression: Results of a randomised controlled trial among 336 Danish women treated for stage I–III breast cancer. *European Journal of Cancer, 49,* 1365–1373. doi:10.1016/j.ejca.2012.10.030

56. Piet, J., Würtzen, H., & Zachariae, R. (2012). The effect of mindfulness-based therapy on symptoms of anxiety and depression in adult cancer patients and survivors: A systematic review and meta-analysis. *Journal of Consulting and Clinical Psychology, 80,* 1007–1020. doi:10.1037/a0028329

57. Bulfone, T., Quattrin, R., Zanotti, R., Regattin, L., & Brusaferro, S. (2009). Effectiveness of music therapy for anxiety reduction in women with breast cancer in chemotherapy treatment. *Holistic Nursing Practice, 23,* 238–242. doi:10.1097/HNP.0b013e3181aeceee

58. Burns, D.S., Azzouz, F., Sledge, R., Rutledge, C., Hincher, K., Monahan, P.O., & Cripe, L.D. (2008). Music imagery for adults with acute leukemia in protective environments: A feasibility study. *Supportive Care in Cancer, 16,* 507–513. doi:10.1007/s00520-007-0330-z

59. Ferrer, A.J. (2007). The effect of live music on decreasing anxiety in patients undergoing chemotherapy treatment. *Journal of Music Therapy, 44,* 242–255. doi:10.1093/jmt/44.3.242

60. Karagozoglu, S., Tekyasar, F., & Yilmaz, F.A. (2013). Effects of music therapy and guided visual imagery on chemotherapy-induced anxiety and nausea-vomiting. *Journal of Clinical Nursing, 22,* 39–50. doi:10.1111/jocn.12030

61. Kwekkeboom, K.L. (2003). Music versus distraction for procedural pain and anxiety in patients with cancer. *Oncology Nursing Forum, 30,* 433–440. doi:10.1188/03.ONF.433-440

62. Li, X.-M., Zhou, K.-N., Yan, H., Wang, D.-L., & Zhang, Y.-P. (2012). Effects of music therapy on anxiety of patients with breast cancer after radical mastectomy: A randomized clinical trial. *Journal of Advanced Nursing, 68,* 1145–1155. doi:10.1111/j.1365-2648.2011.05824.x

63. Nguyen, T.N., Nilsson, S., Hellström, A.-L., & Bengtson, A. (2010). Music therapy to reduce pain and anxiety in children with cancer undergoing lumbar puncture: A randomized clinical trial. *Journal of Pediatric Oncology Nursing, 27,* 146–155. doi:10.1177/1043454209355983

64. Nightingale, C.L., Rodriguez, C., & Carnaby, G. (2013). The impact of music interventions on anxiety for adult cancer patients: A meta-analysis and systematic review. *Integrative Cancer Therapies, 12,* 393–403. doi:10.1177/1534735413485817

65. Tsivian, M., Qi, P., Kimura, M., Chen, V.H., Chen, S.H., Gan, T.J., & Polascik, T.J. (2012). The effect of noise-cancelling headphones or music on pain perception and anxiety in men undergoing transrectal prostate biopsy. *Urology, 79,* 32–36. doi:10.1016/j.urology.2011.09.037

66. Walworth, D., Rumana, C.S., Nguyen, J., & Jarred, J. (2008). Effects of live music therapy sessions on quality of life indicators, medications

administered and hospital length of stay for patients undergoing elective surgical procedures for brain. *Journal of Music Therapy, 45,* 349–359. doi:10.1093/jmt/45.3.349

67. Bradt, J., Dileo, C., Grocke, D., & Magill, L. (2011). Music interventions for improving psychological and physical outcomes in cancer patients. *Cochrane Database of Systematic Reviews, 2011*(8). doi:10.1002/14651858.CD006911.pub2

68. Chan, C.W., Richardson, A., & Richardson, J. (2011). Managing symptoms in patients with advanced lung cancer during radiotherapy: Results of a psychoeducational randomized controlled trial. *Journal of Pain and Symptom Management, 41,* 347–357. doi:10.1016/j.jpainsymman.2010.04.024

69. Cheung, Y.L., Molassiotis, A., & Chang, A.M. (2003). The effect of progressive muscle relaxation training on anxiety and quality of life after stoma surgery in colorectal cancer patients. *Psycho-Oncology, 12,* 254–266. doi:10.1002/pon.638

70. Chien, C.H., Liu, K.L., Chien, H.T., & Liu, H.E. (2014). The effects of psychosocial strategies on anxiety and depression of patients diagnosed with prostate cancer: A systematic review. *International Journal of Nursing Studies, 51,* 28–38. doi:10.1016/j.ijnurstu.2012.12.019

71. Galway, K., Black, A., Cantwell, M., Cardwell, C.R., Mills, M., & Donnelly, M. (2012). Psychosocial interventions to improve quality of life and emotional wellbeing for recently diagnosed cancer patients. *Cochrane Database of Systematic Reviews, 2012*(11). doi:10.1002/14651858.CD007064.pub2

72. Goerling, U., Foerg, A., Sander, S., Schramm, N., & Schlag, P.M. (2011). The impact of short-term psycho-oncological interventions on the psychological outcome of cancer patients of a surgical-oncology department—A randomised controlled study. *European Journal of Cancer, 47,* 2009–2014. doi:10.1016/j.ejca.2011.04.031

73. Hirai, K., Motooka, H., Ito, N., Wada, N., Yoshizaki, A., Shiozaki, M., ... Akechi, T. (2012). Problem-solving therapy for psychological distress in Japanese early-stage breast cancer patients. *Japanese Journal of Clinical Oncology, 42,* 1168–1174. doi:10.1093/jjco/hys158

74. Jones, R.B., Pearson, J., Cawsot, A.J., Bental, D., Barrett, A., White, J., ... Gilmour, W.H. (2006). Effect of different forms of information produced for cancer patients on their use of the information, social support, and anxiety: Randomised trial. *BMJ, 332,* 942–948. doi:10.1136/bmj.38807.571042.68

75. Katz, M.R., Irish, J.C., & Devins, G.M. (2004). Development and pilot testing of a psychoeducational intervention for oral cancer patients. *Psycho-Oncology, 13,* 642–653. doi:10.1002/pon.767

76. Kim, H.S., Shin, S.J., Kim, S.C., An, S., Rha, S.Y., Ahn, J.B., ... Lee, S. (2013). Randomized controlled trial of standardized education and telemonitoring for pain in outpatients with advanced solid tumors. *Supportive Care in Cancer, 21,* 1751–1759. doi:10.1007/s00520-013-1722-x

77. Krischer, M.M., Xu, P., Meade, C.D., & Jacobsen, P.B. (2007). Self-administered stress management training in patients undergoing radiotherapy. *Journal of Clinical Oncology, 25,* 4657–4662. doi:10.1200/JCO.2006.09.0126

78. Lindemalm, C., Mozaffari, F., Choudhury, A., Granstam-Björneklett, H., Lekander, M., Nilsson, B., ... Mellstedt, H. (2008). Immune response, depression and fatigue in relation to support intervention in mammary cancer patients. *Supportive Care in Cancer, 16,* 57–65. doi:10.1007/s00520-007-0275-2

79. Liu, C.-J., Hsiung, P.-C., Chang, K.-J., Liu, Y.-F., Wang, K.-C., Hsiao, F.-H., ... Chan, C.L.W. (2008). A study on the efficacy of body-mind-spirit group therapy for patients with breast cancer. *Journal of Clinical Nursing, 17,* 2539–2549. doi:10.1111/j.1365-2702.2008.02296.x

80. Oh, P.J., & Kim, S.H. (2010). Effects of a brief psychosocial intervention in patients with cancer receiving adjuvant therapy [Online publication]. *Oncology Nursing Forum, 37,* E98–E104. doi:10.1188/10.ONF.E98-E104

81. Preyde, M., & Synnott, E. (2009). Psychosocial intervention for adults with cancer: A meta-analysis. *Journal of Evidence-Based Social Work, 6,* 321–347. doi:10.1080/15433710903126521

82. Rawl, S.M., Given, B.A., Champion, V.L., Kozachik, S.L., Barton, D., Emsley, C.L., & Williams, S.D. (2002). Intervention to improve psychological functioning for newly diagnosed patients with cancer. *Oncology Nursing Forum, 29,* 967–975. doi:10.1188/02.ONF.967-975

83. Schofield, P., Jefford, M., Carey, M., Thomson, K., Evans, M., Baravelli, C., & Aranda, S. (2008). Preparing patients for threatening medical treatments: Effects of a chemotherapy educational DVD on anxiety, unmet needs, and self-efficacy. *Supportive Care in Cancer, 16,* 37–45. doi:10.1007/s00520-007-0273-4

84. Targ, E.F., & Levine, E.G. (2002). The efficacy of a mind-body-spirit group for women with breast cancer: A randomized controlled trial. *General Hospital Psychiatry, 24,* 238–248. doi:10.1016/S0163-8343(02)00191-3

85. Ando, M., Morita, T., Okamoto, T., & Ninosaka, Y. (2008). One-week Short-Term Life Review interview can improve spiritual well-being of terminally ill cancer patients. *Psycho-Oncology, 17,* 885–890. doi:10.1002/pon.1299

86. Cameron, L.D., Booth, R.J., Schlatter, M., Ziginskas, D., & Harman, J.E. (2007). Changes in emotion regulation and psychological adjustment following use of a group psychosocial support program for women recently diagnosed with breast cancer. *Psycho-Oncology, 16,* 171–180. doi:10.1002/pon.1050

87. Chujo, M., Mikami, I., Takashima, S., Saeki, T., Ohsumi, S., Aogi, K., & Okamura, H. (2005). A feasibility study of psychosocial group intervention for breast cancer patients with first recurrence. *Supportive Care in Cancer, 13,* 503–514. doi:10.1007/s00520-004-0733-z

88. Liao, M.-N., Chen, P.-L., Chen, M.-F., & Chen, S.-C. (2010). Effect of supportive care on the anxiety of women with suspected breast cancer. *Journal of Advanced Nursing, 66,* 49–59. doi:10.1111/j.1365-2648.2009.05139.x

89. Miller, D.K., Chibnall, J.T., Videen, S.D., & Duckro, P.N. (2005). Supportive-affective group experience for persons with life-threatening illness: Reducing spiritual, psychological, and death-related distress in dying patients. *Journal of Palliative Medicine, 8,* 333–343. doi:10.1089/jpm.2005.8.333

90. Cankurtaran, E.S., Ozalp, E., Soygur, H., Akbiyik, D.I., Turhan, L., & Alkis, N. (2008). Mirtazapine improves sleep and lowers anxiety and depression in cancer patients: Superiority over imipramine. *Supportive Care in Cancer, 16,* 1291–1298. doi:10.1007/s00520-008-0425-1

91. Suzuki, N., Ninomiya, M., Maruta, T., Hosonuma, S., Yoshioka, N., Ohara, T., … Ishizuka, D. (2011). Clinical study on the efficacy of fluvoxamine for psychological distress in gynecologic cancer patients. *International Journal of Gynecological Cancer, 21,* 1143–1149. doi:10.1097/IGC.0b013e3181ffbeb9

92. Torta, R., Leombruni, P., Borio, R., & Castelli, L. (2011). Duloxetine for the treatment of mood disorder in cancer patients: A 12-week case-control clinical trial. *Human Psychopharmacology: Clinical and Experimental, 26,* 291–299. doi:10.1002/hup.1202

93. Razavi, D., Allilaire, J.-F., Smith, M., Salimpour, A., Verra, M., Desclaux, B., … Blin, P. (1996). The effect of fluoxetine on anxiety and depression symptoms in cancer patients. *Acta Psychiatrica Scandinavica, 94,* 205–210. doi:10.1111/j.1600-0447.1996.tb09850.x

94. Torta, R., Siri, I., & Caldera, P. (2008). Sertraline effectiveness and safety in depressed oncological patients. *Supportive Care in Cancer, 16,* 83–91. doi:10.1007/s00520-007-0269-0

95. Wald, T.G., Kathol, R.G., Noyes, R., Jr., Carroll, B.T., & Clamon, G.H. (1993). Rapid relief of anxiety in cancer patients with both alprazolam and placebo. *Psychosomatics, 34,* 324–332. doi:10.1016/S0033-3182(93)71866-6

96. Lavigne, J.E., Heckler, C., Mathews, J.L., Palesh, O., Kirshner, J.J., Lord, R., … Mustian, K. (2012). A randomized, controlled, double-blinded clinical trial of gabapentin 300 versus 900 mg versus placebo for anxiety symptoms in breast cancer survivors. *Breast Cancer Research and Treatment, 136,* 479–486. doi:10.1007/s10549-012-2251-x

97. Gehring, K., Patwardhan, S.Y., Collins, R., Groves, M.D., Etzel, C.J., Meyers, C.A., & Wefel, J.S. (2012). A randomized trial on the efficacy of methyl-

phenidate and modafinil for improving cognitive functioning and symptoms in patients with a primary brain tumor. *Journal of Neuro-Oncology, 107,* 165–174. doi:10.1007/s11060-011-0723-1

98. Mañas, A., Ciria, J.P., Fernández, M.C., Gonzálvez, M.L., Morillo, V., Pérez, M., … López-Gómez, V. (2011). Post hoc analysis of pregabalin vs. non-pregabalin treatment in patients with cancer-related neuropathic pain: Better pain relief, sleep and physical health. *Clinical and Translational Oncology, 13,* 656–663. doi:10.1007/s12094-011-0711-0

99. Grob, C.S., Danforth, A.L., Chopra, G.S., Hagerty, M., McKay, C.R., Halberstadt, A.L., & Greer, G.R. (2011). Pilot study of psilocybin treatment for anxiety in patients with advanced-stage cancer. *JAMA Psychiatry, 68,* 71–78. doi:10.1001/archgenpsychiatry.2010.116

100. Girgis, A., Breen, S., Stacey, F., & Lecathelinais, C. (2009). Impact of two supportive care interventions on anxiety, depression, quality of life, and unmet needs in patients with nonlocalized breast and colorectal cancers. *Journal of Clinical Oncology, 27,* 6180–6190. doi:10.1200/JCO.2009.22.8718

101. Gravis, G., Protière, C., Eisinger, F., Boher, J.M., Tarpin, C., Coso, D., … Viens, P. (2011). Full access to medical records does not modify anxiety in cancer patients: Results of a randomized study. *Cancer, 117,* 4796–4804. doi:10.1002/cncr.26083

102. Ferrante, J.M., Chen, P.-H., & Kim, S. (2008). The effect of patient navigation on time to diagnosis, anxiety, and satisfaction in urban minority women with abnormal mammograms: A randomized controlled trial. *Journal of Urban Health: Bulletin of the New York Academy of Medicine, 85,* 114–124. doi:10.1007/s11524-007-9228-9

103. Skrutkowski, M., Saucier, A., Eades, M., Swidzinski, M., Ritchie, J., Marchionni, C., & Ladouceur, M. (2008). Impact of a pivot nurse in oncology on patients with lung or breast cancer: Symptom distress, fatigue, quality of life, and use of healthcare resources. *Oncology Nursing Forum, 35,* 948–954. doi:10.1188/08.ONF.948-954

104. Fukui, S., Ogawa, K., Ohtsuka, M., & Fukui, N. (2008). A randomized study assessing the efficacy of communication skill training on patients' psychologic distress and coping: Nurses' communication with patients just after being diagnosed with cancer. *Cancer, 113,* 1462–1470. doi:10.1002/cncr.23710

105. D'Souza, V., Blouin, E., Zeitouni, A., Muller, K., & Allison, P.J. (2013). An investigation of the effect of tailored information on symptoms of anxiety and depression in head and neck cancer patients. *Oral Oncology, 49,* 431–437. doi:10.1016/j.oraloncology.2012.12.001

106. Deng, G., Chan, Y., Sjoberg, D., Vickers, A., Yeung, K.S., Kris, M., … Cassileth, B. (2013). Acupuncture for the treatment of post-chemotherapy chronic fatigue: A randomized, blinded, sham-controlled trial. *Supportive Care in Cancer, 21,* 1735–1741. doi:10.1007/s00520-013-1720-z

107. Molassiotis, A., Bardy, J., Finnegan-John, J., Mackereth, P., Ryder, W.D., Filshie, J., … Richardson, A. (2013). A randomized, controlled trial of acupuncture self-needling as maintenance therapy for cancer-related fatigue after therapist-delivered acupuncture. *Annals of Oncology, 24,* 1645–1652. doi:10.1093/annonc/mdt034

108. Garcia, M.K., McQuade, J., Haddad, R., Patel, S., Lee, R., Yang, P., … Cohen, L. (2013). Systematic review of acupuncture in cancer care: A synthesis of the evidence. *Journal of Clinical Oncology, 31,* 952–960. doi:10.1200/JCO.2012.43.5818

109. Weller, M., Cosmos, E., DeBruyn, J., & Brader, K. (2008). Complementary treatment in gynecologic oncology: The use of energy healing for ovarian cancer patients. *Journal of Gynecologic Oncology Nursing, 18*(4), 29–33.

110. Bar-Sela, G., Atid, L., Danos, S., Gabay, N., & Epelbaum, R. (2007). Art therapy improved depression and influenced fatigue levels in cancer patients on chemotherapy. *Psycho-Oncology, 16,* 980–984. doi:10.1002/pon.1175

111. Lawson, L.M., Williams, P., Glennon, C., Carithers, K., Schnabel, E., Andrejack, A., & Wright, N. (2012). Effect of art making on cancer-related

symptoms of blood and marrow transplantation recipients [Online exclusive]. *Oncology Nursing Forum, 39,* E353–E360. doi:10.1188/12.ONF .E353-E360

112. Nainis, N., Paice, J.A., Ratner, J., Wirth, J.H., Lai, J., & Shott, S. (2005). Relieving symptoms in cancer: Innovative use of art therapy. *Journal of Pain and Symptom Management, 31,* 162–169. doi:10.1016/j.jpainsymman .2005.07.006

113. Thyme, K.E., Sundin, E.C., Wiberg, B., Öster, I., Åström, S., & Lindh, J. (2009). Individual brief art therapy can be helpful for women with breast cancer: A randomized controlled clinical study. *Palliative and Supportive Care, 7,* 87–95. doi:10.1017/S147895150900011X

114. Cochrane, B.B., Lewis, F.M., & Griffith, K.A. (2011). Exploring a diffusion of benefit: Does a woman with breast cancer derive benefit from an intervention delivered to her partner? *Oncology Nursing Forum, 38,* 207–214. doi:10.1188/11.ONF.207-214

115. Manne, S.L., Ostroff, J.S., Winkel, G., Fox, K., Grana, G., Miller, E., ... Frazier, T. (2005). Couple-focused group intervention for women with early stage breast cancer. *Journal of Consulting and Clinical Psychology, 73,* 634–646. doi:10.1037/0022-006X.73.4.634

116. Jensen-Johansen, M.B., Christensen, S., Valdimarsdottir, H., Zakowski, S., Jensen, A.B., Bovbjerg, D.H., & Zachariae, R. (2012). Effects of an expressive writing intervention on cancer-related distress in Danish breast cancer survivors—Results from a nationwide randomized clinical trial. *Psycho-Oncology, 22,* 1492–1500. doi:10.1002/pon.3193

117. Mosher, C.E., DuHamel, K.N., Lam, J., Dickler, M., Li, Y., Massie, M.J., & Norton, L. (2012). Randomised trial of expressive writing for distressed metastatic breast cancer patients. *Psychology and Health, 27,* 88–100. doi:10.1080/08870446.2010.551212

118. Pilkington, K., Kirkwood, G., Rampes, H., Fisher, P., & Richardson, J. (2006). Homeopathy for anxiety and anxiety disorders: A systematic review of the research. *Homeopathy, 95,* 151–162. doi:10.1016/j.homp.2006.05.005

119. Schnur, J.B., Bovbjerg, D.H., Daniel, D., Tatrow, K., Goldfarb, A.B., Silverstein, J.H., ... Montgomery, G.H. (2008). Hypnosis decreases presurgical distress in excisional breast biopsy patients. *Anesthesia and Analgesia, 106,* 440–444. doi:10.1213/ane.0b013e31815edb13

120. Snow, A., Dorfman, D., Warbet, R., Cammarata, M., Eisenman, S., Zilberfein, F., ... Navada, S. (2012). A randomized trial of hypnosis for relief of pain and anxiety in adult cancer patients undergoing bone marrow procedures. *Journal of Psychosocial Oncology, 30,* 281–293. doi:10.1080/ 0734332.2012.664261

121. Ando, M., Morita, T., Akechi, T., Ito, S., Tanaka, M., Ifuku, Y., & Nakayama, T. (2009). The efficacy of mindfulness-based meditation therapy on anxiety, depression, and spirituality in Japanese patients with cancer. *Journal of Palliative Medicine, 12,* 1091–1094. doi:10.1089/jpm.2009.0143

122. Hidderley, M., & Holt, M. (2004). A pilot randomized trial assessing the effects of autogenic training in early stage cancer patients in relation to psychological status and immune system responses. *European Journal of Oncology Nursing, 8,* 61–65. doi:10.1016/j.ejon.2003.09.003

123. Ramachandra, P., Booth, S., Pieters, T., Vrotsou, K., & Huppert, F.A. (2009). A brief self-administered psychological intervention to improve well-being in patients with cancer: Results from a feasibility study. *Psycho-Oncology, 18,* 1323–1326. doi:10.1002/pon.1516

124. Nunes, D.F.T., Rodriquez, A.L., Hoffman, F.D., Luz, C., Braga Filho, A.P.F., Muller, M.C., & Bauer, M.E. (2007). Relaxation and guided imagery program in patients with breast cancer undergoing radiotherapy is not associated with neuroimmunomodulatory effects. *Journal of Psychosomatic Research, 63,* 647–655. doi:10.1016/j.jpsychores.2007.07.004

125. Sloman, R. (2002). Relaxation and imagery for anxiety and depression control in community patients with advanced cancer. *Cancer Nursing, 25,* 432–435. doi:10.1097/00002820-200212000-00005

126. Quattrin, R., Zanini, A., Buchini, S., Turello, D., Annunziata, M.A., Vidotti, C., ... Brusaferro, S. (2006). Use of reflexology foot massage to reduce anxiety in hospitalized cancer patients in chemotherapy treatment: Methodology and outcomes. *Journal of Nursing Management, 14,* 96–105. doi:10.1111/j.1365-2934.2006.00557.x

127. Sharp, D.M., Walker, M.B., Chaturvedi, A., Upadhyay, S., Hamid, A., Walker, A.A., ... Walker, L.G. (2010). A randomised, controlled trial of the psychological effects of reflexology in early breast cancer. *European Journal of Cancer, 46,* 312–322. doi:10.1016/j.ejca.2009.10.006

128. Stephenson, N.L.N., Swanson, M., Dalton, J., Keefe, F.J., & Engelke, M. (2007). Partner-delivered reflexology: Effects on cancer pain and anxiety. *Oncology Nursing Forum, 34,* 127–132. doi:10.1188/07.ONF.127-132

129. Wyatt, G., Sikorskii, A., Rahbar, M.H., Victorson, D., & You, M. (2012). Health-related quality-of-life outcomes: A reflexology trial with patients with advanced-stage breast cancer. *Oncology Nursing Forum, 39,* 568–577. doi:10.1188/12.ONF.568-577

130. Birocco, N., Guillame, C., Storto, S., Ritorto, G., Catino, C., Gir, N., ... Ciuffreda, L. (2012). The effects of Reiki therapy on pain and anxiety in patients attending a day oncology and infusion services unit. *American Journal of Hospice and Palliative Care, 29,* 290–294. doi:10.1177/1049909111420859

131. Potter, P.J. (2007). Breast biopsy and distress: Feasibility of testing a Reiki intervention. *Journal of Holistic Nursing, 25,* 238–248. doi:10.1177/0898010107301618

132. Tsang, K.L., Carlson, L.E., & Olson, K. (2007). Pilot crossover trial of Reiki versus rest for treating cancer-related fatigue. *Integrative Cancer Therapies, 6,* 25–35. doi:10.1177/1534735406298986

133. Hayama, Y., & Inoue, T. (2012). The effects of deep breathing on 'tension-anxiety' and fatigue in cancer patients undergoing adjuvant chemotherapy. *Complementary Therapies in Clinical Practice, 18,* 94–98. doi:10.1016/j.ctcp.2011.10.001

134. Kim, S.-D., & Kim, H.-S. (2005). Effects of a relaxation breathing exercise on anxiety, depression, and leukocyte in hemopoietic stem cell transplantation patients. *Cancer Nursing, 28,* 79–83. doi:10.1097/00002820-200501000-00012

135. Serra, D., Parris, C.R., Carper, E., Homel, P., Fleishman, S.B., Harrison, L.B., & Chadha, M. (2012). Outcomes of guided imagery in patients receiving radiation therapy for breast cancer. *Clinical Journal of Oncology Nursing, 16,* 617–623. doi:10.1188/12.CJON.617-623

136. Hanssens, S., Luyten, R., Watthy, C., Fontaine, C., Decoster, L., Baillon, C., ... De Grève, J. (2011). Evaluation of a comprehensive rehabilitation program for post-treatment patients with cancer [Online exclusive]. *Oncology Nursing Forum, 38,* E418–E424. doi:10.1188/11.ONF.E418-E424

137. Khan, F., Amatya, B., Pallant, J.F., Rajapaksa, I., & Brand, C. (2012). Multidisciplinary rehabilitation in women following breast cancer treatment: A randomized controlled trial. *Journal of Rehabilitation Medicine, 44,* 788–794. doi:10.2340/16501977-1020

138. Rottmann, N., Dalton, S.O., Bidstrup, P.E., Wurtzen, H., Hoybye, M.T., Ross, L., ... Johansen, C. (2012). No improvement in distress and quality of life following psychosocial cancer rehabilitation: A randomised trial. *Psycho-Oncology, 21,* 505–514. doi:10.1002/pon.1924

139. Schneider, S.M., & Hood, L.E. (2007). Virtual reality: A distraction intervention for chemotherapy. *Oncology Nursing Forum, 34,* 39–46. doi:10.1188/07.ONF.39-46

140. Li, W.H.C., Chung, J.O.K., & Ho, E.K.Y. (2011). The effectiveness of therapeutic play, using virtual reality computer games, in promoting the psychological well-being of children hospitalised with cancer. *Journal of Clinical Nursing, 20,* 2135–2143. doi:10.1111/j.1365-2702.2011.03733.x

141. Banerjee, B., Vadiraj, H.S., Ram, A., Rao, R., Jayapal, M., Gopinath, K.S., ... Hande, M.P. (2007). Effects of an integrated yoga program in modulating psychosocial stress and radiation-induced genotoxic stress in breast cancer

patients undergoing radiotherapy. *Integrative Cancer Therapies, 6,* 242–250. doi:10.1177/1534735407306214

142. Cohen, L., Warneke, C., Foulacli, R.T., Rodriguez, M.A., & Chaoul-Reich, A. (2004). Psychological adjustment and sleep quality in a randomized trial of the effects of a Tibetan yoga intervention in patients with lymphoma. *Cancer, 100,* 2253–2260. doi:10.1002/cncr.20236

143. Dhruva, A., Miaskowski, C., Abrams, D., Acree, M., Cooper, B., Goodman, S., & Hecht, F.M. (2012). Yoga breathing for cancer chemotherapy-associated symptoms and quality of life: Results of a pilot randomized controlled trial. *Journal of Alternative and Complementary Medicine, 18,* 473–479. doi:10.1089/acm.2011.0555

144. Rao, M.R., Raghuram, N., Nagendra, H.R., Gopinath, K.S., Srinath, B.S., Diwakar, R.B., … Varambally, S. (2009). Anxiolytic effects of a yoga program in early breast cancer patients undergoing conventional treatment: A randomized controlled trial. *Complementary Therapies in Medicine, 17,* 1–8. doi:10.1016/j.ctim.2008.05.005

145. Ülger, O., & Yağli, N.V. (2010). Effects of yoga on the quality of life in cancer patients. *Complementary Therapies in Clinical Practice, 16,* 60–63. doi:10.1016/j.ctcp.2009.10.007

146. Vadiraja, H.S., Raghavendra, R.M., Nagarathna, R., Nagendra, H.R., Rekha, M., Vanitha, N., … Kumar, V. (2009). Effects of a yoga program on cortisol rhythm and mood states in early breast cancer patients undergoing adjuvant radiotherapy: A randomized controlled trial. *Integrative Cancer Therapies, 8,* 37–46. doi:10.1177/1534735409331456

147. Deshler, A.M.B., Fee-Schroeder, K.C., Dowdy, J.L., Mettler, T.A., Novotny, P., Zhao, X., & Frost, M.H. (2006). A patient orientation program at a comprehensive cancer center. *Oncology Nursing Forum, 33,* 569–578. doi:10.1188/06.ONF.569-578

148. Hoff, A.C., & Haaga, D.A. (2005). Effects of an education program on radiation oncology patients and families. *Journal of Psychosocial Oncology, 23,* 61–79. doi:10.1300/J077v23n04_04

149. Wysocki, W.M., Mituś, J., Komorowski, A.L., & Karolewski, K. (2012). Impact of preoperative information on anxiety and disease-related knowledge in women undergoing mastectomy for breast cancer: A randomized clinical trial. *Acta Chirurgica Belgica, 112,* 111–115.

150. Chan, R.J., Webster, J., & Marquart, L. (2011). Information interventions for orienting patients and their carers to cancer care facilities. *Cochrane Database of Systematic Reviews, 2011*(12). doi:10.1002/14651858. CD008273.pub2

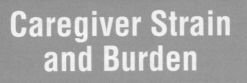

Caregiver Strain and Burden

*Margaret Irwin, PhD, RN, MN,
and Ahlam Jadalla, PhD, RN*

Problem and Incidence

Caregiver strain and burden refers to the psychological, emotional, physical, social, financial, and spiritual distress felt by caregivers as a result of providing care for a family member, a friend, or a loved one. The National Alliance for Caregiving estimates that about four million Americans are caring for an adult with cancer; the value of this care provided by informal caregivers in the United States is estimated between $306 billion and $375 billion.[1] Numerous physical, social, emotional, and health problems among cancer caregivers have been identified.[2] A recent review revealed that 20%–73% of cancer caregivers were depressed, 33% of caregivers still needed help with their own distress two years after diagnosis, and 12% still needed help five years after diagnosis.[2] In other studies, anxiety and depression among partners and caregivers ranged from 10% to 56%.[3,4] A recent meta-analysis showed that risk of anxiety was higher among cancer survivors and caregivers than among the general population.[5]

Risk Factors and Assessment

Caregivers at greatest risk are those whose situations and attributes have been correlated with increased strain and burden, including the following.[2,6-8]

- Need to provide assistance with more symptoms; patient symptoms associated with greater caregiver strain and burden are urinary, bowel, and cognitive impairment problems.[7]
- Low income or financial burden of caregiving

- Inadequate communication between patient and caregiver partners
- Caregiver physical and psychological health problems
- High competing demands (e.g., childcare needs, job responsibilities)
- Barriers in use of resources because of lack of availability of outside help, lack of trust in providers, and misconceptions about the role of services such as hospice; the National Cancer Institute[9] describes the ethnic barriers in these areas.
- Female spousal caregiver[10]

Assessment for caregiver strain and burden includes the following.

- Identification of caregivers and evaluation of their willingness, as well as their physical and mental abilities, to provide needed care[11]
- Identification of individuals at risk and assessment of these factors for the individual
- Exploration of the caregivers' experiences in the caregiving role by asking open-ended questions and providing active listening. Caregivers may not disclose problems unless asked. The nurse can inform the caregiver that it is not unusual for individuals in this role to experience problems like disruption of sleep and usual activities or anxiety and feelings of isolation and should ask the caregivers what types of issues they are experiencing.

Some practical tools to measure and objectively assess severity of strain and burden are

- The Modified Caregiver Strain Index (open access)[12]
- The Caregiver Health Self-Assessment Questionnaire[13]
- The Zarit Burden Interview (open access).[14]

What interventions are effective in preventing and managing strain and burden for caregivers of people with cancer?

Evidence retrieved through July 31, 2013

Recommended for Practice

Cognitive behavioral therapy (CBT) interventions to help restructure thinking and develop problem-solving behaviors have been provided to individuals or patient/caregiver dyads. Significant effects were not shown in a few studies.[15-18] Several large studies showed lower negative reactions among caregivers,[19] as well as improvement in distress,[20] sleep problems,[21,22] and coping and self-efficacy[23] and less decline in quality of life.[24]

Psychoeducation did not improve caregiver symptoms in some studies.[6,22,25-28] However, self-efficacy was shown to be significantly improved in several studies.[21,29-35] Psychoeducation improved caregiver depression,[33,36-38] decreased burden,[8,18] improved well-being,[39] improved quality of life,[40] and had positive effects on coping.[41] One systematic review[37] suggested that dyad-focused interventions had better results.

Likely to Be Effective

Caregiver training and skills development is necessary to assume a caregiving role. Skills training improved self-efficacy and reduced caregiver anxiety.[42,43]

Couples therapy to improve communication and emotional disclosure improved marital function, relationships, and intimacy.[44,45]

Decision aids including a video and workbook reduced decisional conflict and depression for caregivers in one large multisite randomized controlled trial.[46]

Multicomponent interventions such as assistance with transportation, respite care, psychotherapy, education, and other components showed benefit in systematic reviews[21,47-52] and individual research studies.[53,54]

Supportive care/support interventions delivered by phone, in person, or in support groups demonstrated mixed findings in individual studies.[53,55-57] Two systematic reviews[21,58] reported beneficial effects on caregiver burden, although effect sizes were small. Studies demonstrating effectiveness focused on mastery of skills to provide care.[58]

Effectiveness Not Established

Several interventions have shown mixed results in studies, or relevant studies were small or findings were inconclusive due to study limitations. These included the following interventions.

- **Art making/art therapy**[59,60]
- **Caregiver-provided massage** aimed at improving caregiver attitude and self-esteem[61]
- **Family-focused grief therapy** incorporated into hospice care[62]—Family functioning deteriorated in hostile families who received the intervention.
- **Massage/aromatherapy massage** for the caregiver[61,63,64]
- **Mindfulness-based stress reduction**[65]
- **Music/music therapy**[66]
- **Palliative care advisor services** added to usual palliative care staff[67]
- **Provider communication skills training** in which physicians completed a program to improve patient/caregiver communication[68]
- **Structured assessment** with standardized instruments[69]

Application to Practice

Caregiver and patient information and education needs can be met with interventions that have strong supportive evidence, including

- Ensuring that caregivers have the knowledge and skills to provide the required technical and direct assistance. Approaches such as direct observation of caregiver care provision with repeat demonstration and "testing" knowledge through caregiver repeat-back of information provide reinforcement of training and evaluation of efficacy.
- Providing psychoeducation that combines information and education with counseling and assistance in problem solving.

Cognitive behavioral approaches can be helpful to assist caregivers to identify unhelpful thoughts and behaviors and develop more effective coping strategies. Nurses can incorporate CBT principles into psychoeducational interventions.

Individuals and couples who demonstrate significant effects of strain and burden may need referral to qualified providers for full CBT or couples therapy.

Nurses can provide patients and caregivers with information about sources of support in the community and Internet resources. Collaboration with social workers, case managers, or patient navigators can facilitate identification of financial and other supportive resources available. Numerous Internet resources may be helpful to caregivers, including the following.
- American Cancer Society: Coping as a Caregiver[70]
- LIVESTRONG: Navigation Services[71]
- CancerCare: Caregiving[72]
- Today's Caregiver: Local Resources[73]
- National Cancer Institute: Caring for the Caregiver[74]

Nurses can encourage and educate caregivers in health promotion and maintaining treatment for their own health concerns.

Referral for home care, palliative care, hospice, respite care, and other services to meet multiple needs is an intervention that has strong evidence of effectiveness and should be used where appropriate.

Caregiver Strain and Burden Resource Contributors
*Topic leader: Margaret F. Bevans, PhD, RN, AOCN®
Carolyn Spence Cagle, PhD, RNC-OB, Mary Ellen Haisfield-Wolfe,
PhD, RN, OCN®, Ahlam Jadalla, PhD, RN, Margaretta S. Page, MS, RN,
and Thiruppavai Sundaramurthi, MSN, RN, CCRN*

References

1. Gibson, M.J., & Houser, A.N. (2007). *Valuing the invaluable: A new look at the economic value of family caregiving* (Issue Brief No. 82). Washington, DC: AARP Public Policy Institute.

2. Stenberg, U., Ruland, C.M., & Miaskowski, C. (2010). Review of the literature on the effects of caring for a patient with cancer. *Psycho-Oncology, 19,* 1013–1025. doi:10.1002/pon.1670

3. Braun, M., Mikulincer, M., Rydall, A., Walsh, A., & Rodin, G. (2007). Hidden morbidity in cancer: Spouse caregivers. *Journal of Clinical Oncology, 25,* 4829–4834. doi:10.1200/JCO.2006.10.0909

4. Janda, M., Steginga, S., Dunn, J., Langbecker, D., Walker, D., & Eakin, E. (2008). Unmet supportive care needs and interest in services among patients with a brain tumour and their carers. *Patient Education and Counseling, 71,* 251–258. doi:10.1016/j.pec.2008.01.020

5. Mitchell, A.J., Ferguson, D.W., Gill, J., Paul, J., & Symonds, P. (2013). Depression and anxiety in long-term cancer survivors compared with spouses and healthy controls: A systematic review and meta-analysis. *Lancet Oncology, 14,* 721–732. doi:10.1016/S1470-2045(13)70244-4

6. Sherwood, P.R., Given, B.A., Given, C.W., Sikorskii, A., You, M., & Prince, J. (2012). The impact of a problem-solving intervention on increasing caregiver assistance and improving caregiver health. *Supportive Care in Cancer, 20,* 1937–1947. doi:10.1007/s00520-011-1295-5

7. Song, L., Northouse, L.L., Braun, T.M., Zhang, L., Cimprich, B., Ronis, D.L., & Mood, D.W. (2011). Assessing longitudinal quality of life in prostate cancer patients and their spouses: A multilevel modeling approach. *Quality of Life Research, 20,* 371–381. doi:10.1007/s11136-010-9753-y

8. Waldron, E.A., Janke, E.A., Bechtel, C.F., Ramirez, M., & Cohen, A. (2013). A systematic review of psychosocial interventions to improve cancer caregiver quality of life. *Psycho-Oncology, 22,* 1200–1207. doi:10.1002/pon.3118

9. National Cancer Institute. (2014, February 21). Family caregivers in cancer: Roles and challenges (PDQ®)—Factors to consider in caregiver assessment [Health professional version]. Retrieved from http://www.cancer.gov/cancertopics/pdq/supportivecare/caregivers/healthprofessional/page6

10. Li, Q.P., Mak, Y.W., & Loke, A.Y. (2013). Spouses' experience of caregiving for cancer patients: A literature review. *International Nursing Review, 60,* 178–187. doi:10.1111/inr.12000

11. Northouse, L., Williams, A., Given, B., & McCorkle, R. (2012). Psychosocial care for family caregivers of patients with cancer. *Journal of Clinical Oncology, 30,* 1227–1234. doi:10.1200/JCO.2011.39.5798

12. Onega, L.L. (2008). Helping those who help others: The Modified Caregiver Strain Index. *American Journal of Nursing, 108*(9), 62–69. doi:10.1097/01.NAJ.0000334528.90459.9a

13. American Medical Association. (n.d.). Caregiver self-assessment questionnaire: How are you? Retrieved from http://www.caregiving.org/wp-content/uploads/2010/11/caregiverselfassessment_english.pdf

14. University of Iowa. (n.d.). Geriatric assessment tools: Caregivers. Retrieved from http://www.healthcare.uiowa.edu/igec/tools/categoryMenu.asp?categoryID=6

15. Bevans, M., Castro, K., Prince, P., Shelburne, N., Prachenko, O., Loscalzo, M., … Zabora, J. (2010). An individualized dyadic problem-solving education intervention for patients and family caregivers during allogeneic hematopoietic stem cell transplantation: A feasibility study. *Cancer Nursing, 33*(2), E24–E32. doi:10.1097/NCC.0b013e3181be5e6d

16. Campbell, L.C., Keefe, F.J., Scipio, C., McKee, D.C., Edwards, C.L., Herman, S.H., … Donatucci, C. (2007). Facilitating research participation and improving quality of life for African American prostate cancer survivors and their intimate partners. A pilot study of telephone-based coping skills training. *Cancer, 109*(Suppl. 2), 414–424. doi:10.1002/cncr.22355

17. Carter, P.A. (2006). A brief behavioral sleep intervention for family caregivers of persons with cancer. *Cancer Nursing, 29,* 95–103. doi:10.1097/00002820-200603000-00003

18. McMillan, S.C., Small, B.J., Weitzner, M., Schonwetter, R., Tittle, M., Moody, L., … Haley, W.E. (2006). Impact of coping skills intervention with family

caregivers of hospice patients with cancer: A randomized clinical trial. *Cancer, 106,* 214–222. doi:10.1002/cncr.21567

19. Given, B., Given, C.W., Sikorski, A., Jeon, S., Sherwood, P., & Rahbar, M. (2006). The impact of providing symptom management assistance on caregiver reaction: Results of a randomized trial. *Journal of Pain and Symptom Management, 32,* 433–443. doi:10.1016/j.jpainsymman.2006.05 .019

20. Manne, S.L., Kissane, D.W., Nelson, C.J., Mulhall, J.P., Winkel, G., & Zaider, T. (2011). Intimacy-enhancing psychological intervention for men diagnosed with prostate cancer and their partners: A pilot study. *Journal of Sexual Medicine, 8,* 1197–1209. doi:10.1111/j.1743-6109.2010.02163.x

21. Cohen, M., & Kuten, A. (2006). Cognitive-behavior group intervention for relatives of cancer patients: A controlled study. *Journal of Psychosomatic Research, 61,* 187–196. doi:10.1016/j.jpsychores.2005.08.014

22. Langford, D.J., Lee, K., & Miaskowski, C. (2012). Sleep disturbance interventions in oncology patients and family caregivers: A comprehensive review and meta-analysis. *Sleep Medicine Reviews, 16,* 397–414. doi:10.1016/ j.smrv.2011.07.002

23. Northouse, L.L., Katapodi, M.C., Song, L., Zhang, L., & Mood, D.W. (2010). Interventions with family caregivers of cancer patients: Meta-analysis of randomized trials. *CA: A Cancer Journal for Clinicians, 60,* 317–339. doi:10.3322/caac.20081

24. Meyers, F.J., Carducci, M., Loscalzo, M.J., Linder, J., Greasby, T., & Beckett, L.A. (2011). Effects of a problem-solving intervention (COPE) on quality of life for patients with advanced cancer on clinical trials and their caregivers: Simultaneous care educational intervention (SCEI): Linking palliation and clinical trials. *Journal of Palliative Medicine, 14,* 465–473. doi:10.1089/jpm.2010.0416

25. Harding, R., List, S., Epiphaniou, E., & Jones, H. (2012). How can informal caregivers in cancer and palliative care be supported? An updated systematic literature review of interventions and their effectiveness. *Palliative Medicine, 26,* 7–22. doi:10.1177/0269216311409613

26. Hudson, P.L., Aranda, S., & Hayman-White, K. (2005). A psycho-educational intervention for family caregivers of patients receiving palliative care: A randomized controlled trial. *Journal of Pain and Symptom Management, 30,* 329–341. doi:10.1016/j.jpainsymman.2005.04.006

27. Jepson, C., McCorkle, R., Adler, D., Nuamah, I., & Lusk, E. (1999). Effects of home care on caregivers' psychosocial status. *Image: The Journal of Nursing Scholarship, 31,* 115–120. doi:10.1111/j.1547-5069.1999.tb00444.x

28. Keefe, F.J., Ahles, T.A., Sutton, L., Dalton, J., Baucom, D., Pope, M.S., ... Scipio, C. (2005). Partner-guided cancer pain management at the end of life: A preliminary study. *Journal of Pain and Symptom Management, 29,* 263–272. doi:10.1016/j.jpainsymman.2004.06.014

29. Applebaum, A.J., & Breitbart, W. (2013). Care for the cancer caregiver: A systematic review. *Palliative and Supportive Care, 11,* 231–252. doi:10.1017/S1478951512000594

30. Cameron, J.I., Shin, J.L., Williams, D., & Stewart, D.E. (2004). A brief problem-solving intervention for family caregivers to individuals with advanced cancer. *Journal of Psychosomatic Research, 57,* 137–143. doi:10.1016/ S0022-3999(03)00609-3

31. Hudson, P., Trauer, T., Kelly, B., O'Connor, M., Thomas, K., Summers, M., ... White, V. (2013). Reducing the psychological distress of family caregivers of home-based palliative care patients: Short-term effects from a randomised controlled trial. *Psycho-Oncology, 22,* 1987–1993. doi:10.1002/pon.3242

32. Jones, J.M., Lewis, F.M., Griffith, K., Cheng, T., Secord, S. Walton, T., ... Catton, P. (2013). Helping Her Heal-Group: A pilot study to evaluate a group delivered educational intervention for male spouses of women with breast cancer. *Psycho-Oncology,* 2102–2109. doi:10.1002/pon.3263

33. Lewis, F.M., Cochrane, B.B., Fletcher, K.A., Zahlis, E.H., Shands, M.E., Gralow, J.R., ... Schmitz, K. (2008). Helping Her Heal: A pilot study of an

educational counseling intervention for spouses of women with breast cancer. *Psycho-Oncology, 17,* 131–137. doi:10.1002/pon.1203

34. Mokuau, N., Braun, K.L., Wong, L.K., Higuchi, P., & Gotay, C.C. (2008). Development of a family intervention for Native Hawaiian women with cancer: A pilot study. *Social Work, 53,* 9–19. doi:10.1093/sw/53.1.9

35. Pasacreta, J.V., Barg, F., Nuamah, I., & McCorkle, R. (2000). Participant characteristics before and 4 months after attendance at a family caregiver cancer education program. *Cancer Nursing, 23,* 295–303. doi:10.1097/00002820-200008000-00007

36. Badger, T.A., Segrin, C., Figueredo, A.J., Harrington, J., Sheppard, K., Passalacqua, S., ... Bishop, M. (2011). Psychosocial interventions to improve quality of life in prostate cancer survivors and their intimate or family partners. *Quality of Life Research, 20,* 833–844. doi:10.1007/s11136-010-9822-2

37. Hopkinson, J.B., Brown, J.C., Okamoto, I., & Addington-Hall, J.M. (2012). The effectiveness of patient-family carer (couple) intervention for the management of symptoms and other health-related problems in people affected by cancer: A systematic literature search and narrative review. *Journal of Pain and Symptom Management, 43,* 111–142. doi:10.1016/j.jpainsymman.2011.03.013

38. Northouse, L., Kershaw, T., Mood, D., & Schafenacker, A. (2005). Effects of a family intervention on the quality of life of women with recurrent breast cancer and their family caregivers. *Psycho-Oncology, 14,* 478–491. doi:10.1002/pon.871

39. Budin, W.C., Hoskins, C.N., Haber, J., Sherman, D.W., Maislin, G., Cater, J.R., ... Shukla, S. (2008). Breast cancer: Education, counseling, and adjustment among patients and partners: A randomized clinical trial. *Nursing Research, 57,* 199–213. doi:10.1097/01.NNR.0000319496.67369.37

40. Ferrell, B.R., Grant, M., Chan, J., Ahn, C., & Ferrell, B.A. (1995). The impact of cancer pain education on family caregivers of elderly patients. *Oncology Nursing Forum, 22,* 1211–1218.

41. Heinrichs, N., Zimmermann, T., Huber, B., Herschbach, P., Russell, D.W., & Baucom, D.H. (2012). Cancer distress reduction with a couple-based skills training: A randomized controlled trial. *Annals of Behavioral Medicine, 43,* 239–252. doi:10.1007/s12160-011-9314-9

42. Hendrix, C.C., Abernethy, A., Sloane, R., Misuraca, J., & Moore, J. (2009). A pilot study on the influence of an individualized and experiential training on cancer caregiver's self-efficacy in home care and symptom management. *Home Healthcare Nurse, 27,* 271–278. doi:10.1097/01.NHH.0000356777.70503.62

43. Hendrix, C.C., Landerman, R., & Abernethy, A.P. (2013). Effects of an individualized caregiver training intervention on self-efficacy of cancer caregivers. *Western Journal of Nursing Research, 35,* 590–610. doi:10.1177/0193945911420742

44. McLean, L.M., Walton, T., Rodin, G., Esplen, M.J., & Jones, J.M. (2013). A couple-based intervention for patients and caregivers facing end-stage cancer: Outcomes of a randomized controlled trial. *Psycho-Oncology, 22,* 28–38. doi:10.1002/pon.2046

45. Porter, L.S., Keefe, F.J., Baucom, D.H., Hurwitz, H., Moser, B., Patterson, E., & Kim, H.J. (2012). Partner-assisted emotional disclosure for patients with GI cancer: 8-week follow-up and processes associated with change. *Supportive Care in Cancer, 20,* 1755–1762. doi:10.1007/s00520-011-1272-z

46. Yun, Y.H., Lee, M.K., Park, S., Lee, J.L., Choi, J., Choi, Y.S., ... Hong, Y.S. (2011). Use of a decision aid to help caregivers discuss terminal disease status with a family member with cancer: A randomized controlled trial. *Journal of Clinical Oncology, 29,* 4811–4819. doi:10.1200/JCO.2011.35.3870

47. Caress, A., Chalmers, K., & Luker, K. (2009). A narrative review of interventions to support family carers who provide physical care to family members with cancer. *International Journal of Nursing Studies, 46,* 1516–1527. doi:10.1016/j.ijnurstu.2009.03.008

48. Harding, R., & Higginson, I.J. (2003). What is the best way to help caregivers in cancer and palliative care? A systematic literature review of interventions and their effectiveness. *Palliative Medicine, 17,* 63–74. doi:10.1191/0269216303pm667oa

49. Martire, L.M., Lustig, A.P., Schulz, R., Miller, G.E., & Helgeson, V.S. (2004). Is it beneficial to involve a family member? A meta-analysis of psychosocial interventions for chronic illness. *Health Psychology, 23,* 599–611. doi:10.1037/0278-6133.23.6.599

50. Mattila, E., Leino, K., Paavilainen, E., & AstedtKurki, P. (2009). Nursing intervention studies on patients and family members: A systematic literature review. *Scandinavian Journal of Caring Sciences, 23,* 611–622. doi:10.1111/j.1471-6712.2008.00652.x

51. Pasacreta, J.V., & McCorkle, R. (2000). Cancer care: Impact of interventions on caregiver outcomes. *Annual Review of Nursing Research, 18,* 127–148.

52. Sörensen, S., Pinquart, M., & Duberstein, P. (2002). How effective are interventions with caregivers? An updated meta-analysis. *Gerontologist, 42,* 356–372. doi:10.1093/geront/42.3.356

53. Harding, R., Higginson, I.J., Leam, C., Donaldson, N., Pearce, A., George, R., ... Taylor, L. (2004). Evaluation of a short-term group intervention for informal carers of patients attending a home palliative care service. *Journal of Pain and Symptom Management, 27,* 396–408. doi:10.1016/j.jpainsymman.2003.09.012

54. Hutchison, S.D., Sargeant, H., Morris, B.A., Hawkes, A.L., Clutton, S., & Chambers, S.K. (2011). A community-based approach to cancer counseling for patients and carers: A preliminary study. *Psycho-Oncology, 20,* 897–901. doi:10.1002/pon.1786

55. McCorkle, R., Siefert, M.L., Dowd, M.F., Robinson, J.P., & Pickett, M. (2007). Effects of advanced practice nursing on patient and spouse depressive symptoms, sexual function, and marital interaction after radical prostatectomy. *Urologic Nursing, 27,* 65–77. Retrieved from http://www.medscape.com/viewarticle/555708

56. Namkoong, K., DuBenske, L.L., Shaw, B.R., Gustafson, D.H., Hawkins, R.P., Shah, D.V., ... Cleary, J.F. (2012). Creating a bond between caregivers online: Effect on caregivers' coping strategies. *Journal of Health Communication: International Perspectives, 17,* 125–140. doi:10.1080/10810730.2011.585687

57. Toseland, R.W., Blanchard, C.G., & McCallion, P. (1995). A problem solving intervention for caregivers of cancer patients. *Social Science and Medicine, 40,* 517–528. doi:10.1016/0277-9536(94)E0093-8

58. Glasdam, S., Timm, H., & Vittrup, R. (2010). Support efforts for caregivers of chronically ill persons. *Clinical Nursing Research, 19,* 233–265. doi:10.1177/1054773810369683

59. Walsh, S.M., Martin, S.C., & Schmidt, L.A. (2004). Testing the efficacy of a creative-arts intervention with family caregivers of patients with cancer. *Journal of Nursing Scholarship, 36,* 214–219. doi:10.1111/j.1547-5069.2004.04040.x

60. Walsh, S.M., Radcliffe, R.S., Castillo, L.C., Kumar, A.M., & Broschard, D.M. (2007). A pilot study to test the effects of art-making classes for family caregivers of patients with cancer [Online exclusive]. *Oncology Nursing Forum, 34,* E9–E16. doi:10.1188/07.ONF.E9-E16

61. Collinge, W., Kahn, J., Walton, T., Kozak, L., Bauer-Wu, S., Fletcher, K., ... Soltysik, R. (2013). Touch, caring, and cancer: Randomized controlled trial of a multimedia caregiver education program. *Supportive Care in Cancer, 21,* 1405–1414. doi:10.1007/s00520-012-1682-6

62. Kissane, D.W., McKenzie, M., Bloch, S., Moskowitz, C., McKenzie, D.P., & O'Neill, I. (2006). Family focused grief therapy: A randomized, controlled trial in palliative care and bereavement. *American Journal of Psychiatry, 163,* 1208–1218. doi:10.1176/appi.ajp.163.7.1208

63. Cronfalk, B.S., Ternestedt, B., & Strang, P. (2010). Soft tissue massage: Early intervention for relatives whose family members died in palliative

cancer care. *Journal of Clinical Nursing, 19,* 1040–1048. doi:10.1111/j.1365 -2702.2009.02985.x

64. Rexilius, S.J., Mundt, C., Megel, M.E., & Agrawal, S. (2002). Therapeutic effects of massage therapy and healing touch on caregivers of patients undergoing autologous hematopoietic stem cell transplant [Online exclusive]. *Oncology Nursing Forum, 29,* E35–E44. doi:10.1188/02.ONF.E35-E44

65. Birnie, K., Garland, S.N., & Carlson, L.E. (2010). Psychological benefits for cancer patients and their partners participating in mindfulness-based stress reduction (MBSR). *Psycho-Oncology, 19,* 1004–1009. doi:10.1002/pon.1651

66. Lai, H.L., Li, Y.M., & Lee, L.H. (2012). Effects of music intervention with nursing presence and recorded music on psycho-physiological indices of cancer patient caregivers. *Journal of Clinical Nursing, 21,* 745–756. doi:10.1111/j.1365-2702.2011.03916.x

67. Walsh, K., Jones, L., Tookman, A., Mason, C., McLoughlin, J., Blizard, R., & King, M. (2007). Reducing emotional distress in people caring for patients receiving specialist palliative care. Randomised trial. *British Journal of Psychiatry, 190,* 142–147. doi:10.1192/bjp.bp.106.023960

68. Lienard, A., Merckaert, I., Libert, Y., Delvaux, N., Marchal, S., Boniver, J., ... Razavi, D. (2008). Factors that influence cancer patients' and relatives' anxiety following a three-person medical consultation: Impact of a communication skills training program for physicians. *Psycho-Oncology, 17,* 488–496. doi:10.1002/pon.1262

69. McMillan, S.C., Small, B.J., & Haley, W.E. (2011). Improving hospice outcomes through systematic assessment: A clinical trial. *Cancer Nursing, 34,* 89–97. doi:10.1097/NCC.0b013e3181f70aee

70. American Cancer Society. (n.d.). Coping as a caregiver. Retrieved from http://www.cancer.org/treatment/caregivers/copingasacaregiver/index

71. LIVESTRONG. (n.d.). Navigation services. Retrieved from http://www.livestrong.org/we-can-help/navigation-services

72. CancerCare. (n.d.). Caregiving. Retrieved from http://www.cancercare.org/tagged/caregiving

73. Today's Caregiver. (n.d.). Local resources. http://caregiver.com/regional resources/index.htm

74. National Cancer Institute. (2007, June 29). Caring for the caregiver. Retrieved from http://www.cancer.gov/cancertopics/coping/caring-for-the -caregiver

Chemotherapy-Induced Nausea and Vomiting

Catherine Cherwin, MS, RN,
Dwanna M. Ward-Boahen RN, BSN, MSN, AOCNP®,
Stacy Whiteside, RN, MS, CPNP-AC/PC, CPON®,
Colleen Lewis, MSN, ANP-BC, AOCNP®, and
Deborah L. Selm-Orr, RN, MS, DNP(c), CRNP, AOCN®

Problem and Incidence

Nausea is the subjective sensation felt with the urge to vomit. Vomiting is the actual expulsion of stomach contents. These are two distinct symptoms, though they most often occur together. Despite advances in management, at least two-thirds of patients receiving chemotherapy will experience chemotherapy-induced nausea and vomiting (CINV).[1] Nausea and vomiting remain the most feared and unpleasant side effects of chemotherapy.[2] The incidence and severity of CINV are affected by the emetogenicity of the chemotherapy agents used; the dose, schedule, and route of administration; and individual patient variability. CINV may occur in the acute phase (within 24 hours of chemotherapy) and/or delayed phase (24 hours to several days after chemotherapy administration). Anticipatory CINV may occur before chemotherapy. Breakthrough and refractory CINV can occur at any time after chemotherapy. Uncontrolled CINV can have severe consequences, such as dehydration, electrolyte imbalance, and malnutrition. Uncontrolled CINV also increases the cost of care, may result in the need for emergency department care or hospitalization,[3] and can lead to discontinuation of treatment.[4-6]

Risk Factors and Assessment

The major determinant of CINV risk is the emetogenic potential of the chemotherapy used. National Comprehensive Cancer Network guidelines identify the emetogenic potential of various agents according to the frequency of observed CINV.[7,8]

- Drugs with high emetogenic potential, depending on dose level, include doxorubicin, epirubicin, platinum-based agents, carmustine, cyclophosphamide, dacarbazine, ifosfamide, mechlorethamine, and streptozocin.
- Oral agents with moderate-to-high emetogenicity include altretamine, busulfan, cyclophosphamide, procarbazine, estramustine, etoposide, lomustine, temozolomide, and hexamethylmelamine.

Patients who experienced CINV with previous treatment are at risk for anticipatory CINV. Factors such as female gender and younger age may also increase risk.[9]

CINV assessment includes the symptoms of both nausea and vomiting, the stage (e.g., acute, delayed, anticipatory, breakthrough), frequency, intensity, and the use and effects of antiemetics.

Assessment tools include
- National Cancer Institute Cancer Therapy Evaluation Program *Common Terminology Criteria for Adverse Events* (open access)[10]
- Multinational Association of Supportive Care in Cancer Antiemesis Tool (open access)[11]
- Numeric rating scale.

What interventions are effective in preventing and treating CINV?

Evidence retrieved through July 31, 2013

Recommended for Practice

Cannabinoids reduced both acute and delayed CINV in studies[12,13] and systematic reviews.[14-18] Laws regarding medical use of cannabinoids are inconsistent.

Neurokinin (NK₁) receptor antagonists are effective and recommended in professional guidelines.[7,8,19,20]
- **Aprepitant** is effective for acute and delayed CINV.[21-38]
- **Fosaprepitant** is as effective as aprepitant.[39,40]
- Use of NK₁ receptor antagonists in children has not been well studied.[41]

Serotonin (5-HT₃) receptor antagonists are effective[18,42-44] and have been recommended in professional guidelines.[8,20,45,46]
- **Granisetron** appears to be most effective for acute-phase CINV. The addition of dexamethasone improved delayed CINV results[42,45,47-50] and improved results with highly emetogenic chemotherapy.[4H] **Transdermal granisetron** was as effective as oral granisetron.[51,52]
- **Ondansetron** was effective in the acute phase. The addition of dexamethasone can improve delayed-phase results.[18,42,53-56] An oral formulation of ondansetron was as effective as intramuscular administration.[56]
- **Palonosetron** was demonstrated to be effective in several studies.[57-71]
  - Studies examining comparative effectiveness of various 5-HT₃ receptor antagonist drugs showed mixed results.[29,72-75] Two meta-analyses suggested that palonosetron may be more effective than other 5-HT₃ receptor antagonist drugs.[76,77]
  - Palonosetron may be more effective than other 5-HT₃ receptor antagonist drugs to prevent delayed nausea.[43,66,77-82]
  - Palonosetron has been recommended for children.[20,41,83,84]

Triple-drug regimens consisting of 5-HT₃ receptor antagonists, NK₁ receptor antagonists, and dexamethasone are effective[8,20,25-27,30,32,34,35,40,70,85-95] and recommended in guidelines[7] for adults and children receiving highly emetogenic therapy.

Likely to Be Effective

Dexamethasone used as a single agent is recommended for chemotherapy with low emetogenic potential.[7,96-98]

Gabapentin as an adjunct to standard antiemetics reduced acute-phase CINV.[99]

Hypnosis for anticipatory CINV was effective in one small study[100] and was evaluated in systematic reviews of nonpharmacologic interventions.[101-103]

Managing patient expectations about CINV demonstrated benefit, particularly for anticipatory nausea.[104-106]

Megestrol/megestrol acetate reduced nausea but not vomiting.[107]

Olanzapine for breakthrough CINV was effective in the majority of patients.[108,109]

Progressive muscle relaxation and guided imagery with antiemetics showed benefit.[110,111] However, systematic reviews concluded that the evidence was weak.[101,102,112]

Benefits Balanced With Harms

Virtual reality decreased postinfusion emesis in a small study but may cause motion sickness.[113]

Effectiveness Not Established

A number of pharmacologic and nonpharmacologic interventions have been studied for the prevention or reduction of CINV. Evidence was insufficient to show effectiveness because of study limitations, lack of effects in small studies, or inconsistent results.
- **Pharmacologic interventions**
  - **Haloperidol**[16]

- **Mirtazapine**[114]
- **Olanzapine** as a primary antiemetic with a **5-HT₃ receptor antagonist** and **dexamethasone**[115]
- **Prochlorperazine** for breakthrough CINV[116]
- **Prophylactic metoclopramide** as an adjunct to standard antiemetics[117]
- **Thalidomide**[118]
- **Nonpharmacologic interventions**
  - **Acupressure** applied to the P6 point on the wrist[105,119-133]—Systematic reviews did not show effectiveness.[103,134-137]
  - **Acupuncture, electroacupuncture, and acustimulation**[103,125,128,129,133-136,138-144]
  - **Exercise**[145,146]
  - **Ginger**[147-152]—Systematic reviews[153,154] and a meta-analysis[155] did not support use of ginger.
  - **Grape juice** in addition to standard antiemetics[156]
  - **Herbal medicine**[157]
  - **Massage/aromatherapy massage**[158-162]
  - **Progressive muscle relaxation**[163]
  - **Psychoeducational interventions**[103,164-166]
  - **Visual imagery**, with and without music[167-169]
  - **Yoga**[170]—A systematic review concluded evidence was weak.[103]

Effectiveness Unlikely

Cocculine, a mixture of homeopathic components, added to standard antiemetics did not reduce CINV.[171]

Expert Opinion

Dietary approaches that may be helpful include eating smaller meals, avoiding food and other stimuli with strong odors, avoiding spicy and fatty foods, and avoiding an empty stomach before chemotherapy.[172]

Lorazepam has been suggested to reduce anticipatory CINV.[8,19]

Application to Practice

CINV prevention needs to be the goal. Ongoing evaluation of antiemetic effectiveness for all phases of CINV is essential to refine management approaches and to identify and implement the optimal combination of pharmacologic and nonpharmacologic interventions.

Patients need to be educated in using antiemetics on a regular schedule for prevention.

Patients receiving chemotherapy that is highly or moderately emetogenic need effective prophylactic antiemetic regimens. Emerging evidence also suggests benefit of aggressive prophylaxis with chemotherapy of low emetogenicity.

Nurses need to assess effectiveness of antiemetics and occurrence of delayed or breakthrough CINV. It is useful for patients to have medication available in case of breakthrough CINV. When delayed CINV is expected, agents shown to reduce delayed symptoms should be considered. Cannabinoids may be helpful as an adjunct to standard antiemetics and as a rescue medication for patients with refractory CINV.

Patients at risk for anticipatory CINV can benefit from interventions to manage expectations, as well as interventions such as hypnosis, relaxation, and anxiolytics before treatment.

Control of nausea is more difficult than control of vomiting. Inclusion of interventions shown to reduce nausea needs to be considered in antiemetic regimens.

Nurses can educate patients regarding dietary interventions that might be helpful.

Chemotherapy-Induced Nausea and Vomiting Resource Contributors

*Topic leader: Cynthia R. King, PhD, NP, MSN, RN, FAAN
Catherine Cherwin, MS, RN, Lynn M. Czaplewski, MS, RN, ACNS-BC,
CRNI, AOCNS®, Rasha Dabbour, PhD, Myrna Doumit, PhD, RN,
Beyhan Duran, RN, MS, Patricia Jakel, RN, MN, AOCN®, Jiyeon
Lee, PhD, RN, Colleen Lewis, MSN, ANP-BC, AOCNP®,*

Cheryl C. Rodgers, PhD, RN, CPNP, CPON®, Deborah L. Selm-Orr, RN, MS, DNP(c), CRNP, AOCN®, Patricia C. Starr, RN, MSN, OCN®, Pam Stephenson, RN, PhD, AOCNS®, PMHCNS-BC, Dwanna M. Ward-Boahen, RN, BSN, MSN, AOCNP®, Joan L. Ralph Webber, RN, MSN, CNS, CRNI, OCN®, Susan Wesmiller, PhD, RN, and Stacy Whiteside, RN, MS, CPNP-AC/PC, CPON®

References

1. Molassiotis, A., Stamataki, Z., & Kontopantelis, E. (2013). Development and preliminary validation of a risk prediction model for chemotherapy-related nausea and vomiting. *Supportive Care in Cancer, 21*, 2759–2767. doi:10.1007/s00520-013-1843-2

2. Hesketh, P.J. (2009). Penny wise, dollar foolish approach to antiemetic use may compromise patient care. *Journal of Oncology Practice, 5*, 221–222. doi:10.1200/JOP.091026

3. Carlotto, A., Hogsett, V.L., Maiorini, E.M., Razulis, J.G., & Sonis, S.T. (2013). The economic burden of toxicities associated with cancer treatment: Review of the literature and analysis of nausea and vomiting, diarrhoea, oral mucositis and fatigue. *PharmacoEconomics, 31*, 753–766. doi:10.1007/s40273-013-0081-2

4. Davidson, W., Teleni, L., Muller, J., Ferguson, M., McCarthy, A.L., Vick, J., & Isenring, E. (2012). Malnutrition and chemotherapy-induced nausea and vomiting: Implications for practice [Online exclusive]. *Oncology Nursing Forum, 39*, E340–E345. doi:10.1188/12.ONF.E340-E345

5. Tong, H.T., Isenring, E.A., & Yates, P. (2009). The prevalence of nutrition impact symptoms and their relationship to quality of life and clinical outcomes in medical oncology patients. *Supportive Care in Cancer, 17*, 83–90. doi:10.1007/s00520-008-0472-7

6. Van Cutsem, E., & Arends, J. (2005). The causes and consequences of cancer-associated malnutrition. *European Journal of Oncology Nursing, 9*(Suppl. 2), S51–S63. doi:10.1016/j.ejon.2005.09.007

7. Gralla, R.J., Roila F., Tonato, M., & Herrstedt, J. (2013). MASCC/ESMO antiemetic guideline 2013 [Slide presentation]. Retrieved from http://www.mascc.org/assets/documents/mascc_guidelines_english_2013.pdf

8. National Comprehensive Cancer Network. (2013). *NCCN Clinical Practice Guidelines in Oncology: Antiemesis* [v.1.2014]. Retrieved from http://www.nccn.org/professionals/physician_gls/pdf/antiemesis.pdf

9. Irwin, M.M., Lee, J., Rodgers, C., Starr, P., & Webber, J.R. (2012). *Putting evidence into practice: Improving oncology patient outcomes. Chemotherapy-induced nausea and vomiting resource.* Pittsburgh, PA: Oncology Nursing Society.

10. National Cancer Institute Cancer Therapy Evaluation Program. (2010, June 14). *Common terminology criteria for adverse events* [v.4.03]. Retrieved from http://evs.nci.nih.gov/ftp1/CTCAE/CTCAE_4.03_2010-06-14_QuickReference_5x7.pdf

11. Multinational Association of Supportive Care in Cancer. (2004). MASCC Antiemesis Tool (MAT). Retrieved from http://www.mascc.org/mat

12. Duran, M., Pérez, E., Abanades, S., Vidal, X., Saura, C., Majem, M., ... Capellà, D. (2010). Preliminary efficacy and safety of an oromucosal standardized cannabis extract in chemotherapy-induced nausea and vomiting. *British Journal of Clinical Pharmacology, 70*, 656–663. doi:10.1111/j.1365-2125.2010.03743.x

13. Meiri, E., Jhangiani, H., Vredenburgh, J.J., Barbato, L.M., Carter, F.J., Yang, H.M., & Baranowski, V. (2007). Efficacy of dronabinol alone and

in combination with ondansetron versus ondansetron alone for delayed chemotherapy-induced nausea and vomiting. *Current Medical Research and Opinion, 23,* 533–543. doi:10.1185/030079907X167525

14. Cotter, J. (2009). Efficacy of crude marijuana and synthetic delta-9-tetrahydrocannabinol as treatment for chemotherapy-induced nausea and vomiting: A systematic literature review. *Oncology Nursing Forum, 36,* 345–352. doi:10.1188/09.ONF.345-352

15. Davis, M.P. (2008). Oral nabilone capsules in the treatment of chemotherapy-induced nausea and vomiting and pain. *Expert Opinion on Investigational Drugs, 17,* 85–95. doi:10.1517/13543784.17.1.85

16. Keeley, P.W. (2009). Nausea and vomiting in people with cancer and other chronic diseases. *BMJ Clinical Evidence, 2009,* 2406. Retrieved from http://www.ncbi.nlm.nih.gov/pmc/articles/PMC2907825

17. Machado Rocha, F.C., Stefano, S.C., De Cassia Haiek, R., Rosa Oliveira, L.M., & Da Silveira, D.X. (2008). Therapeutic use of *Cannabis sativa* on chemotherapy-induced nausea and vomiting among cancer patients: Systematic review and meta-analysis. *European Journal of Cancer Care, 17,* 431–443. doi:10.1111/j.1365-2354.2008.00917.x

18. Phillips, R.S., Gopaul, S., Gibson, F., Houghton, E., Craig, J.V., Light, K., & Pizer, B. (2010). Antiemetic medication for prevention and treatment of chemotherapy induced nausea and vomiting in childhood. *Cochrane Database of Systematic Reviews, 2010*(9). doi:10.1002/14651858.CD007786.pub2

19. Herrstedt, J., & Roila, F. (2008). Chemotherapy-induced nausea and vomiting: ESMO clinical recommendations for prophylaxis. *Annals of Oncology, 19*(Suppl. 2), ii110–ii112. doi:10.1093/annonc/mdn105

20. Roila, F., Herrstedt, J., Aapro, M., Gralla, R.J., Einhorn, L.H., Ballatori, E., ... Warr, D. (2010). Guideline update for MASCC and ESMO in the prevention of chemotherapy- and radiotherapy-induced nausea and vomiting: Results of the Perugia consensus conference. *Annals of Oncology, 21*(Suppl. 5), v232–v243. doi:10.1093/annonc/mdq194

21. Abidi, M.H., Tageja, N., Ayash, L., Abrams, J., Ratanatharathorn, V., Al-Kadhimi, Z., ... Uberti, J. (2012). Aprepitant for prevention of nausea and vomiting secondary to high-dose cyclophosphamide administered to patients undergoing autologous peripheral blood stem cells mobilization: A phase II trial. *Supportive Care in Cancer, 20,* 2363–2369. doi:10.1007/s00520-011-1341-3

22. Choi, M.R., Jiles, C., & Seibel, N.L. (2010). Aprepitant use in children, adolescents, and young adults for the control of chemotherapy-induced nausea and vomiting (CINV). *Journal of Pediatric Hematology/Oncology, 32,* e268–e271. doi:10.1097/MPH.0b013e3181e5e1af

23. dos Santos, L.V., Souza, F.H., Brunetto, A.T., Sasse, A.D., & da Silveira Nogueira Lima, J.P. (2012). Neurokinin-1 receptor antagonists for chemotherapy-induced nausea and vomiting: A systematic review. *Journal of the National Cancer Institute, 104,* 1280–1292. doi:10.1093/jnci/djs335

24. Gore, L., Chawla, S., Petrilli, A., Hemenway, M., Schissel, D., Chua, V., ... Oxenius, B. (2009). Aprepitant in adolescent patients for prevention of chemotherapy-induced nausea and vomiting: A randomized, double-blind, placebo-controlled study of efficacy and tolerability. *Pediatric Blood and Cancer, 52,* 242–247. doi:10.1002/pbc.21811

25. Herrington, J.D., Jaskiewicz, A.D., & Song, J. (2008). Randomized, placebo-controlled, pilot study evaluating aprepitant single dose plus palonosetron and dexamethasone for the prevention of acute and delayed chemotherapy-induced nausea and vomiting. *Cancer, 112,* 2080–2087. doi:10.1002/cncr.23364

26. Herrstedt, J., & Roila, F. (2009). Chemotherapy-induced nausea and vomiting: ESMO clinical recommendations for prophylaxis. *Annals of Oncology, 20*(Suppl. 4), iv156–iv158. doi:10.1093/annonc/mdp160

27. Hesketh, P.J., Grunberg, S.M., Herrstedt, J., de Wit, R., Gralla, R.J., Carides, A.D., ... Horgan, K.J. (2006). Combined data from two phase III trials of the NK$_1$ antagonist aprepitant plus a 5HT$_3$ antagonist and a corticosteroid

for prevention of chemotherapy-induced nausea and vomiting: Effect of gender on treatment response. *Supportive Care in Cancer, 14*, 354–360. doi:10.1007/s00520-005-0914-4

28. Hesketh, P.J., Warr, D.G., Street, J.C., & Carides, A.D. (2011). Differential time course of action of 5-HT_3 and NK_1 receptor antagonists when used with highly and moderately emetogenic chemotherapy (HEC and MEC). *Supportive Care in Cancer, 19*, 1297–1302. doi:10.1007/s00520-010-0944-4

29. Jin, Y., Wu, X., Guan, Y., Gu, D., Shen, Y., Xu, Z., … Chen, J. (2012). Efficacy and safety of aprepitant in the prevention of chemotherapy-induced nausea and vomiting: A pooled analysis. *Supportive Care in Cancer, 20*, 1815–1822. doi:10.1007/s00520-011-1280-z

30. Jordan, K., Kinitz, I., Voigt, W., Behlendorf, T., Wolf, H., & Schmoll, H. (2009). Safety and efficacy of a triple antiemetic combination with the NK-1 antagonist aprepitant in highly and moderately emetogenic multiple-day chemotherapy. *European Journal of Cancer, 45*, 1184–1187. doi:10.1016/j.ejca.2008.11.046

31. Rapoport, B.L., Jordan, K., Boice, J.A., Taylor, A., Brown, C., Hardwick, J.S., … Schmoll, H.J. (2010). Aprepitant for the prevention of chemotherapy-induced nausea and vomiting associated with a broad range of moderately emetogenic chemotherapies and tumor types: A randomized, double-blind study. *Supportive Care in Cancer, 18*, 423–431. doi:10.1007/s00520-009-0680-9

32. Stiff, P.J., Fox-Geiman, M.P., Kiley, K., Rychlik, K., Parthasarathy, M., Fletcher-Gonzalez, D., … Rodriguez, T.E. (2013). Prevention of nausea and vomiting associated with stem cell transplant: Results of a prospective, randomized trial of aprepitant used with highly emetogenic preparative regimens. *Biology of Blood and Marrow Transplantation, 19*, 49.e1–55.e1. doi:10.1016/j.bbmt.2012.07.019

33. Takahashi, T., Hoshi, E., Takagi, M., Katsumata, N., Kawahara, M., & Eguchi, K. (2010). Multicenter, phase II, placebo-controlled, double-blind, randomized study of aprepitant in Japanese patients receiving high-dose cisplatin. *Cancer Science, 101*, 2455–2461. doi:10.1111/j.1349-7006.2010.01689.x

34. Uchida, M., Ikesue, H., Kato, K., Ichinose, K., Hiraiwa, H., Sakurai, A., … Oishi, R. (2013). Antiemetic effectiveness and safety of aprepitant in patients with hematologic malignancy receiving multiday chemotherapy. *American Journal of Health-System Pharmacy, 70*, 343–349. doi:10.2146/ajhp120363

35. Uchino, J., Hirano, R., Tashiro, N., Yoshida, Y., Ushijima, S., Matsumoto, T., … Watanabe, K. (2012). Efficacy of aprepitant in patients with advanced or recurrent lung cancer receiving moderately emetogenic chemotherapy. *Asian Pacific Journal of Cancer Prevention, 13*, 4187–4190. doi:10.7314/APJCP.2012.13.8.4187

36. Warr, D.G., Street, J.C., & Carides, A.D. (2011). Evaluation of risk factors predictive of nausea and vomiting with current standard-of-care antiemetic treatment: Analysis of phase 3 trial of aprepitant in patients receiving adriamycin-cyclophosphamide-based chemotherapy. *Supportive Care in Cancer, 19*, 807–813. doi:10.1007/s00520-011-0899-5

37. Wu, C.-E., & Liaw, C.-C. (2012). Using aprepitant as secondary antiemetic prophylaxis for cancer patients with cisplatin-induced emesis. *Supportive Care in Cancer, 20*, 2357–2361. doi:10.1007/s00520-011-1345-z

38. Yeo, W., Mo, F.K.F., Suen, J.J.S., Ho, W.M., Chan, S.L., Lau, W., … Zee, B. (2009). A randomized study of aprepitant, ondansetron and dexamethasone for chemotherapy-induced nausea and vomiting in Chinese breast cancer patients receiving moderately emetogenic chemotherapy. *Breast Cancer Research and Treatment, 113*, 529–535. doi:10.1007/s10549-008-9957-9

39. Grunberg, S., Chua, D., Maru, A., Dinis, J., DeVandry, S., Boice, J.A., … Herrstedt, J. (2011). Single-dose fosaprepitant for the prevention of chemotherapy-induced nausea and vomiting associated with cisplatin therapy: Randomized, double-blind study protocol—EASE. *Journal of Clinical Oncology, 29*, 1495–1501. doi:10.1200/JCO.2010.31.7859

40. Saito, H., Yoshizawa, H., Yoshimori, K., Katakami, N., Katsumata, N., Kawahara, M., & Eguchi, K. (2013). Efficacy and safety of single-dose fosaprepitant in the prevention of chemotherapy-induced nausea and vomiting in patients receiving high-dose cisplatin: A multicentre, randomised, double-blind, placebo-controlled phase 3 trial. *Annals of Oncology, 24,* 1067–1073. doi:10.1093/annonc/mds541

41. Jordan, K., Roila, F., Molassiotis, A., Maranzano, E., Clark-Snow, R.A., & Feyer, P. (2011). Antiemetics in children receiving chemotherapy: MASCC/ESMO guideline update 2009. *Supportive Care in Cancer, 19*(Suppl. 1), 37–42. doi:10.1007/s00520-010-0994-7

42. Billio, A., Morello, E., & Clarke, M.J. (2010). Serotonin receptor antagonists for highly emetogenic chemotherapy in adults. *Cochrane Database of Systematic Reviews, 2010*(1). doi:10.1002/14651858.CD006272.pub2

43. Hesketh, P.J., Bosnjak, S.M., Nikolic, V., & Rapoport, B. (2011). Incidence of delayed nausea and vomiting in patients with colorectal cancer receiving irinotecan-based chemotherapy. *Supportive Care in Cancer, 19,* 2063–2066. doi:10.1007/s00520-011-1286-6

44. Naeim, A., Dy, S.M., Lorenz, K.A., Sanati, H., Walling, A., & Asch, S.M. (2008). Evidence-based recommendations for cancer nausea and vomiting. *Journal of Clinical Oncology, 26,* 3903–3910. doi:10.1200/JCO.2007.15.9533

45. Einhorn, L.H., Grunberg, S.M., Rapoport, B., Rittenberg, C., & Feyer, P. (2011). Antiemetic therapy for multiple-day chemotherapy and additional topics consisting of rescue antiemetics and high-dose chemotherapy with stem cell transplant: Review and consensus statement. *Supportive Care in Cancer, 19*(Suppl. 1), S1–S4. doi:10.1007/s00520-010-0920-z

46. Kris, M.G., Hesketh, P.J., Somerfield, M.R., Feyer, P., Clark-Snow, R., Koeller, J.M., … Grunberg, S.M. (2006). American Society of Clinical Oncology guideline for antiemetics in oncology: Update 2006. *Journal of Clinical Oncology, 24,* 2932–2947. doi:10.1200/JCO.2006.06.9591

47. Keat, C.H., Phua, G., Abdul Kassim, M.S., Poh, W.K., & Sriraman, M. (2013). Can granisetron injection used as primary prophylaxis improve the control of nausea and vomiting with low-emetogenic chemotherapy? *Asian Pacific Journal of Cancer Prevention, 14,* 469–473. doi:10.7314/APJCP.2013.14.1.469

48. Keyhanian, S., Taziki, O., Saravi, M.M., & Fotokian, Z. (2009). A randomized comparison of granisetron plus dexamethasone with granisetron alone for the control of acute chemotherapy-induced emesis and nausea. *International Journal of Hematology-Oncology and Stem Cell Research, 3*(2), 27–30. Retrieved from http://ijhoscr.tums.ac.ir/index.php/ijhoscr/article/view/213/124

49. Tsuji, D., Kim, Y.-I., Taku, K., Nakagaki, S., Ikematsu, Y., Tsubota, H., … Daimon, T. (2011). Comparative trial of two intravenous doses of granisetron (1 versus 3 mg) in the prevention of chemotherapy-induced acute emesis: A double-blind, randomized, non-inferiority trial. *Supportive Care in Cancer, 20,* 1057–1064. doi:10.1007/s00520-011-1185-x

50. Yonemura, M., Katsumata, N., Hashimoto, H., Satake, S., Kaneko, M., Kobayashi, Y., … Hojo, T. (2009). Randomized controlled study comparing two doses of intravenous granisetron (1 and 3 mg) for acute chemotherapy-induced nausea and vomiting in cancer patients: A non-inferiority trial. *Japanese Journal of Clinical Oncology, 3,* 443–448. doi:10.1093/jjco/hyp036

51. Boccia, R., Gordan, L.N., Clark, G., Howell, J.D., & Grunberg, S.M. (2011). Efficacy and tolerability of transdermal granisetron for the control of chemotherapy-induced nausea and vomiting associated with moderately and highly emetogenic multi-day chemotherapy: A randomized, double-blind, phase III study. *Supportive Care in Cancer, 19,* 1609–1617. doi:10.1007/s00520-010-0990-y

52. Tuca, A. (2009). Use of granisetron transdermal system in the prevention of chemotherapy-induced nausea and vomiting: A review. *Cancer Management and Research, 2,* 1–12. doi:10.2147/CMAR.S4953

53. Kaushal, J., Gupta, M.C., Kaushal, V., Bhutani, G., Dhankar, R., Atri, R., & Verma, S. (2010). Clinical evaluation of two antiemetic combinations palonosetron dexamethasone versus ondansetron dexamethasone in chemotherapy of head and neck cancer. *Singapore Medical Journal, 51*, 871–875.

54. Lajolo, P.P., De Camargo, B., & Del Giglio, A. (2009). Omission of day 2 of antiemetic medications is a cost saving strategy for improving chemotherapy-induced nausea and vomiting control results of a randomized phase III trial. *American Journal of Clinical Oncology, 32,* 23–26. doi:10.1097/COC.0b013e318178e4fe

55. Ng, W., & Della-Fiorentina, S. (2010). The efficacy of oral ondansetron and dexamethasone for the prevention of acute chemotherapy-induced nausea and vomiting associated with moderately emetogenic chemotherapy—A retrospective audit. *European Journal of Cancer Care, 19,* 403–407. doi:10.1111/j.1365-2354.2009.01068.x

56. Fabi, A., Ciccarese, M., Metro, G., Savarese, A., Giannarelli, D., Nuzzo, C.M., … Cognetti, F. (2008). Oral ondansetron is highly active as rescue antiemetic treatment for moderately emetogenic chemotherapy: Results of a randomized phase II study. *Supportive Care in Cancer, 16,* 1375–1380. doi:10.1007/s00520-008-0438-9

57. Blazer, M., Phillips, G., Reardon, J., Efries, D., Smith, Y., Weatherby, L., … Bekaii-Saab, T. (2012). Antiemetic control with palonosetron in patients with gastrointestinal cancer receiving a fluoropyrimidine-based regimen in addition to either irinotecan or oxaliplatin: A retrospective study. *Oncology, 83,* 135–140. doi:10.1159/000339145

58. Boccia, R., Grunberg, S., Franco-Gonzales, E., Rubenstein, E., & Voisin, D. (2013). Efficacy of oral palonosetron compared to intravenous palonosetron for the prevention of chemotherapy-induced nausea and vomiting associated with moderately emetogenic chemotherapy: A phase 3 trial. *Supportive Care in Cancer, 21,* 1453–1460. doi:10.1007/s00520-012-1691-5

59. Botrel, T.E.A., Clark, O.A.C., Clark, L., Paladini, L., Faleiros, E., & Pegoretti, B. (2010). Efficacy of palonosetron (PAL) compared to other serotonin inhibitors (5-HT₃R) in preventing chemotherapy-induced nausea and vomiting (CINV) in patients receiving moderately or highly emetogenic (MoHE) treatment: Systematic review and meta-analysis. *Supportive Care in Cancer, 19,* 823–832. doi:10.1007/s00520-010-0908-8

60. Brugnatelli, S., Gattoni, E., Grasso, D., Rossetti, F., Perrone, T., & Danova, M. (2011). Single-dose palonosetron and dexamethasone in preventing nausea and vomiting induced by moderately emetogenic chemotherapy in breast and colorectal cancer patients. *Tumori, 97,* 362–366. doi:10.1700/912.10035

61. Celio, L., Denaro, A., Agustoni, F., & Bajetta, E. (2012). Palonosetron plus 1-day dexamethasone for the prevention of nausea and vomiting due to moderately emetogenic chemotherapy: Effect of established risk factors on treatment outcome in a phase III trial. *Journal of Supportive Oncology, 10,* 65–71. doi:10.1016/j.suponc.2011.06.007

62. Celio, L., Frustaci, S., Denaro, A., Buonadonna, A., Ardizzoia, A., Piazza, E., … Bajetta, E. (2011). Palonosetron in combination with 1-day versus 3-day dexamethasone for prevention of nausea and vomiting following moderately emetogenic chemotherapy: A randomized, multicenter, phase III trial. *Supportive Care in Cancer, 19,* 1217–1225. doi:10.1007/s00520-010-0941-7

63. Craver, C., Gayle, J., Balu, S., & Buchner, D. (2011). Palonosetron versus other 5-HT₃ receptor antagonists for prevention of chemotherapy-induced nausea and vomiting in patients with hematologic malignancies treated with emetogenic chemotherapy in a hospital outpatient setting in the United States. *Journal of Medical Economics, 14,* 341–349. doi:10.3111/13696998.2011.582908

64. Di Renzo, N., Montanini, A., Mannina, D., Dondi, A., Muci, S., Mancuso, S., … Federico, M. (2011). Single-dose palonosetron for prevention of chemotherapy-induced nausea and vomiting in patients with aggressive non-Hodgkin's lymphoma receiving moderately emetogenic chemotherapy

containing steroids: Results of a phase II study from the Gruppo Italiano per lo Studio dei Linfomi (GISL). *Supportive Care in Cancer, 19,* 1505–1510. doi:10.1007/s00520-010-0974-y

65. Feinberg, B., Gilmore, J., Haislip, S., Jackson, J., Jain, G., Balu, S., & Buchner, D. (2012). Impact of initiating antiemetic prophylaxis with palonosetron versus ondansetron on risk of uncontrolled chemotherapy-induced nausea and vomiting in patients with lung cancer receiving multi-day chemotherapy. *Supportive Care in Cancer, 20,* 615–623. doi:10.1007/s00520-011-1140-x

66. Ghosh, S., & Dey, S. (2010). Comparing different antiemetic regimens for chemotherapy induced nausea and vomiting. *International Journal of Collaborative Research on Internal Medicine and Public Health, 2,* 142–156. Retrieved from http://www.iomcworld.com/ijcrimph/ijcrimph-v02-n05-03-f.htm

67. Giralt, S.A., Mangan, K.F., Maziarz, R.T., Bubalo, J.S., Beveridge, R., Hurd, D.D., … Schuster, M.W. (2011). Three palonosetron regimens to prevent CINV in myeloma patients receiving multiple-day high-dose melphalan and hematopoietic stem cell transplantation. *Annals of Oncology, 22,* 939–946. doi:10.1093/annonc/mdq457

68. Hatoum, H.T., Lin, S.-J., Buchner, D., & Cox, D. (2012). Comparative clinical effectiveness of various 5-HT₃ RA antiemetic regimens on chemotherapy-induced nausea and vomiting associated with hospital and emergency department visits in real world practice. *Supportive Care in Cancer, 20,* 941–949. doi:10.1007/s00520-011-1165-1

69. Hesketh, P.J., Morrow, G., Komorowski, A.W., Ahmed, R., & Cox, D. (2012). Efficacy and safety of palonosetron as salvage treatment in the prevention of chemotherapy-induced nausea and vomiting in patients receiving low emetogenic chemotherapy (LEC). *Supportive Care in Cancer, 20,* 2633–2637. doi:10.1007/s00520-012-1527-3

70. Longo, F., Mansueto, G., Lapadula, V., De Sanctis, R., Quadrini, S., Grande, R., … Di Seri, M. (2011). Palonosetron plus 3-day aprepitant and dexamethasone to prevent nausea and vomiting in patients receiving highly emetogenic chemotherapy. *Supportive Care in Cancer, 19,* 1159–1164. doi:10.1007/s00520-010-0930-x

71. Rozzi, A., Nardoni, C., Corona, M., Restuccia, M.R., Fabi, A., Bria, E., … Lanzetta, G. (2011). Palonosetron for the prevention of chemotherapy-induced nausea and vomiting in glioblastoma patients treated with te-mozolomide: A phase II study. *Supportive Care in Cancer, 19,* 697–701. doi:10.1007/s00520-010-0893-y

72. Lin, S.J., Hatoum, H.T., Buchner, D., Cox, D., & Balu, S. (2012). Impact of 5-HT₃ receptor antagonists on chemotherapy-induced nausea and vomiting: A retrospective cohort study. *BMC Health Services Research, 12,* 215. doi:10.1186/1472-6963-12-215

73. Schwartzberg, L., Morrow, G., Balu, S., Craver, C., Gayle, J., & Cox, D. (2011). Chemotherapy-induced nausea and vomiting and antiemetic prophylaxis with palonosetron versus other 5-HT₃ receptor antagonists in patients with cancer treated with low emetogenic chemotherapy in a hospital outpatient setting in the United States. *Current Medical Research and Opinion, 27,* 1613–1622. doi:10.1185/03007995.2011.596201

74. Tian, W., Wang, Z., Zhou, J., Zhang, S., Wang, J., Chen, Q., … Lin, T. (2011). Randomized, double-blind, crossover study of palonosetron compared with granisetron for the prevention of chemotherapy-induced nausea and vomiting in a Chinese population. *Medical Oncology, 28,* 71–78. doi:10.1007/s12032-009-9398-2

75. Yu, Z., Liu, W., Wang, L., Liang, H., Huang, Y., Si, X., … Zhang, H. (2009). The efficacy and safety of palonosetron compared with granisetron in preventing highly emetogenic chemotherapy-induced vomiting in the Chinese cancer patients: A phase II, multicenter, randomized, double-blind, parallel, comparative clinical trial. *Supportive Care in Cancer, 17,* 99–102. doi:10.1007/s00520-008-0503-4

76. Jin, Y., Sun, W., Gu, D., Yang, J., Xu, Z., & Chen, J. (2013). Comparative efficacy and safety of palonosetron with the first 5-HT₃ receptor antagonists for the chemotherapy-induced nausea and vomiting: A meta-analysis. *European Journal of Cancer Care, 22,* 41–50. doi:10.1111/j.1365-2354.2012.01353.x

77. Likun, Z., Xiang, J., Yi, B., Xin, D., & Tao, Z.L. (2011). A systematic review and meta-analysis of intravenous palonosetron in the prevention of chemotherapy-induced nausea and vomiting in adults. *Oncologist, 16,* 207–216. doi:10.1634/theoncologist.2010-0198

78. Dong, X., Huang, J., Cao, R., & Liu, L. (2010). Palonosetron for prevention of acute and delayed nausea and vomiting in non-small-cell lung carcinoma patients. *Medical Oncology, 28,* 1425–1429. doi:10.1007/s12032-010-9608-y

79. Massa, E., Astara, G., Madeddu, C., Dessi, M., Loi, C., Lepori, S., & Mantovani, G. (2009). Palonosetron plus dexamethasone effectively prevents acute and delayed chemotherapy-induced nausea and vomiting following highly or moderately emetogenic chemotherapy in pre-treated patients who have failed to respond to a previous antiemetic treatment: Comparison between elderly and non-elderly patient response. *Critical Reviews in Oncology/Hematology, 70,* 83–91. doi:10.1016/j.critrevonc.2008.07.002

80. Mattiuzzi, G.N., Cortes, J.E., Blamble, D.A., Bekele, B.N., Xiao, L., Cabanillas, M., … Kantarjian, H. (2010). Daily palonosetron is superior to ondansetron in the prevention of delayed chemotherapy-induced nausea and vomiting in patients with acute myelogenous leukemia. *Cancer, 116,* 5659–5666. doi:10.1002/cncr.25365

81. Saito, M., & Tsukuda, M. (2010). Review of palonosetron: Emerging data distinguishing it as a novel 5HT₃ receptor antagonist for chemotherapy induced nausea and vomiting. *Expert Opinion on Pharmacotherapy, 11,* 1003–1014. doi:10.1517/14656561003705746

82. Schwartzberg, L., Jackson, J., Jain, G., Balu, S., & Buchner, D. (2011). Impact of 5-HT₃ RA selection within triple antiemetic regimens on uncontrolled highly emetogenic chemotherapy-induced nausea/vomiting. *Expert Review of Pharmacoeconomics and Outcomes Research, 11,* 401–408. doi:10.1586/erp.11.47

83. Nadaraja, S., Mamoudou, A.D., Thomassen, H., Wehner, P.S., Rosthoej, S., & Schroeder, H. (2012). Palonosetron for the prevention of nausea and vomiting in children with acute lymphoblastic leukemia treated with high dose methotrexate. *Pediatric Blood and Cancer, 59,* 870–873. doi:10.1002/pbc.24068

84. Sepúlveda-Vildósola, A.C., Betanzos-Cabrera, Y., Gascón Lastiri, G., Rivera-Márquez, H., Villasis-Keever, M.A., Wanzke Del Angel, V., … López-Aguilar, E. (2008). Palonosetron hydrochloride is an effective and safe option to prevent chemotherapy-induced nausea and vomiting in children. *Archives of Medical Research, 39,* 601–606. doi:10.1016/j.arcmed.2008.04.007

85. Aapro, M.S., Schmoll, H.J., Jahn, F., Carides, A.D., & Webb, R.T. (2013). Review of the efficacy of aprepitant for the prevention of chemotherapy-induced nausea and vomiting in a range of tumor types. *Cancer Treatment Reviews, 39,* 113–117. doi:10.1016/j.ctrv.2012.09.002

86. Gao, H.F., Liang, Y., Zhou, N.N., Zhang, D.S., & Wu, H.Y. (2013). Aprepitant plus palonosetron and dexamethasone for prevention of chemotherapy-induced nausea and vomiting in patients receiving multiple-day cisplatin-based chemotherapy. *Internal Medicine Journal, 43,* 73–76. doi:10.1111/j.1445-5994.2011.02637.x

87. García Gómez, J., Pérez López, M.E., García Mata, J., & Isla Casado, D. (2010). SEOM clinical guidelines for the treatment of antiemetic prophylaxis in cancer patients receiving chemotherapy. *Clinical and Translational Oncology, 12,* 770–774. doi:10.1007/s12094-010-0594-5

88. Grunberg, S.M., Dugan, M., Muss, H., Wood, M., Burdette-Radoux, S., Weisberg, T., & Siebel, M. (2009). Effectiveness of a single-day three-drug regimen of dexamethasone, palonosetron, and aprepitant for the prevention

of acute and delayed nausea and vomiting caused by moderately emetogenic chemotherapy. *Supportive Care in Cancer, 17,* 589–594. doi:10.1007/s00520-008-0535-9

89. Herrstedt, J. (2008). Antiemetics: An update and the MASCC guidelines applied in clinical practice. *Nature Clinical Practice Oncology, 5,* 32–43. doi:10.1038/ncponc1021

90. Hesketh, P.J., & Sanz-Altamira, P. (2012). Aprepitant, dexamethasone, and palonosetron in the prevention of doxorubicin/cyclophosphamide-induced nausea and vomiting. *Supportive Care in Cancer, 20,* 653–656. doi:10.1007/s00520-011-1312-8

91. Jordan, K., Jahn, F., Jahn, P., Behlendorf, T., Stein, A., Ruessel, J., ... Schmoll, H.J. (2011). The NK-1 receptor-antagonist aprepitant in high-dose chemotherapy (high-dose melphalan and high-dose T-ICE: paclitaxel, ifosfamide, carboplatin, etoposide): Efficacy and safety of a triple antiemetic combination. *Bone Marrow Transplantation, 46,* 784–789. doi:10.1038/bmt.2010.205

92. Longo, F., Mansueto, G., Lapadula, V., Stumbo, L., DelBene, G., Adua, D., ... Quadrini, S. (2012). Combination of aprepitant, palonosetron and dexamethasone as antiemetic prophylaxis in lung cancer patients receiving multiple cycles of cisplatin-based chemotherapy. *International Journal of Clinical Practice, 66,* 753–757. doi:10.1111/j.1742-1241.2012.02969.x

93. Olver, I.N., Grimison, P., Chatfield, M., Stockler, M.R., Toner, G.C., Gebski, V., ... Thomson, D. (2013). Results of a 7-day aprepitant schedule for the prevention of nausea and vomiting in 5-day cisplatin-based germ cell tumor chemotherapy. *Supportive Care in Cancer, 21,* 1561–1568. doi:10.1007/s00520-012-1696-0

94. Pielichowski, W., Barzal, J., Gawronski, K., Mlot, B., Oborska, S., Wasko-Grabowska, A., & Rzepecki, P. (2011). A triple-drug combination to prevent nausea and vomiting following BEAM chemotherapy before autologous hematopoietic stem cell transplantation. *Transplantation Proceedings, 43,* 3107–3110. doi:10.1016/j.transproceed.2011.08.010

95. Roila, F., Warr, D., Aapro, M., Clark-Snow, R.A., Einhorn, L., Gralla, R.J., ... Tonato, M. (2011). Delayed emesis: Moderately emetogenic chemotherapy (single-day chemotherapy regimens only). *Supportive Care in Cancer, 19*(Suppl. 1), S57–S62. doi:10.1007/s00520-010-1039-y

96. Hayashi, T., Ikesue, H., Esaki, T., Fukazawa, M., Abe, M., Ohno, S., ... Oishi, R. (2012). Implementation of institutional antiemetic guidelines for low emetic risk chemotherapy with docetaxel: A clinical and cost evaluation. *Supportive Care in Cancer, 20,* 1805–1810. doi:10.1007/s00520-011-1278-6

97. Kawazoe, H., Mutoki, Y., Takechi, Y., Shishino, Y., Ido, K., Suemaru, K., & Araki, H. (2010). Comparison of antiemetic efficacy between single and repeat treatment with dexamethasone in patients receiving carboplatin-based combination chemotherapy. *Methods and Findings in Experimental and Clinical Pharmacology, 32,* 499–505. doi:10.1358/mf.2010.32.7.1501438

98. Olver, I., Clark-Snow, R.A., Ballatori, E., Espersen, B.T., Bria, E., & Jordan, K. (2011). Guidelines for the control of nausea and vomiting with chemotherapy of low or minimal emetic potential. *Supportive Care in Cancer, 19*(Suppl. 1), S33–S36. doi:10.1007/s00520-010-0985-8

99. Cruz, F.M., Cubero, D.D.G.C., Taranto, P., Lerner, T., Lera, A.T., Miranda, M.D., ... del Giglio, A. (2012). Gabapentin for the prevention of chemotherapy-induced nausea and vomiting: A pilot study. *Supportive Care in Cancer, 20,* 601–606. doi:10.1007/s00520-011-1138-4

100. Marchioro, G., Azzarello, G., Viviani, F., Barbato, F., Pavanetto, M., Rosetti, F., ... Vinante, O. (2000). Hypnosis in the treatment of anticipatory nausea and vomiting in patients receiving cancer chemotherapy. *Oncology, 59,* 100–104. doi:10.1159/000012144

101. Luebbert, K., Dahme, B., & Hasenbring, M. (2001). The effectiveness of relaxation training in reducing treatment-related symptoms and improving emotional adjustment in acute non-surgical cancer treatment: A meta-analytical review. *Psycho-Oncology, 10,* 490–502. doi:10.1002/pon.537

102. Redd, W.H., Montgomery, G.H., & DuHamel, K.N. (2001). Behavioral intervention for cancer treatment side effects. *Journal of the National Cancer Institute, 93,* 810–823. doi:10.1093/jnci/93.11.810

103. Silva, D.R.F., dos Reis, P.E.D., Gomes, I.P., Funghetto, S.S., & Ponce de Leon, C.G.R.M. (2009). Non pharmacological interventions for chemotherapy induced nausea and vomits: Integrative review. *Online Brazilian Journal of Nursing, 8.* doi:10.5935/1676-4285.20092098

104. Colagiuri, B., & Zachariae, R. (2010). Patient expectancy and post-chemotherapy nausea: A meta-analysis. *Annals of Behavioral Medicine, 40,* 3–14. doi:10.1007/s12160-010-9186-4

105. Roscoe, J.A., O'Neill, M., Jean-Pierre, P., Heckler, C.E., Kaptchuk, T.J., Bushunow, P., … Smith, B. (2010). An exploratory study on the effects of an expectancy manipulation on chemotherapy-related nausea. *Journal of Pain and Symptom Management, 40,* 379–390. doi:10.1016/j.jpainsymman .2009.12.024

106. Shelke, A.R., Roscoe, J.A., Morrow, G.R., Colman, L.K., Banerjee, T.K., & Kirshner, J.J. (2008). Effect of a nausea expectancy manipulation on chemotherapy-induced nausea: A University of Rochester Cancer Center Community Clinical Oncology Program study. *Journal of Pain and Symptom Management, 35,* 381–387. doi:10.1016/j.jpainsymman.2007.05.008

107. Zang, J., Hou, M., Gou, H.F., Qiu, M., Wang, J., Zhou, X.J., … Yi, C. (2011). Antiemetic activity of megestrol acetate in patients receiving chemotherapy. *Supportive Care in Cancer, 19,* 667–673. doi:10.1007/s00520-010-0886-x

108. Navari, R.M., Einhorn, L.H., Loehrer, P.J., Sr., Passik, S.D., Vinson, J., McClean, J., … Johnson, C.S. (2007). A phase II trial of olanzapine, dexamethasone, and palonosetron for the prevention of chemotherapy-induced nausea and vomiting: A Hoosier oncology group study. *Supportive Care in Cancer, 15,* 1285–1291. doi:10.1007/s00520-007-0248-5

109. Navari, R.M., Nagy, C.K., & Gray, S.E. (2013). The use of olanzapine versus metoclopramide for the treatment of breakthrough chemotherapy-induced nausea and vomiting in patients receiving highly emetogenic chemotherapy. *Supportive Care in Cancer, 21,* 1655–1663. doi:10.1007/ s00520-012-1710-6

110. Arakawa, S. (1997). Relaxation to reduce nausea, vomiting, and anxiety induced by chemotherapy in Japanese patients. *Cancer Nursing, 20,* 342–349. doi:10.1097/00002820-199710000-00005

111. Molassiotis, A., Yung, H.P., Yam, B.M.C., Chan, F.Y.S., & Mok, T.S.K. (2002). The effectiveness of progressive muscle relaxation training in managing chemotherapy-induced nausea and vomiting in Chinese breast cancer patients: A randomised controlled trial. *Supportive Care in Cancer, 10,* 237–246. doi:10.1007/s00520-001-0329-9

112. Miller, M., & Kearney, N. (2004). Chemotherapy-related nausea and vomiting—Past reflections, present practice and future management. *European Journal of Cancer Care, 13,* 71–81. doi:10.1111/j.1365-2354.2004.00446.x

113. Oyama, H., Kaneda, M., Katsumata, N., Akechi, T., & Ohsuga, M. (2000). Using the bedside wellness system during chemotherapy decreases fatigue and emesis in cancer patients. *Journal of Medical Systems, 24,* 173–182. doi:10.1023/A:1005591626518

114. Kim, S.-W., Shin, I.-S., Kim, J.-M., Kim, Y.-C., Kim, K.-S., Kim, K.-M., … Yoon, J.-S. (2008). Effectiveness of mirtazapine for nausea and insomnia in cancer patients with depression. *Psychiatry and Clinical Neurosciences, 62,* 75–83. doi:10.1111/j.1440-1819.2007.01778.x

115. Tan, L., Liu, J., Liu, X., Chen, J., Yan, Z., Yang, H., & Zhang, D. (2009). Clinical research of olanzapine for prevention of chemotherapy-induced nausea and vomiting. *Journal of Experimental and Clinical Cancer Research, 28,* 131. doi:10.1186/1756-9966-28-131

116. Jones, J.M., Qin, R., Bardia, A., Linquist, B., Wolf, S., & Loprinzi, C.L. (2011). Antiemetics for chemotherapy-induced nausea and vomiting occurring despite prophylactic antiemetic therapy. *Journal of Palliative Medicine, 14,* 810–814. doi:10.1089/jpm.2011.0058

117. Ithimakin, S., Runglodvatana, K., Nimmannit, A., Akewanlop, C., Srimuninnimit, V., Keerativitayanan, N., … Laocharoenkeat, A. (2012). Randomized, double-blinded, placebo-controlled trial of ondansetron plus dexamethasone with or without metoclopramide as antiemetic prophylaxis in patients receiving high-dose cisplatin in medical practice. *Supportive Care in Cancer, 20,* 849–855. doi:10.1007/s00520-011-1162-4

118. Liu, Y., Zhang, J., Teng, Y., Zhang, L., Yu, P., Jin, B., … Li, Z. (2009). Thalidomide improves prevention of chemotherapy-induced gastrointestinal side effects following a modified FOLFOX7 regimen: Results of a prospective randomized crossover study. *Tumori, 95,* 691–696.

119. Dibble, S.L., Chapman, J., Mack, K.A., & Shih, A.S. (2000). Acupressure for nausea: Results of a pilot study. *Oncology Nursing Forum, 27,* 41–47.

120. Dibble, S.L., Luce, J., Cooper, B.A., Israel, J., Cohen, M., Nussey, B., & Rugo, H. (2007). Acupressure for chemotherapy-induced nausea and vomiting: A randomized clinical trial. *Oncology Nursing Forum, 34,* 813–820. doi:10.1188/07.ONF.813-820

121. Gardani, G., Cerrone, R., Biella, C., Galbiati, G., Proserpio, E., Casiraghi, M., … Lissoni, P. (2007). A progress study of 100 cancer patients treated by acupressure for chemotherapy-induced vomiting after failure of pharmacological approach. *Minerva Medica, 98,* 665–668. Retrieved from http://www.minervamedica.it/en/journals/minerva-medica/article.php?cod=R10Y2007N06A0665

122. Genç, A., Can, G., & Aydiner, A. (2012). The efficiency of the acupressure in prevention of the chemotherapy-induced nausea and vomiting. *Supportive Care in Cancer, 21,* 253–261. doi:10.1007/s00520-012-1519-3

123. Jones, E., Isom, S., Kemper, K.J., & McLean, T.W. (2008). Acupressure for chemotherapy-associated nausea and vomiting in children. *Journal of the Society for Integrative Oncology, 6,* 141–145. Retrieved from https://www.integrativeonc.org/index.php/journal-of-the-society-for-integrative-oncology-jsio/jsio-issues-prior-to-83

124. Lee, J., Dibble, S., Dodd, M., Abrams, D., & Burns, B. (2010). The relationship of chemotherapy-induced nausea to the frequency of pericardium 6 digital acupressure [Online exclusive]. *Oncology Nursing Forum, 37,* E419–E425. doi:10.1188/10.ONF.E419-E425

125. Melchart, D., Ihbe-Heffinger, A., Leps, B., von Schilling, C., & Linde, K. (2006). Acupuncture and acupressure for the prevention of chemotherapy-induced nausea: A randomised cross-over pilot study. *Supportive Care in Cancer, 14,* 878–882. doi:10.1007/s00520-006-0028-7

126. Molassiotis, A., Helin, A.M., Dabbour, R., & Hummerston, S. (2007). The effects of P6 acupressure in the prophylaxis of chemotherapy-related nausea and vomiting in breast cancer patients. *Complementary Therapies in Medicine, 15,* 3–12. doi:10.1016/j.ctim.2006.07.005

127. Molassiotis, A., Russell, W., Hughes, J., Breckons, M., Lloyd-Williams, M., Richardson, J., … Ryder, W.D. (2014). The effectiveness of acupressure for the control and management of chemotherapy-related acute and delayed nausea: A randomized controlled trial. *Journal of Pain and Symptom Management, 47,* 12–25. doi:10.1016/j.jpainsymman.2013.03.007

128. Roscoe, J.A., Matteson, S.E., Morrow, G.R., Hickok, J.T., Bushunow, P., Griggs, J., … Smith, J. (2005). Acustimulation wrist bands are not effective for the control of chemotherapy-induced nausea in women with breast cancer. *Journal of Pain and Symptom Management, 29,* 376–384. doi:10.1016/j.jpainsymman.2004.07.007

129. Roscoe, J.A., Morrow, G.R., Hickok, J.T., Bushunow, P., Pierce, H.I., Flynn, P.J., … Atkins, J.N. (2003). The efficacy of acupressure and acustimulation wrist bands for the relief of chemotherapy-induced nausea and vomiting: A University of Rochester Cancer Center Community Clinical Oncology Program multicenter study. *Journal of Pain and Symptom Management, 26,* 731–740. doi:10.1016/S0885-3924(03)00254-9

130. Shin, Y.H., Kim, T.I., Shin, M.S., & Juon, H.-S. (2004). Effect of acupressure on nausea and vomiting during chemotherapy cycle for Korean postoper-

ative stomach cancer patients. *Cancer Nursing, 27*, 267–274. Retrieved from http://journals.lww.com/cancernursingonline/pages/articleviewer.aspx?year=2004&issue=07000&article=00002&type=abstract

131. Suh, E.E. (2012). The effects of P6 acupressure and nurse-provided counseling on chemotherapy-induced nausea and vomiting in patients with breast cancer [Online exclusive]. *Oncology Nursing Forum, 39*, E1–E9. doi:10.1188/12.ONF.E1-E9

132. Taspinar, A., & Sirin, A. (2010). Effect of acupressure on chemotherapy-induced nausea and vomiting in gynecologic cancer patients in Turkey. *European Journal of Oncology Nursing, 14*, 49–54. doi:10.1016/j.ejon.2009.07.006

133. Treish, I., Shord, S., Valgus, J., Harvey, D., Nagy, J., Stegal, J., & Lindley, C. (2003). Randomized double-blind study of the Reliefband as an adjunct to standard antiemetics in patients receiving moderately-high to highly emetogenic chemotherapy. *Supportive Care in Cancer, 11*, 516–521. doi:10.1007/s00520-004-0467-3

134. Chao, L.F., Zhang, A.L., Liu, H.E., Cheng, M.H., Lam, H.B., & Lo, S.K. (2009). The efficacy of acupoint stimulation for the management of therapy-related adverse events in patients with breast cancer: A systematic review. *Breast Cancer Research and Treatment, 118*, 255–267. doi:10.1007/s10549-009-0533-8

135. Collins, K.B., & Thomas, D.J. (2004). Acupuncture and acupressure for the management of chemotherapy-induced nausea and vomiting. *Journal of the American Association of Nurse Practitioners, 16*, 80–84. doi:10.1111/j.1745-7599.2004.tb00376.x

136. Ezzo, J., Vickers, A., Richardson, M.A., Allen, C., Dibble, S.L., Issell, B., … Zhang, G. (2005). Acupuncture-point stimulation for chemotherapy-induced nausea and vomiting. *Journal of Clinical Oncology, 23*, 7188–7198. doi:10.1200/JCO.2005.06.028

137. Klein, J., & Griffiths, P. (2004). Acupressure for nausea and vomiting in cancer patients receiving chemotherapy. *British Journal of Community Nursing, 9*, 383–387. Retrieved from http://www.internurse.com/cgi-bin/go.pl/library/article.cgi?uid=15936;article=BJCN_9_9_383_388;format=pdf

138. Choo, S.-P., Kong, K.-H., Lim, W.-T., Gao, F., Chua, K., & Leong, S.S. (2006). Electroacupuncture for refractory acute emesis caused by chemotherapy. *Journal of Alternative and Complementary Medicine, 12*, 963–969. doi:10.1089/acm.2006.12.963

139. Garcia, M.K., McQuade, J., Haddad, R., Patel, S., Lee, R., Yang, P., … Cohen, L. (2013). Systematic review of acupuncture in cancer care: A synthesis of the evidence. *Journal of Clinical Oncology, 31*, 952–960. doi:10.1200/JCO.2012.43.5818

140. Gottschling, S., Reindl, T.K., Meyer, S., Berrang, J., Henze, G., Graeber, S., … Graf, N. (2008). Acupuncture to alleviate chemotherapy-induced nausea and vomiting in pediatric oncology—A randomized multicenter crossover pilot trial. *Klinische Padiatrie, 220*, 365–370. doi:10.1055/s-0028-1086039

141. Mayer, D.J. (2000). Acupuncture: An evidence-based review of the clinical literature. *Annual Review of Medicine, 51*, 49–63. doi:10.1146/annurev.med.51.1.49

142. Roscoe, J.A., Morrow, G.R., Matteson, S., Bushunow, P., & Tian, L. (2002). Acustimulation wristbands for the relief of chemotherapy-induced nausea. *Alternative Therapies in Health and Medicine, 8*, 56–57, 59–63. Retrieved from http://www.alternative-therapies.com/index.cfm/fuseaction/archives.main&mode=issue&issueid=7111

143. Shen, J., Wenger, N., Glaspy, J., Hays, R.D., Albert, P.S., Choi, C., & Shekelle, P.G. (2000). Electroacupuncture for control of myeloablative chemotherapy-induced emesis: A randomized controlled trial. *JAMA, 284*, 2755–2761. doi:10.1001/jama.284.21.2755

144. Yeh, C.H., Chien, L.-C., Chiang, Y.C., Lin, S.W., Huang, C.K., & Ren, D. (2012). Reduction in nausea and vomiting in children undergoing cancer chemotherapy by either appropriate or sham auricular acupuncture points

with standard care. *Journal of Alternative and Complementary Medicine, 18*, 334–340. doi:10.1089/acm.2011.0102

145. Andersen, C., Adamsen, L., Moeller, T., Midtgaard, J., Quist, M., Tveteraas, A., & Rorth, M. (2006). The effect of a multidimensional exercise programme on symptoms and side-effects in cancer patients undergoing chemotherapy— The use of semi-structured diaries. *European Journal of Oncology Nursing, 10*, 247–262. doi:10.1016/j.ejon.2005.12.007

146. Winningham, M.L., & MacVicar, M.G. (1988). The effect of aerobic exercise on patient reports of nausea. *Oncology Nursing Forum, 15*, 447–450.

147. Ernst, E., & Pittler, M.H. (2000). Efficacy of ginger for nausea and vomiting: A systematic review of randomized clinical trials. *British Journal of Anaesthesia, 84*, 367–371. doi:10.1093/oxfordjournals.bja.a013442

148. Levine, M.E., Gillis, M.G., Koch, S.Y., Voss, A.C., Stern, R.M., & Koch, K.L. (2008). Protein and ginger for the treatment of chemotherapy-induced delayed nausea. *Journal of Alternative and Complementary Medicine, 14*, 545–551. doi:10.1089/acm.2007.0817

149. Panahi, Y., Saadat, A., Sahebkar, A., Hashemian, F., Taghikhani, M., & Abolhasani, E. (2012). Effect of ginger on acute and delayed chemotherapy-induced nausea and vomiting: A pilot, randomized, open-label clinical trial. *Integrative Cancer Therapies, 11*, 204–211. doi:10.1177/1534735411433201

150. Pillai, A.K., Sharma, K.K., Gupta, Y.K., & Bakhshi, S. (2010). Anti-emetic effect of ginger powder versus placebo as an add-on therapy in children and young adults receiving high emetogenic chemotherapy. *Pediatric Blood and Cancer, 56*, 234–238. doi:10.1002/pbc.22778

151. Ryan, J.L., Heckler, C.E., Roscoe, J.A., Dakhil, S.R., Kirshner, J., Flynn, P.J., … Morrow, G.R. (2012). Ginger (*Zingiber officinale*) reduces acute chemotherapy-induced nausea: A URCC CCOP study of 576 patients. *Supportive Care in Cancer, 20*, 1479–1489. doi:10.1007/s00520-011-1236-3

152. Zick, S.M., Ruffin, M.T., Lee, J., Normolle, D.P., Siden, R., Alrawi, S., & Brenner, D.E. (2009). Phase II trial of encapsulated ginger as a treatment for chemotherapy-induced nausea and vomiting. *Supportive Care in Cancer, 17*, 563–572. doi:10.1007/s00520-008-0528-8

153. Manusirivithaya, S., Sripramote, M., Tangjitgamol, S., Sheanakul, C., Leelahakorn, S., Thavaramara, T., & Tangcharoenpanich, K. (2004). Antiemetic effect of ginger in gynecologic oncology patients receiving cisplatin. *International Journal of Gynecologic Cancer, 14*, 1063–1069. doi:10.1111/j.1048-891X.2004.14603.x

154. Marx, W.M., Teleni, L., McCarthy, A.L., Vitetta, L., McKavanagh, D., Thomson, D., & Isenring, E. (2013). Ginger (*Zingiber officinale*) and chemotherapy-induced nausea and vomiting: A systematic literature review. *Nutrition Reviews, 71*, 245–254. doi:10.1111/nure.12016

155. Lee, J., & Oh, H. (2013). Ginger as an antiemetic modality for chemotherapy-induced nausea and vomiting: A systematic review and meta-analysis. *Oncology Nursing Forum, 40*, 163–170. doi:10.1188/13.ONF.163-170

156. Ingersoll, G.L., Wasilewski, A., Haller, M., Pandya, K., Bennett, J., He, H., … Berry, C. (2010). Effect of Concord grape juice on chemotherapy-induced nausea and vomiting: Results of a pilot study. *Oncology Nursing Forum, 37*, 213–221. doi:10.1188/10.ONF.213-221

157. Mok, T.S., Yeo, W., Johnson, P.J., Hui, P., Ho, W.M., Lam, K.C., … Zee, B. (2007). A double-blind placebo-controlled randomized study of Chinese herbal medicine as complementary therapy for reduction of chemotherapy-induced toxicity. *Annals of Oncology, 18*, 768–774. doi:10.1093/annonc/mdl465

158. Ahles, T.A., Tope, D.M., Pinkson, B., Walch, S., Hann, D., Whedon, M., … Silberfarb, P.M. (1999). Massage therapy for patients undergoing autologous bone marrow transplantation. *Journal of Pain and Symptom Management, 18*, 157–163. doi:10.1016/s0885-3924(99)00061-5

159. Billhult, A., Bergbom, I., & Stener-Victorin, E. (2007). Massage relieves nausea in women with breast cancer who are undergoing chemotherapy. *Journal of Alternative and Complementary Medicine, 13*, 53–58. doi:10.1089/acm.2006.6049

160. Cassileth, B.R., & Vickers, A.J. (2004). Massage therapy for symptom control: Outcome study at a major cancer center. *Journal of Pain and Symptom Management, 28,* 244–249. doi:10.1016/j.jpainsymman.2003.12.016

161. Fellowes, D., Barnes, K., & Wilkinson, S.S.M. (2008). Aromatherapy and massage for symptom relief in patients with cancer. *Cochrane Database of Systematic Reviews, 2008*(4). doi:10.1002/14651858.CD002287.pub3

162. Grealish, L., Lomasney, A., & Whiteman, B. (2000). Foot massage: A nursing intervention to modify the distressing symptoms of pain and nausea in patients hospitalized with cancer. *Cancer Nursing, 23,* 237–243. doi:10.1097/00002820-200006000-00012

163. Campos de Carvalho, E., Martins, F.T., & dos Santos C.B. (2007). A pilot study of a relaxation technique for management of nausea and vomiting in patients receiving cancer chemotherapy. *Cancer Nursing, 30,* 163–167. doi:10.1097/01.NCC.0000265007.87311.d0

164. Chan, C.W., Cheng, K.K.F., Lam, L.W., Li, C.K., Chik, K.W., & Cheung, J.S.S. (2008). Psycho-educational intervention for chemotherapy-associated nausea and vomiting in paediatric oncology patients: A pilot study. *Hong Kong Medical Journal, 14*(Suppl. 5), 32–35. Retrieved from http://www.hkmj.org/article_pdfs/hkm0810sp5p32.pdf

165. Jahn, P., Renz, P., Stukenkemper, J., Book, K., Kuss, O., Jordan, K., ... Landenberger, M. (2009). Reduction of chemotherapy-induced anorexia, nausea, and emesis through a structured nursing intervention: A cluster-randomized multicenter trial. *Supportive Care in Cancer, 17,* 1543–1552. doi:10.1007/s00520-009-0698-z

166. Williams, S.A., & Schreier, A.M. (2004). The effect of education in managing side effects in women receiving chemotherapy for treatment of breast cancer [Online exclusive]. *Oncology Nursing Forum, 31,* E16–E23. doi:10.1188/04.ONF.E16-E23

167. Karagozoglu, S., Tekyasar, F., & Yilmaz, F.A. (2013). Effects of music therapy and guided visual imagery on chemotherapy-induced anxiety and nausea-vomiting. *Journal of Clinical Nursing, 22,* 39–50. doi:10.1111/jocn.12030

168. Sahler, O.J.Z., Hunter, B.C., & Liesveld, J.L. (2003). The effect of using music therapy with relaxation imagery in the management of patients undergoing bone marrow transplantation: A pilot feasibility study. *Alternative Therapies in Health and Medicine, 9,* 70–74.

169. Troesch, L.M., Rodehaver, C.B., Delaney, E.A., & Yanes, B. (1993). The influence of guided imagery on chemotherapy-related nausea and vomiting. *Oncology Nursing Forum, 20,* 1179–1185.

170. Raghavendra, R.M., Nagarathna, R., Nagendra, H.R., Gopinath, K.S., Srinath, B.S., Ravi, B.D., ... Nalini, R. (2007). Effects of an integrated yoga programme on chemotherapy-induced nausea and emesis in breast cancer patients. *European Journal of Cancer Care, 16,* 462–474. doi:10.1111/j.1365-2354.2006.00739.x

171. Pérol, D., Provençal, J., Hardy-Bessard, A.-C., Coeffic, D., Jacquin, J.-P., Agostini, C., ... Ray-Coquard, I. (2012). Can treatment with Cocculine improve the control of chemotherapy-induced emesis in early breast cancer patients? A randomized, multi-centered, double-blind, placebo-controlled phase III trial. *BMC Cancer, 12,* 603. doi:10.1186/1471-2407-12-603

172. Eaton, L.H., & Tipton, J.M. (Eds.). (2009). *Putting evidence into practice: Improving oncology patient outcomes.* Pittsburgh, PA: Oncology Nursing Society.

Cognitive Impairment

Catherine E. Jansen, PhD, RN, AOCNS®,
Deborah H. Allen, PhD, RN, AOCNP®,
Diane Von Ah, PhD, RN,
and Lee Ann Johnson, PhD(c), RN

Problem and Incidence

Cognitive impairment is a symptom that impacts quality of life, social relationships, and activities of everyday function in cancer survivors. Patients have described it as forgetfulness, memory lapses, inability to focus, being easily distracted, difficulties in making decisions, and feeling mentally slow or overwhelmed. Healthy brain functioning involves integration and effective performance of multiple cognitive domains. Cognitive impairment involves a decline in one or more domains.

The incidence of cognitive impairment is difficult to determine because it is multifactorial and related to cancer location, disease stage, and treatment type and intensity. Cognitive impairment may occur at various times during the cancer trajectory and may vary in type and severity. Rates from 11%–35% in patients with breast cancer and up to 80% in patients with brain and lung cancers have been reported.[1-3]

Risk Factors and Assessment

Numerous factions have been proposed that may influence an individual's risk for cognitive impairment.[4,5]
- Factors that place patients at high risk for cognitive impairment include
  - Central nervous system (CNS) primary or metastatic disease

- Intrathecal chemotherapy
- Brain irradiation.
- Factors contributing to risk include
  - Older age
  - Comorbidities
  - Treatment-related side effects
  - Cancer type, staging, and disease trajectory
  - Cancer treatments (e.g., surgery, radiation therapy, chemotherapy, biologic therapy, hormonal therapy)
  - Medications (prescription, over-the-counter, supplements)
  - Psychological distress (e.g., anxiety, depression)
  - Higher symptom burden (e.g., fatigue, sleep disturbances).

Assessment approaches for cognitive impairment include neuropsychological examination (incorporating a comprehensive clinical evaluation and standardized cognitive tests), neuroimaging, and self-report measures (e.g., Functional Assessment of Cancer Therapy–Cognitive Function).

What interventions are effective in preventing and managing cognitive impairment in people with cancer?

Evidence retrieved through March 31, 2013

Likely to Be Effective

Group cognitive training improved memory, cognitive function, neuropsychiatric parameters, and perceived cognitive functioning.[6-9]

Effectiveness Not Established

A number of pharmacologic and nonpharmacologic interventions have had inconsistent results across studies or were studied in small samples.

- **Pharmacologic interventions**
  - **Donepezil**[10,11]
  - **Methylphenidate**[12-20]
  - **Modafinil**[21-23]
- **Nonpharmacologic interventions**
  - **Cognitive behavioral approach interventions**[24-26]
  - **Environmental interventions** involving exposure to a natural environment[27]
  - **Exercise**[19,28-30]
  - **Individual cognitive training**[24,31-33]
  - **Mindfulness-based stress reduction**[34]
  - **Qigong/body-mind-spirit therapy** incorporating approaches from Western medicine and Eastern philosophies[35]
  - **Vitamin E**[10,36]

Effectiveness Unlikely

Ginkgo biloba[37,38]

Not Recommended for Practice

Erythropoiesis-stimulating agents (ESAs) showed mixed results. The U.S. Food and Drug Administration has safety warnings associated with ESAs because of the risk of tumor growth, decreased survival, and increased cardiovascular side effects.[39-45]

Application to Practice

Patients at risk for cognitive impairment need to be identified and assessed throughout cancer treatment and referred for formal neuropsychological assessment if indicated.

Presence of factors contributing to risk should be managed through pharmacologic or nonpharmacologic interventions to determine impact on cognitive function.

Pharmacologic interventions have primarily focused on treatment with psychostimulants, dexmethylphenidate, methylphenidate, and modafinil. Nurses need to assess for effectiveness and side effects of psychostimulants if used, including CNS (e.g., headache, insomnia) and gastrointestinal symptoms (e.g., anorexia, nausea).

Complementary and alternative interventions have primarily focused on cognitive training, cognitive behavioral training, exercise, and mindfulness-based stress reduction.
- Nurses need to identify what coping strategies or nonpharmacologic interventions patients have tried to evaluate effectiveness and promote healthy lifestyle behaviors.
- Group cognitive training is supported by evidence. Referral to appropriate providers for this type of intervention can be beneficial.

Cancer survivors have identified that healthcare providers' validation of their cognitive concerns is vital to adaptation and rehabilitation. Nurses can validate these concerns and monitor patients' progress using rehabilitation interventions.

Cognitive Impairment Resource Contributors
Topic leader: Diane Von Ah, PhD, RN
Deborah H. Allen, PhD, RN, AOCNP®, Catherine E. Jansen, PhD, RN, AOCNS®, and Jennifer Wulff, RN, MN, ARNP, AOCNP®

References

1. Jansen, C.E., Cooper, B.A., Dodd, M.J., & Miaskowski, C.A. (2011). A prospective longitudinal study of chemotherapy-induced cognitive changes in breast cancer patients. *Supportive Care in Cancer, 19,* 1647–1656. doi:10.1007/s00520-010-0997-4
2. Meyers, C.A., Byrne, K.S., & Komaki, R. (1995). Cognitive deficits in patients with small cell lung cancer before and after chemotherapy. *Lung Cancer, 12,* 231–235. doi:10.1016/0169-5002(95)00446-8
3. Tucha, O., Smely, C., Preier, M., & Lange, K.W. (2000). Cognitive deficits before treatment among patients with brain tumors. *Neurosurgery, 47,* 324–334. doi:10.1097/00006123-200008000-00011
4. National Comprehensive Cancer Network. (2013a). *NCCN Clinical Practice Guidelines in Oncology: Senior adult oncology* [v.2.2014]. Retrieved from http://www.nccn.org/professionals/physician_gls/pdf/senior.pdf
5. National Comprehensive Cancer Network. (2013b). *NCCN Clinical Practice Guidelines in Oncology: Survivorship* [v.1.2013]. Retrieved from http://www.nccn.org/professionals/physician_gls/pdf/survivorship.pdf

6. Hassler, M.R., Elandt, K., Preusser, M., Lehrner, J., Binder, P., Dieckmann, K., ... Marosi, C. (2010). Neurocognitive training in patients with high-grade glioma: A pilot study. *Journal of Neuro-Oncology, 97,* 109–115. doi:10.1007/s11060-009-0006-2

7. McDougall, G.J., Jr. (2001). Memory improvement program for elderly cancer survivors. *Geriatric Nursing, 22,* 185–190. doi:10.1067/mgn.2001.117916

8. Poppelreuter, M., Weis, J., & Bartsch, H.H. (2009). Effects of specific neuropsychological training programs for breast cancer patients after adjuvant chemotherapy. *Journal of Psychosocial Oncology, 27,* 274–296. doi:10.1080/07347330902776044

9. Von Ah, D., Carpenter, J.S., Saykin, A., Monahan, P., Wu, J., Yu, M., ... Unverzagt, F. (2012). Advanced cognitive training for breast cancer survivors: A randomized controlled trial. *Breast Cancer Research and Treatment, 135,* 799–809. doi:10.1007/s10549-012-2210-6

10. Jatoi, A., Kahanic, S.P., Frytak, S., Schaefer, P., Foote, R.L., Sloan, J., & Petersen, R.C. (2005). Donepezil and vitamin E for preventing cognitive dysfunction in small cell lung cancer patients: Preliminary results and suggestions for future study designs. *Supportive Care in Cancer, 13,* 66–69. doi:10.1007/s00520-004-0696-0

11. Shaw, E.G., Rosdhal, R., D'Agostino, R.B., Jr., Lovato, J., Naughton, M.J., Robbins, M.E., & Rapp, S.R. (2006). Phase II study of donepezil in irradiated brain tumor patients: Effect on cognitive function, mood, and quality of life. *Journal of Clinical Oncology, 24,* 1415–1420. doi:10.1200/JCO.2005.03.3001

12. Bruera, E., Miller, M.J., Macmillan, K., & Kuehn, N. (1992). Neuropsychological effects of methylphenidate in patients receiving a continuous infusion of narcotics for cancer pain. *Pain, 48,* 163–166. doi:10.1016/0304-3959(92)90053-E

13. Butler, J.M., Jr., Case, L.D., Atkins, J., Frizzell, B., Sanders, G., Griffin, P., ... Shaw, E.G. (2007). A phase III, double-blind, placebo-controlled prospective randomized clinical trial of d-threo-methylphenidate HCl in brain tumor patients receiving radiation therapy. *International Journal of Radiation Oncology, Biology, Physics, 69,* 1496–1501. doi:10.1016/j.ijrobp.2007.05.076

14. Gagnon, B., Low, G., & Schreier, G. (2005). Methylphenidate hydrochloride improves cognitive function in patients with advanced cancer and hypoactive delirium: A prospective clinical study. *Journal of Psychiatry and Neuroscience, 30,* 100–107. Retrieved from http://www.ncbi.nlm.nih.gov/pmc/articles/PMC551162/?tool=pubmed

15. Gehring, K., Patwardhan, S.Y., Collins, R., Groves, M.D., Etzel, C.J., Meyers, C.A., & Wefel, J.S. (2012). A randomized trial on the efficacy of methylphenidate and modafinil for improving cognitive functioning and symptoms in patients with a primary brain tumor. *Journal of Neuro-Oncology, 107,* 165–174. doi:10.1007/s11060-011-0723-1

16. Lower, E.E., Fleishman, S., Cooper, A., Zeldis, J., Faleck, H., Yu, Z., & Manning, D. (2009). Efficacy of dexmethylphenidate for the treatment of fatigue after cancer chemotherapy: A randomized clinical trial. *Journal of Pain and Symptom Management, 38,* 650–662. doi:10.1016/j.jpainsymman.2009.03.011

17. Mar Fan, H.G., Clemons, M., Xu, W., Chemerynsky, I., Breunis, H., Braganza, S., & Tannock, I.F. (2008). A randomised, placebo-controlled, double-blind trial of the effects of d-methylphenidate on fatigue and cognitive dysfunction in women undergoing adjuvant chemotherapy for breast cancer. *Supportive Care in Cancer, 16,* 577–583. doi:10.1007/s00520-007-0341-9

18. Meyers, C.A., Weitzner, M.A., Valentine, A.D., & Levin, V.A. (1998). Methylphenidate therapy improves cognition, mood, and function of brain tumor patients. *Journal of Clinical Oncology, 16,* 2522–2527. Retrieved from http://jco.ascopubs.org/content/16/7/2522.long

19. Schwartz, A.L., Thompson, J.A., & Masood, N. (2002). Interferon-induced fatigue in patients with melanoma: A pilot study of exercise and methylphenidate [Online exclusive]. *Oncology Nursing Forum, 29,* E85–E90. doi:10.1188/02.ONF.E85-E90

20. Stone, P., & Minton, O. (2011). European Palliative Care Research collaborative pain guidelines. Central side-effects management: What is the evidence to support best practice in the management of sedation, cognitive impairment and myoclonus? *Palliative Medicine, 25,* 431–441. doi:10.1177/0269216310380763

21. Blackwell, L., Petroni, G., Shu, J., Baum, L., & Farace, E. (2009). A pilot study evaluating the safety and efficacy of modafinil for cancer-related fatigue. *Journal of Palliative Medicine, 12,* 433–439. doi:10.1089/jpm.2008.0230

22. Kohli, S., Fisher, S.G., Tra, Y., Adams, M.J., Mapstone, M.E., Wesnes, K.A., ... Morrow, G.R. (2009). The effects of modafinil on cognitive function in breast cancer survivors. *Cancer, 115,* 2605–2616. doi:10.1002/cncr.24287

23. Lundorff, L.E., Jønsson, B.H., & Sjøgren, P. (2009). Modafinil for attentional and psychomotor dysfunction in advanced cancer: A double-blind randomised, cross-over trial. *Palliative Medicine, 23,* 731–738. doi:10.1177/0269216309106872

24. Ferguson, R.J., Ahles, T.A., Saykin, A.J., McDonald, B.C., Furstenberg, C.T., Cole, B.F., & Mott, L.A. (2007). Cognitive-behavioral management of chemotherapy-related cognitive change. *Psycho-Oncology, 16,* 772–777. doi:10.1002/pon.1133

25. Ferguson, R.J., McDonald, B.C., Rocque, M.A., Furstenberg, C.T., Horrigan, S., Ahles, T.A., & Saykin, A.J. (2012). Development of CBT for chemotherapy-related cognitive change: Results of a waitlist control trial. *Psycho-Oncology, 21,* 176–186. doi:10.1002/pon.1878

26. Schuurs, A., & Green, H.J. (2013). A feasibility study of group cognitive rehabilitation for cancer survivors: Enhancing cognitive function and quality of life. *Psycho-Oncology, 22,* 1043–1049. doi:10.1002/pon.3102

27. Cimprich, B., & Ronis, D.L. (2003). An environmental intervention to restore attention in women with newly diagnosed breast cancer. *Cancer Nursing, 26,* 284–292. doi:10.1097/00002820-200308000-00005

28. Baumann, F.T., Drosselmeyer, N., Leskaroski, A., Knicker, A., Krakowski-Roosen, H., Zopf, E.M., & Bloch, W. (2011). 12-week resistance training with breast cancer patients during chemotherapy: Effects on cognitive abilities. *Breast Care, 6,* 142–143. doi:10.1159/000327505

29. Korstjens, I., Mesters, I., van der Peet, E., Gijsen, B., & van den Borne, B. (2006). Quality of life of cancer survivors after physical and psychosocial rehabilitation. *European Journal of Cancer Prevention, 15,* 541–547. doi:10.1097/01.cej.0000220625.77857.95

30. Reid-Arndt, S.A., Matsuda, S., & Cox, C.R. (2012). Tai Chi effects on neuropsychological, emotional, and physical functioning following cancer treatment: A pilot study. *Complementary Therapies in Clinical Practice, 18,* 26–30. doi:10.1016/j.ctcp.2011.02.005

31. Gehring, K., Sitskoorn, M.M., Gundy, C.M., Sikkes, S.A.M., Klein, M., Postma, T.J., ... Aaronson, N.K. (2009). Cognitive rehabilitation in patients with gliomas: A randomized, controlled trial. *Journal of Clinical Oncology, 27,* 3712–3722. doi:10.1200/JCO.2008.20.5765

32. McDougall, G.J., Becker, H., Acee, T.W., Vaughan, P.W., & Delville, C.L. (2011). Symptom management of affective and cognitive disturbance with a group of cancer survivors. *Archives of Psychiatric Nursing, 25,* 24–35. doi:10.1016/j.apnu.2010.05.004

33. Sherer, M., Meyers, C.A., & Bergloff, P. (1997). Efficacy of postacute brain injury rehabilitation for patients with primary malignant brain tumors. *Cancer, 80,* 250–257. doi:10.1002/(SICI)1097-0142(19970715)80:2%3C250::AID-CNCR13%3E3.0.CO;2-T

34. Hoffman, C.J., Ersser, S.J., Hopkinson, J.B., Nicholls, P.G., Harrington, J.E., & Thomas, P.W. (2012). Effectiveness of mindfulness-based stress reduction in mood, breast- and endocrine-related quality of life, and well-being in stage 0 to III breast cancer: A randomized, controlled trial. *Journal of Clinical Oncology, 30,* 1335–1342. doi:10.1200/JCO.2010.34.0331

35. Oh, B., Butow, P.N., Mullan, B.A., Clarke, S.J., Beale, P.J., Pavlakis, N., ... Vardy, J. (2012). Effect of medical Qigong on cognitive function, quality

of life, and a biomarker of inflammation in cancer patients: A randomized controlled trial. *Supportive Care in Cancer, 20*, 1235–1242. doi:10.1007/s00520-011-1209-6

36. Chan, A.S., Cheung, M.-C., Law, S.C., & Chan, J.H. (2004). Phase II study of alpha-tocopherol in improving the cognitive function of patients with temporal lobe radionecrosis. *Cancer, 100*, 398–401. doi:10.1002/cncr.11885

37. Attia, A., Rapp, S.R., Case, L.D., D'Agostino, R., Lesser, G., Naughton, M., ... Shaw, E.G. (2012). Phase II study of *Ginkgo biloba* in irradiated brain tumor patients: Effect on cognitive function, quality of life, and mood. *Journal of Neuro-Oncology, 109*, 357–363. doi:10.1007/s11060-012-0901-9

38. Barton, D.L., Burger, K., Novotny, P.J., Fitch, T.R., Kohli, S., Soori, G., ... Loprinzi, C.L. (2012). The use of *Ginkgo biloba* for the prevention of chemotherapy-related cognitive dysfunction in women receiving adjuvant treatment for breast cancer, N00C9. *Supportive Care in Cancer, 21*, 1185–1192. doi:10.1007/s00520-012-1647-9

39. Chang, J., Couture, F.A., Young, S.D., Lau, C.Y., & McWatters, K.L. (2004). Weekly administration of epoetin alfa improves cognition and quality of life in patients with breast cancer receiving chemotherapy. *Supportive Cancer Therapy, 2*, 52–58. doi:10.3816/SCT.2004.n.023

40. Iconomou, G., Koutras, A., Karaivazoglou, K., Kalliolas, G.D., Assimakopoulos, K., Argyriou, A.A., ... Kalofonos, H.P. (2008). Effect of epoetin alpha therapy on cognitive function in anemic patients with solid tumors undergoing chemotherapy. *European Journal of Cancer Care, 17*, 535–541 doi:10.1111/j.1365-2354.2007.00857.x

41. Mancuso, A., Migliorino, M., De Santis, S., Saponiero, A., & De Marinis, F. (2006). Correlation between anemia and functional/cognitive capacity in elderly lung cancer patients treated with chemotherapy. *Annals of Oncology, 17*, 146–150. doi:10.1093/annonc/mdj038

42. Mar Fan, H.G., Park, A., Xu, W., Yi, Q.-L., Braganza, S., Chang, J., ... Tannock, I.F. (2009). The influence of erythropoietin on cognitive function in women following chemotherapy for breast cancer. *Psycho-Oncology, 18*, 156–161. doi:10.1002/pon.1372

43. Massa, E., Madeddu, C., Lusso, M.R., Gramignano, G., & Mantovani, G. (2005). Evaluation of the effectiveness of treatment with erythropoietin on anemia, cognitive functioning and functions studied by comprehensive geriatric assessment in elderly cancer patients with anemia related to cancer chemotherapy. *Critical Reviews in Oncology/Hematology, 57*, 175–182. doi:10.1016/j.critrevonc.2005.06.001

44. O'Shaughnessy, J.A. (2002). Effects of epoetin alfa on cognitive function, mood, asthenia, and quality of life in women with breast cancer undergoing adjuvant chemotherapy. *Clinical Breast Cancer, 3*(Suppl. 3), S116–S120. doi:10.3816/CBC.2002.s.022

45. O'Shaughnessy, J.A., Vukelja, S.J., Holmes, F.A., Savin, M., Jones, M., Royall, D., ... Von Hoff, D. (2005). Feasibility of quantifying the effects of epoetin alpha therapy on cognitive function in women with breast cancer undergoing adjuvant or neoadjuvant chemotherapy. *Clinical Breast Cancer, 5*, 439–446. doi:10.3816/CBC.2005.n.002

7

Constipation

Lee Ann Johnson, PhD(c), RN,
and Margaret Irwin, PhD, RN, MN

Problem and Incidence

Constipation is infrequent passage of hard, dry stool. It may be caused by the disease, treatments, medications, or lifestyle modifications that occur with cancer.[1,2] Constipation may be accompanied by abdominal pain, distention, nausea and vomiting, and loss of appetite.[3-6] Prevalence of constipation in patients with cancer has ranged from 40%–100%, depending on setting.[7-9] In one study, 95% of patients reported constipation as the major side effect of opioid use.[10]

Risk Factors and Assessment

Multiple risk factors contribute to the development of constipation, including the following.
- Continuous use of opioid therapy
- Treatment with vinca alkaloid agents
- Decreased mobility or immobility
- Decreased fluid intake

Assessment tools include
- Constipation Assessment Scale
- National Cancer Institute Cancer Therapy Evaluation Program *Common Terminology Criteria for Adverse Events*
- Modified Constipation Assessment Scale.

What interventions are effective in preventing and managing constipation in people with cancer?

Evidence retrieved through July 31, 2013

Recommended for Practice

Methylnaltrexone reduced opioid-induced constipation in studies[11-15] and systematic reviews[16-18] and is recommended in guidelines.[19-21]

Oxycodone and naloxone relieved constipation in patients taking prolonged-release oxycodone for non–cancer-related pain[22,23] and cancer-related pain.[24-27]

Transdermal fentanyl was associated with less constipation than other opioids.[28-31]

Likely to Be Effective

Alvimopan decreased time to recovery of GI function after surgery[32] and was suggested to reduce constipation in systematic reviews.[16,17]

Amidotrizoate was effective and well tolerated.[33]

Polyethylene glycol reduced constipation in patients without cancer[16,34-36] and in cancer populations.[37] Guidelines recommend use for patients receiving opioids.[20,21]

Prophylactic laxatives for patients on opioids are recommended in guidelines[20] and reduced prevalence of constipation.[34,38,39]

Senna plus docusate reduced constipation in individual studies[40,41] and showed mixed results in systematic reviews.[16,42] Use is recommended in guidelines.[21]

Effectiveness Not Established

Various interventions for constipation have limited evidence of effectiveness for patients with cancer. Evidence is limited because of inconsistent results, small samples, and lack of evidence specific to patients with cancer.

- **Baker's yeast**[43]
- **Biofeedback** for patients with pelvic floor dysfunction[44,45]—A systematic review noted that study quality was poor.[46]
- **Bisacodyl**, a stimulant laxative[16,47,48]
- **Colchicine**[49]
- **Dietary fiber**[50,51]—Increasing fiber in the diet has been recommended in guidelines.[21,52]
- **Konjac glucomannan**, a plant-derived soluble fiber[53]
- **Lactulose**, an osmotic laxative[24,31,35,36,42,54-56]—Most studies were done in palliative care patients.
- **Linaclotide**, which accelerates colonic transit time[57]
- **Lubiprostone**,[58-60] but has not been studied in patients with cancer or on chronic opioid therapy
- **Massage**[61]
- **Naloxone**[16,62,63]
- **Opioid switching** from oral to IV or transdermal formulations[28-31,64]
- **Probiotics**[52,65,66]—A technical review noted data are limited to support their effectiveness.[52]
- **Prucalopride**, a 5-HT_4 receptor agonist[67]
- **Sodium picosulfate**[68]—This was less effective than polyethylene glycol in patients with cancer.[37]
- **Sorbitol**[69]

Expert Opinion

In myelosuppressed patients, rectal manipulation and use of enemas or suppositories should be avoided.[70]

Daily fluid intake of 48 oz is generally recommended for adults; however, no evidence shows that increasing fluid intake improves constipation.[52]

Dietary interventions such as prune, pear, and apple juices may be helpful.[71]

Patients may benefit from nutritional consultation.

Patients should increase physical activity.[52]

Application to Practice

Patients at risk should be routinely assessed for constipation and evaluated for effectiveness of interventions used.

A bowel regimen with prophylactic use of laxatives should be initiated with patients on continuous opioids.

Patients receiving chemotherapy that slows colonic transit time (e.g., vincristine) should be educated regarding potential constipation and measures for prevention.

Nurses can educate patients regarding dietary and activity behaviors from expert opinion that may be helpful for prevention.

In general, evidence and effective interventions for constipation are limited, and even less evidence exists for patients with cancer.

Commonly used medications for constipation may be helpful.

Constipation Resource Contributors

Topic leader: Deborah M. Thorpe, PhD, APRN, ACHPN
Katherine L. Byar, RN, MSN, APN, BC, Arlene B. Davis, RN, MSN,
AOCN®, Jeanne Held-Warmkessel, MSN, RN, AOCN®, ACNS-BC,
and Elizabeth S. Kiker, RN, MSN, OCN®

References

1. Candrilli, S.D., Davis, K.L., & Iyer, S. (2009). Impact of constipation on opioid use patterns, health care resource utilization, and costs in cancer patients on opioid therapy. *Journal of Pain and Palliative Care Pharmacotherapy, 23*, 231–241. doi:10.1080/15360280903098440
2. Bell, T., Annunziata, K., & Leslie, J.B. (2009). Opioid-induced constipation negatively impacts pain management, productivity, and health-related

quality of life: Findings from the National Health and Wellness Survey. *Journal of Opioid Management, 5,* 137.

3. Cope, D.G. (2001). Management of chemotherapy-induced diarrhea and constipation. *Nursing Clinics of North America, 36,* 695–707.

4. Petticrew, M., Rodgers, M., & Booth, A. (2001). Effectiveness of laxatives in adults. *Quality in Health Care, 10,* 268–273. doi:10.1136/qhc.0100268

5. Tamayo, A.C., & Diaz-Zuluaga, P.A. (2004). Management of opioid-induced bowel dysfunction in cancer patients. *Supportive Care in Cancer, 12,* 613–618. doi:10.1007/s00520-004-0649-7

6. Thompson, M.J., Boyd-Carson, W., Trainor, B., & Boyd, K. (2003). Management of constipation. *Nursing Standard, 18*(14–18), 41–42. doi:10.7748/ns2003.12.18.14.41.c3519

7. McMillan, S.C. (2002). Presence and severity of constipation in hospice patients with advanced cancer. *American Journal of Hospice and Palliative Care, 19,* 426–430. doi:10.1177/104990910201900616

8. McMillan, S.C., & Weitzner, M.A. (2000). How problematic are various aspects of quality of life in patients with cancer at the end of life? *Oncology Nursing Forum, 27,* 817–823.

9. Weitzner, M.A., Moody, L.N., & McMillan, S.C. (1997). Symptom management issues in hospice care. *American Journal of Hospice and Palliative Care, 14,* 190–195. doi:10.1177/104990919701400407

10. Robinson, C.B., Fritch, M., Hullett, L., Petersen, M.A., Sikkema, S., Theuninck, L., & Timmer, K. (2000). Development of a protocol to prevent opioid-induced constipation in patients with cancer: A research utilization project. *Clinical Journal of Oncology Nursing, 4,* 79–84.

11. Chamberlain, B.H., Cross, K., Winston, J.L., Thomas, J., Wang, W., Su, C., & Israel, R.J. (2009). Methylnaltrexone treatment of opioid-induced constipation in patients with advanced illness. *Journal of Pain and Symptom Management, 38,* 683–690. doi:10.1016/j.jpainsymman.2009.02.234

12. Lipman, A.G., Karver, S., Cooney, G.A., Stambler, N., & Israel, R.J. (2011). Methylnaltrexone for opioid-induced constipation in patients with advanced illness: A 3-month open-label treatment extension study. *Journal of Pain and Palliative Care Pharmacotherapy, 25,* 136–145. doi:10.3109/15360288.2011.573531

13. Portenoy, R.K., Thomas, J., Moehl Boatwright, M.L., Tran, D., Galasso, F.L., Stambler, N., ... Israel, R.J. (2008). Subcutaneous methylnaltrexone for the treatment of opioid-induced constipation in patients with advanced illness: A double-blind, randomized, parallel group, dose-ranging study. *Journal of Pain and Symptom Management, 35,* 458–468. doi:10.1016/j.jpainsymman.2007.12.005

14. Slatkin, N., Thomas, J., Lipman, A.G., Wilson, G., Boatwright, M.L., Wellman, C., ... Israel, R. (2009). Methylnaltrexone for treatment of opioid-induced constipation in advanced illness patients. *Journal of Supportive Oncology, 7,* 39–46. Retrieved from http://www.oncologypractice.com/jso/journal/articles/0701039.pdf

15. Thomas, J., Karver, S., Cooney, G.A., Chamberlain, B.H., Watt, C.K., Slatkin, N.E., ... Israel, R.J. (2008). Methylnaltrexone for opioid-induced constipation in advanced illness. *New England Journal of Medicine, 358,* 2332–2343. doi:10.1056/NEJMoa0707377

16. Ahmedzai, S.H., & Boland, J. (2010, April). Constipation in people prescribed opioids. *Clinical Evidence, 2010,* 2407. Retrieved from http://www.ncbi.nlm.nih.gov/pmc/articles/PMC2907601

17. Becker, G., Galandi, D., & Blum, H.E. (2007). Peripherally acting opioid antagonists in the treatment of opiate-related constipation: A systematic review. *Journal of Pain and Symptom Management, 34,* 547–565. doi:10.1016/j.jpainsymman.2006.12.018

18. Candy, B., Jones, L., Goodman, M.L., Drake, R., & Tookman, A. (2011). Laxatives or methylnaltrexone for the management of constipation in palliative care patients. *Cochrane Database of Systematic Reviews, 2011*(1). doi:10.1002/14651858.CD003448.pub3

19. Librach, S.L., Bouvette, M., De Angelis, C., Farley, J., Oneschuk, D., & Pereira, J.L. (2010). Consensus recommendations for the management of constipation in patients with advanced, progressive illness. *Journal of Pain and Symptom Management, 40,* 761–773. doi:10.1016/j.jpainsymman.2010.03.026

20. National Comprehensive Cancer Network. (2013). *NCCN Clinical Practice Guidelines in Oncology: Adult cancer pain* [v. 2.2013]. Retrieved from http://www.nccn.org/professionals/physician_gls/pdf/pain.pdf

21. National Comprehensive Cancer Network. (2013). *NCCN Clinical Practice Guidelines in Oncology: Palliative care* [v.2.2013]. Retrieved from http://www.nccn.org/professionals/physician_gls/pdf/palliative.pdf

22. Löwenstein, O., Leyendecker, P., Hopp, M., Schutter, U., Rogers, P.D., Uhl, R., ... Reimer, K. (2009). Combined prolonged-release oxycodone and naloxone improves bowel function in patients receiving opioids for moderate-to-severe non-malignant chronic pain: A randomised controlled trial. *Expert Opinion on Pharmacotherapy, 10,* 531–543. doi:10.1517/14656560902796798

23. Simpson, K., Leyendecker, P., Hopp, M., Müller-Lissner, S., Löwenstein, O., De Andrés, J., ... Reimer, K. (2008). Fixed-ratio combination oxycodone/naloxone compared with oxycodone alone for the relief of opioid-induced constipation in moderate-to-severe noncancer pain. *Current Medical Research and Opinion, 24,* 3503–3512. doi:10.1185/03007990802584454

24. Ahmedzai, S.H., Nauck, F., Bar-Sela, G., Bosse, B., Leyendecker, P., & Hopp, M. (2012). A randomized, double-blind, active-controlled, double-dummy, parallel-group study to determine the safety and efficacy of oxycodone/naloxone prolonged-release tablets in patients with moderate/severe, chronic cancer pain. *Palliative Medicine, 26,* 50–60. doi:10.1177/0269216311418869

25. Meissner, W., Schmidt, U., Hartmann, M., Kath, R., & Reinhart, K. (2000). Oral naloxone reverses opioid-associated constipation. *Pain, 84,* 105–109. doi:10.1016/S0304-3959(99)00185-2

26. Nadstawek, J., Leyendecker, P., Hopp, M., Ruckes, C., Wirz, S., Fleischer, W., & Reimer, K. (2008). Patient assessment of a novel therapeutic approach for the treatment of severe, chronic pain. *International Journal of Clinical Practice, 62,* 1159–1167. doi:10.1111/j.1742-1241.2008.01820.x

27. Schutter, U., Grunert, S., Meyer, C., Schmidt, T., & Nolte, T. (2010). Innovative pain therapy with a fixed combination of prolonged-release oxycodone/naloxone: A large observational study under conditions of daily practice. *Current Medical Research and Opinion, 26,* 1377–1387. doi:10.1185/03007991003787318

28. Ahmedzai, S., & Brooks, D. (1997). Transdermal fentanyl versus sustained-release oral morphine in cancer pain: Preference, efficacy, and quality of life. *Journal of Pain and Symptom Management, 13,* 254–261. doi:10.1016/S0885-3924(97)00082-1

29. Radbruch, L., Sabatwski, R., Loick, G., Kulbe, C., & Casper, M. (2000). Constipation and the use of laxatives: A comparison between transdermal fentanyl and oral morphine. *Palliative Medicine, 13,* 111–119. doi:10.1191/026921600671594561

30. Tassinari, D., Sartori, S., Tamburini, E., Scarpi, E., Tombesi, P., Santelmo, C., & Maltoni, M. (2009). Transdermal fentanyl as a front-line approach to moderate-severe pain: A meta-analysis of randomized clinical trials. *Journal of Palliative Care, 25,* 172–180.

31. Wirz, S., Wittmann, M., Schenk, M., Schroeck, A., Schaefer, N., Mueller, M., ... Nadstawek, J. (2009). Gastrointestinal symptoms under opioid therapy: A prospective comparison of oral sustained-release hydromorphone, transdermal fentanyl, and transdermal buprenorphine. *European Journal of Pain, 13,* 737–743. doi:10.1016/j.ejpain.2008.09.005

32. Taguchi, A., Sharma, N., Saleem, R.M., Sessler, D.I., Carpenter, R.L., Seyedsadr, M., & Kurz, A. (2001). Selective postoperative inhibition of gastrointestinal opioid receptors. *New England Journal of Medicine, 345,* 935–940. doi:10.1056/NEJMoa010564

33. Mercadante, S., Ferrera, P., & Casuccio, A. (2010). Effectiveness and tolerability of amidotrizoate for the treatment of constipation resistant to laxatives in advanced cancer patients. *Journal of Pain and Symptom Management, 41*, 421–425. doi:10.1016/j.jpainsymman.2010.04.022

34. Larkin, P.J., Sykes, N.P., Centeno, C., Ellershaw, J.E., Elsner, F., Eugene, B., ... Zuurmond, W.W.A. (2008). The management of constipation in palliative care: Clinical practice recommendations. *Palliative Medicine, 22*, 796–807. doi:10.1177/0269216308096908

35. Lee-Robichaud, H., Thomas, K., Morgan, J., & Nelson, R.L. (2010). Lactulose versus polyethylene glycol for chronic constipation. *Cochrane Database of Systematic Reviews, 2010*(7). doi:10.1002/14651858.CD007570.pub2

36. van der Spoel, J.I., Oudemans-van Straaten, H.M., Kuiper, M.A., van Roon, E.N., Zandstra, D.F., & van der Voort, P.H. (2007). Laxation of critically ill patients with lactulose or polyethylene glycol: A two-center randomized, double-blind, placebo-controlled trial. *Critical Care Medicine, 35*, 2726–2731. doi:10.1097/01.CCM.0000287526.08794.29

37. Wirz, S., Nadstawek, J., Elsen, C., Junker, U., & Wartenberg, H.C. (2012). Laxative management in ambulatory cancer patients on opioid therapy: A prospective, open-label investigation of polyethylene glycol, sodium picosulphate and lactulose. *European Journal of Cancer Care, 21*, 131–140. doi:10.1111/j.1365-2354.2011.01286.x

38. Ishihara, M., Iihara, H., Okayasu, S., Yasuda, K., Matsuura, K., Suzui, M., & Itoh, Y. (2010). Pharmaceutical interventions facilitate premedication and prevent opioid-induced constipation and emesis in cancer patients. *Supportive Care in Cancer, 18*, 1531–1538. doi:10.1007/s00520-009-0775-3

39. Ishihara, M., Ikesue, H., Matsunaga, H., Suemaru, K., Kitaichi, K., Suetsugu, K., ... Itoh, Y. (2012). A multi-institutional study analyzing effect of prophylactic medication for prevention of opioid-induced gastrointestinal dysfunction. *Clinical Journal of Pain, 28*, 373–381. doi:10.1097/AJP.0b013e318237d626

40. Hawley, P.H., & Byeon, J.J. (2008). A comparison of sennosides-based bowel protocols with and without docusate in hospitalized patients with cancer. *Journal of Palliative Medicine, 11*, 575–581. doi:10.1089/jpm.2007.0178

41. Patel, M., Schimpf, M.O., O'Sullivan, D.M., & LaSala, C.A. (2010). The use of senna with docusate for postoperative constipation after pelvic reconstructive surgery: A randomized, double-blind, placebo-controlled trial. *American Journal of Obstetrics and Gynecology, 202*, 479.e1–479.e5. doi:10.1016/j.ajog.2010.01.003

42. Miles, C.L., Fellowes, D., Goodman, M.L., & Wilkinson, S.S.M. (2009). Laxatives for the management of constipation in palliative care patients. *Cochrane Database of Systematic Reviews, 2009*(1). doi:10.1002/14651858.CD003448.pub2

43. Wenk, R., Bertolino, M., Ochoa, J., Cullen, C., Bertucelli, N., & Bruera, E. (2000). Laxative effects of fresh baker's yeast. *Journal of Pain and Symptom Management, 19*, 163–164. doi:10.1016/S0885-3924(99)00159-1

44. Chiarioni, G., Salandini, L., & Whitehead, W.E. (2005). Biofeedback benefits only patients with outlet dysfunction, not patients with isolated slow transit constipation. *Gastroenterology, 129*, 86–97. doi:10.1053/j.gastro.2005.05.015

45. Chiarioni, G., Whitehead, W.E., Pezza, V., Morelli, A., & Bassotti, G. (2006). Biofeedback is superior to laxatives for normal transit constipation due to pelvic floor dyssynergia. *Gastroenterology, 130*, 657–664. doi:10.1053/j.gastro.2005.11.014

46. Koh, C.E., Young, C.J., Young, J.M., & Solomon, M.J. (2008). Systematic review of randomized controlled trials of the effectiveness of biofeedback for pelvic floor dysfunction. *British Journal of Surgery, 95*, 1079–1087. doi:10.1002/bjs.6303

47. Kienzle-Horn, S., Vix, J.-M., Schuijt, C., Peil, H., Jordan, C.C., & Kamm, M.A. (2006). Efficacy and safety of bisacodyl in acute treatment of constipation: A double-blind, randomized, placebo-controlled study. *Alimentary*

Pharmacology and Therapeutics, 23, 1479–1488. doi:10.1111/j.1365-2036.2006.02903.x

48. Kienzle-Horn, S., Vix, J.-M., Schuijt, C., Peil, H., Jordan, C.C., & Kamm, M.A. (2007). Comparison of bisacodyl and sodium picosulfate in the treatment of chronic constipation. *Current Medical Research and Opinion, 23,* 691–699. doi:10.1185/030079907X178865

49. Taghavi, S.A., Shabani, S., Mehramiri, A., Eshraghian, A., Kazemi, S.M., Moeini, M., ... Mostaghni, A.A. (2010). Colchicine is effective for short-term treatment of slow transit constipation: A double-blind placebo-controlled clinical trial. *International Journal of Colorectal Disease, 25,* 389–394. doi:10.1007/s00384-009-0794-z

50. Griffenberg, L., Morris, M., Atkinson, N., & Levenback, C. (1997). The effect of dietary fiber on bowel function following radical hysterectomy: A randomized trial. *Gynecologic Oncology, 66,* 417–424. doi:10.1006/gyno.1997.4797

51. Holma, R., Hongisto, S.M., Saxelin, M., & Korpela, R. (2010). Constipation is relieved more by rye bread than wheat bread or laxatives without increased adverse gastrointestinal effects. *Journal of Nutrition, 140,* 534–541. doi:10.3945/jn.109.118570

52. Bharucha, A.E., Pemberton, J.H., & Locke, G.R., III. (2013). American Gastroenterological Association technical review on constipation. *Gastroenterology, 144,* 218–238. doi:10.1053/j.gastro.2012.10.028

53. Chen, H.L., Cheng, H.C., Wu, W.T., Liu, Y.J., & Liu, S.Y. (2008). Supplementation of konjac glucomannan into a low-fiber Chinese diet promoted bowel movement and improved colonic ecology in constipated adults: A placebo-controlled, diet-controlled trial. *Journal of the American College of Nutrition, 27,* 102–108. doi:10.1080/07315724.2008.10719681

54. Agra, Y., Sacristan, A., Gonzalez, M., Ferrari, M., Portugues, A., & Calvo, M.J. (1998). Efficacy of senna versus lactulose in terminal cancer patients treated with opioids. *Journal of Pain and Symptom Management, 15,* 1–7. doi:10.1016/S0885-3924(97)00276-5

55. Candy, D., & Belsey, J. (2009). Macrogol (polyethylene glycol) laxatives in children with functional constipation and faecal impaction: A systematic review. *Archives of Disease in Childhood, 94,* 156–160. doi:10.1136/adc.2007.128769

56. Harris, A.C., & Jackson, J.M. (1977). Lactulose in vincristine-induced constipation. *Medical Journal of Australia, 2,* 573–574.

57. Johnston, J.M., Kurtz, C.B., Drossman, D.A., Lembo, A.J., Jeglinski, B.I., MacDougall, J.E., ... Currie, M.G. (2009). Pilot study on the effect of linaclotide in patients with chronic constipation. *American Journal of Gastroenterology, 104,* 125–132. doi:10.1038/ajg.2008.59

58. Baker, D.E. (2007). Lubiprostone: A new drug for the treatment of chronic idiopathic constipation. *Reviews in Gastroenterological Disorders, 7,* 214–222. Retrieved from http://www.medreviews.com/issue.cfm?toLogin=Log+In&issue=211

59. Barish, C.F., Drossman, D., Johanson, J.F., & Ueno, R. (2010). Efficacy and safety of lubiprostone in patients with chronic constipation. *Digestive Diseases and Sciences, 55,* 1090–1097. doi:10.1007/s10620-009-1068-x

60. Johanson, J.F., Morton, D., Geenen, J., & Ueno, R. (2008). Multicenter, 4-week, double-blind, randomized, placebo-controlled trial of lubiprostone, a locally-acting type-2 chloride channel activator, in patients with chronic constipation. *American Journal of Gastroenterology, 103,* 170–177. doi:10.1111/j.1572-0241.2007.01524.x

61. Lai, T.K.T., Cheung, M.C., Lo, C.K., Ng, K.L., Fung, Y.H., Tong, M., & Yau, C.C. (2011). Effectiveness of aroma massage on advanced cancer patients with constipation: A pilot study. *Complementary Therapies in Clinical Practice, 17,* 37–43. doi:10.1016/j.ctcp.2010.02.004

62. Meissner, W., Leyendecker, P., Mueller-Lissner, S., Nadstawek, J., Hopp, M., Ruckes, C., ... Reimer, K. (2009). A randomised controlled trial with prolonged-release oral oxycodone and naloxone to prevent and reverse

opioid-induced constipation. *European Journal of Pain, 13,* 56–64. doi:10.1016/j.ejpain.2008.06.012

63. Tofil, N.M., Benner, K.W., Faro, S.J., & Winkler, M.K. (2006). The use of enteral naloxone to treat opioid-induced constipation in a pediatric intensive care unit. *Pediatric Critical Care Medicine, 7,* 252–254. doi:10.1097/01 .PCC.0000216421.72002.09

64. Mazumdar, A., Mishra, S., Bhatnagar, S., & Gupta, D. (2008). Intravenous morphine can avoid distressing constipation associated with oral morphine: A retrospective analysis of our experience in 11 patients in the palliative care in-patient unit. *American Journal of Hospice and Palliative Care, 25,* 282–284. doi:10.1177/1049909108315913

65. Higashikawa, F., Noda, M., Awaya, T., Nomura, K., Oku, H., & Sugiyama, M. (2010). Improvement of constipation and liver function by plant-derived lactic acid bacteria: A double-blind, randomized trial. *Nutrition, 26,* 367–374. doi:10.1016/j.nut.2009.05.008

66. Ohigashi, S., Hoshino, Y., Ohde, S., & Onodera, H. (2011). Functional outcome, quality of life, and efficacy of probiotics in postoperative patients with colorectal cancer. *Surgery Today, 41,* 1200–1206. doi:10.1007/s00595-010-4450-6

67. Quigley, E.M.M., Vandeplassche, L., Kerstens, R., & Ausma, J. (2009). Clinical trial: The efficacy, impact on quality of life, and safety and tolerability of prucalopride in severe chronic constipation—A 12-week, randomized, double-blind, placebo-controlled study. *Alimentary Pharmacology and Therapeutics, 29,* 315–328. doi:10.1111/j.1365-2036.2008.03884.x

68. Mueller-Lissner, S., Kamm, M.A., Wald, A., Hinkel, U., Koehler, U., Richter, E., & Bubeck, J. (2010). Multicenter, 4-week, double-blind, randomized, placebo-controlled trial of sodium picosulfate in patients with chronic constipation. *American Journal of Gastroenterology, 105,* 897–903. doi:10.1038/ajg.2010.41

69. Lederle, F.A., Busch, D.L., Mattox, K.M., West, M.J., & Aske, D.M. (1990). Cost-effective treatment of constipation in the elderly: A randomized double-blind comparison of sorbitol and lactulose. *American Journal of Medicine, 89,* 597–601. doi:10.1016/0002-9343(90)90177-F

70. Bisanz, A.K., Woolery, M.J., Lyons, H.F., Gaido, L., Yenulevich, M., & Fulton, S. (2009). ONS PEP resource: Constipation. In L.H. Eaton & J.M. Tipton (Eds.), *Putting evidence into practice: Improving oncology patient outcomes* (pp. 93–104). Pittsburgh, PA: Oncology Nursing Society.

71. Baker, S.S., Liptak, G.S., Colletti, R.B., Croffie, J.M., Di Lorenzo, C., Ector, W., & Nurko, S. (2006). Evaluation and treatment of constipation in infants and children: Recommendations of the North American Society for Pediatric Gastroenterology, Hepatology, and Nutrition. *Journal of Pediatric Gastroenterology and Nutrition, 43*(3), e1–e13. doi:10.1097/01.mpg .0000233159.97667.c3

Depression

Heeju Kim, PhD, RN, OCN®,
and Caryl D. Fulcher, MSN, RN, CNS-BC

Problem and Incidence

Symptoms such as depressed mood, loss of interest or pleasure in activities that were previously enjoyed, loss of energy, social withdrawal, disturbances in eating and sleeping, difficulty thinking or concentrating, and feelings of worthlessness or guilt are indicative of depression.[1] Depression is often undiagnosed and may be untreated in patients with cancer. It can affect patients' quality of life and acceptance and adherence to cancer treatment.[2,3]

Prevalence of depression varies widely across studies. The variation is associated with different methods of assessment, use of different criteria to define depression, and differences in cancer type, stage, phase of care, and type of treatment. One meta-analysis reported prevalence of 5%–16% among outpatients, 4%–14% among inpatients, and 7%–49% in patients receiving palliative care.[4] Rates of depression also have varied in reports according to cancer type, with highest rates among those with breast, pancreatic, lung, and oropharyngeal cancers.[3,5] Krebber et al.[5] reported a pooled prevalence of 14%–27% in the acute phase of cancer care, 9%–21% in the first year after treatment, and 8%–15% after the first year. Cancer survivors are more likely to experience clinically relevant depression than individuals without cancer.[6]

Risk Factors and Assessment

Risk factors include the following.
- Advanced disease
- Poorly controlled pain

- Increased physical impairment/disability
- Perceived lack of support[7]

Periods of increased vulnerability for depression or distress include the following.
- Hearing the diagnosis
- Ending treatment; discharge from hospital
- Medical follow-up/surveillance
- Disease recurrence/progression
- End of life[8]

Consistent screening is standard for quality cancer care. Assessment should include the following.
- Ask the following questions.[9]
  - Are you feeling down or depressed?
  - Have you lost interest in activities you usually find pleasurable?
- Nurses may notice a patient's inability to smile, to be cheered up, or to respond to good news.
- Family may mention the patient's social withdrawal or poor participation in medical care.[10]
- Symptoms of cancer and its treatment may make it difficult to distinguish depression. Focus on the psychological symptoms,[11,12] including
  - Loss of interest in usually pleasurable activities
  - Hopelessness
  - Worthlessness
  - Low mood
  - Sense of guilt
  - Lack of control
  - Loss of confidence
  - Irritability.

Self-assessment tools include
- Hospital Depression and Anxiety Scale
- Patient Health Questionnaire-9 (open access)[13,14]
- Beck Depression Inventory.

What interventions are effective in managing depression in people with cancer?

Evidence retrieved through June 30, 2013

Recommended for Practice

Antidepressants (sertraline, mirtazapine, fluoxetine, fluvoxamine, escitalopram, paroxetine, citalopram, and duloxetine) reduced depression in patients with cancer.[15-27] One meta-analysis showed both short- and long-term response to antidepressants.[21] Professional guidelines support use of antidepressants.[8,28]

Cognitive-behavioral approach interventions showed moderate to strong effects in two meta-analyses.[29,30] Individual studies had mixed results.[31-41]

Mindfulness-based stress reduction provided over six to eight weeks reduced depression.[42-47] Meta-analyses reported low to moderate effect sizes.[48,49]

Psychoeducational interventions in various cancer types were beneficial with small effect sizes.[50-61] No one type of intervention eclipsed others.[62,63] Effectiveness of psychoeducation was reported in multiple other systematic reviews[21,23,39,64]; however, mixed results were seen in other studies.[65-69] Psychoeducation is recommended in professional guidelines.[28,70]

Likely to Be Effective

Individual psychotherapy improved symptoms of depression[71,72] and demonstrated effects in two meta-analyses.[30,73]

Peer counseling provided by trained prostate cancer survivors to newly diagnosed patients reduced depression.[74]

Relaxation therapy demonstrated positive effects.[75,76] One study in 17 patients did not show an effect.[77]

Effectiveness Not Established

A number of interventions have shown conflicting results, were only studied in small samples, or were evaluated in studies with multiple design limitations. Rigorously designed studies are needed to determine their effectiveness. These include pharmacologic interventions, psychosocial interventions, and a variety of other nonpharmacologic interventions.

- **Pharmacologic interventions**
  - **Infliximab**, a monoclonal antibody directed at inflammatory cytokines[78]
  - **Stimulants**, methylphenidate and modafinil[79]
- **Psychosocial interventions**
  - **Group psychotherapy**[80,81]—One meta-analysis showed short-term benefit in patients with advanced disease.[30]
  - **Hypnosis/hypnotherapy**[82]
  - **Narrative interviewing**, in which patients were encouraged to discuss meaning, sense of suffering, and well-being[83]
  - **Online support groups**, which showed inconsistent results across studies[84,85]
- **Nonpharmacologic interventions**
  - **Acupuncture**[86-89]—A systematic review of acupuncture in patients with cancer was inconclusive.[90]
  - **Aromatherapy**[91]
  - **Art making/art therapy**[92,93]
  - **Body-mind-spirit therapy/Qigong**, incorporating gentle exercise and Eastern philosophies[94,95]
  - **Early palliative care** provided proactively, rather than by patient request[96]
  - **Exercise**[97-105]—One meta-analysis showed a small effect size.[106]
  - **Guarana**, an herbal medicine[107]
  - **Healing touch**[77,108]
  - **Massage/aromatherapy massage**[91,109]
  - **Music/music therapy**[110]—A meta-analysis reported no significant effects of music for depression.[111]
  - **Reiki**[112]
  - **Relaxation and visual imagery**[113]
  - **Structured assessment**, including screening for depression[114]—A meta-analysis did not show improved depression outcomes with screening.[115]
  - **Structured rehabilitation services**[116,117]
  - **Supportive care/support interventions** provided by telephone or Internet or via support groups[81,84,85,118-121]—

A systematic review suggested support groups may be beneficial.[27]

- **Tailored information** provided via a multimedia tool to educate patients[122]
- **Virtual reality games** for hospitalized pediatric patients[123]
- **Yoga** and similar mind-body therapies[124-127]

Effectiveness Unlikely

Beauty treatments were evaluated for impact on body image and distress in women who had undergone mastectomy. Depression and anxiety declined over time in both treatment and control groups with no difference between groups.[128]

Expressive writing to facilitate emotional disclosure did not have an effect.[129-132]

Orientation and information provision via written materials, in person, or by video disc showed no benefit for depression in one randomized controlled trial (RCT)[133] and two systematic reviews.[134,135]

Reflexology had no effect on depressive symptoms in two large RCTs.[136,137]

Application to Practice

Nurses need to develop a relationship in which patients feel comfortable sharing feelings and understand that their emotional reactions are of interest. Screening for distress[138] and identifying contributing factors can pinpoint those patients who need in-depth assessment and intervention for depression.

- Nurses can implement interventions that have strong evidence of effectiveness within their individual scope of practice, such as
  - Prescribing or advocating use of antidepressants, educating about antidepressant medications, and monitoring patients for side effects if these are prescribed

- Referring patients to advanced practice providers for psychotherapy, cognitive behavioral therapy, and mindfulness-based stress reduction
- Educating and counseling about depression and incorporating cognitive behavioral therapy approaches in psychoeducational interventions by helping patients to identify unhelpful thoughts and behaviors and plan approaches to solve problems and cope more effectively
- Promoting peer support, including available support groups and disease-based organizations
- Teaching patients relaxation therapy.
- Because depression frequently coexists with pain, fatigue, sleep disturbance, and anxiety, those symptoms must also be addressed.[139]

Depression Resource Contributors

*Topic leader: Caryl D. Fulcher, MSN, RN, CNS-BC
Angelia Berkowitz, MSN, APRN, FNP-BC, Diane G. Cope, RN,
PhD, ARNP-BC, AOCNP®, Patricia J. Friend, PhD, APRN, AOCN®,
Heeju Kim, PhD, RN, OCN® Tammie L. Sherner, MSN, APRN-CNS,
Patsy Smith, RN, PhD, Thiruppavai Sundaramurthi, MSN, RN,
CCRN, Meghan L. Underhill, PhD, RN, AOCNS®, and Deborah K.
Walker, DNP, FNP-BC, AOCN®*

References

1. American Psychiatric Association. (2013). *Diagnostic and statistical manual of mental disorders* (5th ed.). Washington, DC: Author.
2. Colleoni, M., Mandala, M., Peruzzotti, G., Robertson, C., Bredart, A., & Goldhirsch, A. (2000). Depression and degree of acceptance of adjuvant cytotoxic drugs. *Lancet, 356*, 1326–1327. doi:10.1016/S0140-6736(00)02821-X
3. Sharpe, M., Strong, V., Allen, K., Rush, R., Postma, K., Tulloh, A., … Cull, A. (2004). Major depression in outpatients attending a regional cancer centre: Screening and unmet treatment needs. *British Journal of Cancer, 90*, 314–320. doi:10.1038/sj.bjc.6601578
4. Walker, J., Holm Hansen, C., Martin, P., Sawhney, A., Thekkumpurath, P., Beale, C., … Sharpe, M. (2013). Prevalence of depression in adults with cancer: A systematic review. *Annals of Oncology, 24*, 895–900. doi:10.1093/annonc/mds575
5. Krebber, A.M.H., Buffart, L.M., Kleijn, G., Riepma, I.C., de Bree, R., Leemans, C.R., … Verdonck-de Leeuw, I.M. (2014). Prevalence of depression in cancer patients: A meta-analysis of diagnostic interviews and self-report instruments. *Psycho-Oncology, 23*, 121–130. doi:10.1002/pon.3409
6. Schumacher, J.R., Palta, M., LoConte, N.K., Trentham-Dietz, A., Witt, W.P., Heidrich S.M., & Smith, M.A. (2013). Characterizing the psychological distress response before and after a cancer diagnosis. *Journal of Behavioral Medicine, 6*, 591–600. doi:10.1007/s10865-012-9453-x

7. Miller, K., & Massie, M.J. (2010). Depressive disorders. In J.C. Holland, W.S. Breitbart, P.B. Jacobsen, M.S. Lederberg, M.J. Loscalzo, & R.S. McCorkle (Eds.), *Psycho-oncology* (2nd ed., pp. 311–318). New York, NY: Oxford University Press.

8. National Comprehensive Cancer Network. (2012). *NCCN Clinical Practice Guidelines in Oncology: Distress management* [v.2.2013]. Retrieved from http://www.nccn.org/professionals/physician_gls/pdf/distress.pdf

9. Kroenke, K., Spitzer, R.L., & Williams, J.B.W. (2003). The Patient Health Questionnaire-2: Validity of a two-item depression screener. *Journal of General Internal Medicine, 14,* 1284–1292. doi:10.1097/01.MLR.0000093487.78664.3C

10. Akechi, T., Ietsugu, T., Sukigara, M., Okamura, H.L., Nakano, T., Akizuki, N., … Uchetomi, Y. (2009). Symptom indicator of severity of depression in cancer patients: A comparison of the *DSM-IV* criteria with alternative diagnostic criteria. *General Hospital Psychiatry, 31,* 225–232. doi:10.1016/j.genhosppsych.2008.12.004

11. Kleiboer, A., Bennett, F., Hodges, L., Walker, J., Thekkumpurath, P., & Sharpe, M. (2011). The problems reported by cancer patients with major depression. *Psycho-Oncology, 20,* 62–68. doi:10.1002/pon.1708

12. Miller, K., & Massie, M.J. (2006). Depression and anxiety. *Cancer Journal, 12,* 388–397. doi:10.1097/00130404-200609000-00008

13. Pfizer. (1999). Patient Health Questionnaire (PHQ-9). Retrieved from http://www.integration.samhsa.gov/images/res/PHQ%20-%20Questions.pdf

14. Spitzer, R.L., Williams, J.B.W., & Kroenke, K. (n.d.). Patient Health Questionnaire-9. Retrieved from http://www.phqscreeners.com/pdfs/02_PHQ-9/English.pdf

15. Amodeo, L., Castelli, L., Leombruni, P., Cipriani, D., Biancofiore, A., & Torta, R. (2012). Slow versus standard up-titration of paroxetine for the treatment of depression in cancer patients: A pilot study. *Supportive Care in Cancer, 20,* 375–384. doi:10.1007/s00520-011-1118-8

16. Cankurtaran, E.S., Ozalp, E., Soygur, H., Akbiyik, D.I., Turhan, L., & Alkis, N. (2008). Mirtazapine improves sleep and lowers anxiety and depression in cancer patients: Superiority over imipramine. *Supportive Care in Cancer, 16,* 1291–1298. doi:10.1007/s00520-008-0425-1

17. Ersoy, M.A., Noyan, A.M., & Elbi, H. (2008). An open-label long-term naturalistic study of mirtazapine treatment for depression in cancer patients. *Clinical Drug Investigation, 28,* 113–120. doi:10.2165/00044011-200828020-00005

18. Lydiatt, W.M., Denman, D., McNeilly, D.P., Puumula, S.E., & Burke, W.J. (2008). A randomized, placebo-controlled trial of citalopram for the prevention of major depression during treatment for head and neck cancer. *Archives of Otolaryngology, 134,* 528–535. doi:10.1001/archotol.134.5.528

19. Navari, R.M., Brenner, M.C., & Wilson, M.N. (2008). Treatment of depressive symptoms in patients with early stage breast cancer undergoing adjuvant therapy. *Breast Cancer Research and Treatment, 112,* 197–201. doi:10.1007/s10549-007-9841-z

20. Park, H.Y., Lee, B.-J., Kim, J.-H., Bae, J.-N., & Hahm, B.-J. (2012). Rapid improvement of depression and quality of life with escitalopram treatment in outpatients with breast cancer: A 12-week, open-label prospective trial. *Progress in Neuro-Psychopharmacology and Biological Psychiatry, 30,* 318–323. doi:10.1016/j.pnpbp.2011.11.010

21. Pirl, W.F. (2004). Evidence report on the occurrence, assessment, and treatment of depression in cancer patients. *Journal of the National Cancer Institute Monographs, 2004,* 2–39. doi:10.1093/jncimonographs/lgh026

22. Rayner, L., Price, A., Evans, A., Valsraj, K., Higginson, I.J., & Hotopf, M. (2010). Antidepressants for depression in physically ill people. *Cochrane Database of Systematic Reviews, 2010*(3). doi:10.1002/14651858.CD007503.pub2

23. Rodin, G., Lloyd, N., Katz, M., Green, E., Mackay, J.A., & Wong, R.K.S. (2007). The treatment of depression in cancer patients: A systematic

review. *Supportive Care in Cancer, 15,* 123–136. doi:10.1007/s00520-006 -0145-3

24. Suzuki, N., Ninomiya, M., Maruta, T., Hosonuma, S., Yoshioka, N., Ohara, T., ... Ishizuka, B. (2011). Clinical study on the efficacy of fluvoxamine for psychological distress in gynecologic cancer patients. *International Journal of Gynecological Cancer, 21,* 1143–1149. doi:10.1097/IGC.0b013e3181ffbeb9

25. Torta, R., Leombruni, P., Borio, R., & Castelli, L. (2011). Duloxetine for the treatment of mood disorder in cancer patients: A 12-week case-control clinical trial. *Human Psychopharmacology, 26,* 291–299. doi:10.1002/hup.1202

26. Torta, R., Siri, I., & Caldera, P. (2008). Sertraline effectiveness and safety in depressed oncological patients. *Supportive Care in Cancer, 16,* 83–91. doi:10.1007/s00520-007-0269-0

27. Williams, S., & Dale, J. (2006). The effectiveness of treatment for depression/ depressive symptoms in adults with cancer: A systematic review. *British Journal of Cancer, 94,* 372–390. doi:10.1038/sj.bjc.6602949

28. Qaseem, A., Snow, V., Shekelle, P., Casey, D.E., Jr., Cross, J.T., Jr., Owens, D.K., ... Shekelle, P. (2008). Evidence-based interventions to improve the palliative care of pain, dyspnea, and depression at the end of life: A clinical practice guideline from the American College of Physicians. *Annals of Internal Medicine, 148,* 141–146. doi:10.7326/0003-4819-148 -2-200801150-00009

29. Hart, S.L., Hoyt, M.A., Diefenbach, M., Anderson, D.R., Kilbourn, K.M., Craft, L.L., ... Stanton, A.L. (2012). Meta-analysis of efficacy of interventions for elevated depressive symptoms in adults diagnosed with cancer. *Journal of the National Cancer Institute, 104,* 990–1004. doi:10.1093/jnci/djs256

30. Naaman, S.C., Radwan, K., Fergusson, D., & Johnson, S. (2009). Status of psychological trials in breast cancer patients: A report of three meta-analyses. *Psychiatry, 70,* 50–69. doi:10.1521/psyc.2009.72.1.50

31. Boesen, E.H., Karlsen, R., Christensen, J., Paaschburg, B., Nielsen, D., Bloch, I.S., ... Johansen, C. (2011). Psychosocial group intervention for patients with primary breast cancer: A randomised trial. *European Journal of Cancer, 47,* 1363–1372. doi:10.1016/j.ejca.2011.01.002

32. Given, C., Given, B., Rahbar, M., Jeon, S., McCorkle, R., Cimprich, B., ... Bowie, E. (2004). Does a symptom management intervention affect depression among cancer patients: Results from a clinical trial. *Psycho-Oncology, 13,* 818–830. doi:10.1002/pon.807

33. Greer, J.A., Traeger, L., Bemis, H., Solis, J., Hendriksen, E.S., Park, E.R., ... Safren, S.A. (2012). A pilot randomized controlled trial of brief cognitive-behavioral therapy for anxiety in patients with terminal cancer. *Oncologist, 17,* 1337–1345. doi:10.1634/theoncologist.2012-0041

34. Hopko, D.R., Bell, J.L., Armento, M., Robertson, S., Mullane, C., Wolf, N., & Lejuez, C.W. (2008). Cognitive-behavior therapy for depressed cancer patients in a medical care setting. *Behavior Therapy, 39,* 126–136. doi:10.1016/j.beth.2007.05.007

35. Hunter, M.S., Coventry, S., Hamed, H., Fentiman, I., & Grunfeld, E.A. (2009). Evaluation of a group cognitive behavioural intervention for women suffering from menopausal symptoms following breast cancer treatment. *Psycho-Oncology, 18,* 560–563. doi:10.1002/pon.1414

36. Kangas, M., Milross, C., Taylor, A., & Bryant, R.A. (2013). A pilot randomized controlled trial of a brief early intervention for reducing posttraumatic stress disorder, anxiety and depressive symptoms in newly diagnosed head and neck cancer patients. *Psycho-Oncology, 22,* 1665–1673. doi:10.1002/pon.3208

37. Korstjens, I., Mesters, I., May, A.M., van Weert, E., van den Hout, J.H., Ros, W., ... van den Borne, B. (2011). Effects of cancer rehabilitation on problem-solving, anxiety and depression: A RCT comparing physical and cognitive-behavioural training versus physical training. *Psychology and Health, 26*(Suppl. 1), 63–82. doi:10.1080/08870441003611569

38. Lewis, F.M., Casey, S.M., Brandt, P.A., Shands, M.E., & Zahlis, E.H. (2006). The enhancing connections program: Pilot study of a cognitive-behavioral

intervention for mothers and children affected by breast cancer. *Psycho-Oncology, 15,* 486–497. doi:10.1002/pon.979

39. Osborn, R.L., Demoncada, A.C., & Feuerstein, M. (2006). Psychosocial interventions for depression, anxiety, and quality of life in cancer survivors: Meta-analyses. *International Journal of Psychiatry in Medicine, 36,* 13–34. doi:10.2190/EUFN-RV1K-Y3TR-FK0L

40. Pitceathly, C., Maguire, P., Fletcher, I., Parle, M., Tomenson, B., & Creed, F. (2009). Can a brief psychological intervention prevent anxiety or depressive disorders in cancer patients? A randomised controlled trial. *Annals of Oncology, 20,* 928–934. doi:10.1093/annonc/mdn708

41. Serfaty, M., Wilkinson, S., Freeman, C., Mannix, K., & King, M. (2012). The ToT study: Helping with touch or talk (ToT): A pilot randomised controlled trial to examine the clinical effectiveness of aromatherapy massage versus cognitive behaviour therapy for emotional distress in patients in cancer/palliative care. *Psycho-Oncology, 21,* 563–569. doi:10.1002/pon.1921

42. Ando, M., Morita, T., Akechi, T., Ito, S., Tanaka, M., Ifuku, Y., & Nakayama, T. (2009). The efficacy of mindfulness-based meditation therapy on anxiety, depression, and spirituality in Japanese patients with cancer. *Journal of Palliative Medicine, 12,* 1091–1094. doi:10.1089/jpm.2009.0143

43. Hoffman, C.J., Ersser, S.J., Hopkinson, J.B., Nicholls, P.G., Harrington, J.E., & Thomas, P.W. (2012). Effectiveness of mindfulness-based stress reduction in mood, breast- and endocrine-related quality of life, and well-being in stage 0 to III breast cancer: A randomized, controlled trial. *Journal of Clinical Oncology, 31,* 1–9. doi:10.1200/JCO.2010.34.0331

44. Lengacher, C.A., Johnson-Mallard, V., Post-White, J., Moscoso, M.S., Jacobsen, P.B., Klein, T.W., … Kip, K.E. (2009). Randomized controlled trial of mindfulness-based stress reduction (MBSR) for survivors of breast cancer. *Psycho-Oncology, 18,* 1261–1272. doi:10.1002/pon.1529

45. Lengacher, C.A., Reich, R.R., Post-White, J., Moscoso, M., Shelton, M.M., Barta, M., … Budhrani, P. (2012). Mindfulness based stress reduction in post-treatment breast cancer patients: An examination of symptoms and symptom clusters. *Journal of Behavioral Medicine, 35,* 86–94. doi:10.1007/s10865-011-9346-4

46. Sharplin, G.R., Jones, S.B., Hancock, B., Knott, V.E., Bowden, J.A., & Whitford, H.S. (2010). Mindfulness-based cognitive therapy: An efficacious community-based group intervention for depression and anxiety in a sample of cancer patients. *Medical Journal of Australia, 193*(Suppl. 5), S79–S82.

47. Würtzen, H., Dalton, S.O., Elsass, P., Sumbundu, A.D., Steding-Jensen, M., Karlsen, R.V., … Johansen, C. (2013). Mindfulness significantly reduces self-reported levels of anxiety and depression: Results of a randomized controlled trial among 336 Danish women treated for stage I–III breast cancer. *European Journal of Cancer, 49,* 1365–1373. doi:10.1016/j.ejca.2012.10.030

48. Hofmann, S.G., Sawyer, A.T., Witt, A.A., & Oh, D. (2010). The effect of mindfulness-based therapy on anxiety and depression: A meta-analytic review. *Journal of Consulting and Clinical Psychology, 78,* 169–183. doi:10.1037/a0018555

49. Piet, J., Würtzen, H., & Zachariae, R. (2012). The effect of mindfulness-based therapy on symptoms of anxiety and depression in adult cancer patients and survivors: A systematic review and meta-analysis. *Journal of Consulting and Clinical Psychology, 80,* 1007–1020. doi:10.1037/a0028329

50. Badger, T.A., Segrin, C., Figueredo, A.J., Harrington, J., Sheppard, K., Passalacqua, S., … Bishop, M. (2011). Psychosocial interventions to improve quality of life in prostate cancer survivors and their intimate or family partners. *Quality of Life Research, 20,* 833–844. doi:10.1007/s11136-010-9822-2

51. Chien, C.-H., Liu, K.-L., Chien, H.-T., & Liu, H.-E. (2014). The effects of psychosocial strategies on anxiety and depression of patients diagnosed with prostate cancer: A systematic review. *International Journal of Nursing Studies, 51,* 28–38. doi:10.1016/j.ijnurstu.2012.12.019

52. Ell, K., Xie, B., Quon, B., Quinn, D.I., Dwight-Johnson, M., & Lee, P.-J. (2008). Randomized controlled trial of collaborative care management of depression among low-income patients with cancer. *Journal of Clinical Oncology, 26,* 4488–4496. doi:10.1200/JCO.2008.16.6371

53. Ell, K., Aranda, M.P., Xie, B., Lee, P.-J., & Chou, C.-P. (2010). Collaborative depression treatment in older and younger adults with physical illness: Pooled comparative analysis of three randomized clinical trials. *American Journal of Geriatric Psychiatry, 18,* 520–530. doi:10.1097/JGP.0b013e3181cc0350

54. Ell, K., Xie, B., Kapetanovic, S., Quinn, D.I., Lee, P.J., Wells, A., & Chou, C.P. (2011). One-year follow-up of collaborative depression care for low-income, predominantly Hispanic patients with cancer. *Psychiatric Services, 62,* 162–170. doi:10.1176/appi.ps.62.2.162

55. Galway, K., Black, A., Cantwell, M., Cardwell, C.R., Mills, M., & Donnelly, M. (2012). Psychosocial interventions to improve quality of life and emotional wellbeing for recently diagnosed cancer patients. *Cochrane Database of Systematic Reviews, 2012*(11). doi:10.1002/14651858.CD007064.pub2

56. Jacobsen, P.B., & Jim, H.S. (2008). Psychosocial interventions for anxiety and depression in adult cancer patients: Achievements and challenges. *CA: A Cancer Journal for Clinicians, 58,* 214–230. doi:10.3322/CA.2008.0003

57. Kim, H.S., Shin, S.J., Kim, S.C., An, S., Rha, S.Y., Ahn, J.B., ... Lee, S. (2013). Randomized controlled trial of standardized education and telemonitoring for pain in outpatients with advanced solid tumors. *Supportive Care in Cancer, 21,* 1751–1759. doi:10.1007/s00520-013-1722-x

58. Rottmann, N., Dalton, S.O., Bidstrup, P.E., Würtzen, H., Høybye, M.T., Ross, L., ... Johansen, C. (2012). No improvement in distress and quality of life following psychosocial cancer rehabilitation: A randomised trial. *Psycho-Oncology, 21,* 505–514. doi:10.1002/pon.1924

59. Van der Meulen, I.C., May, A.M., Ros, W.J., Oosterom, M., Hordijk, G.-J., Koole, R., & de Leeuw, J.R.J. (2013). One-year effect of a nurse-led psychosocial intervention on depressive symptoms in patients with head and neck cancer: A randomized controlled trial. *Oncologist, 18,* 336–344. doi:10.1634/theoncologist.2012-0299

60. Vilela, L.D., Nicolau, B., Mahmud, S., Edgar, L., Hier, M., Black, M., ... Allison, P.J. (2006). Comparison of psychosocial outcomes in head and neck cancer patients receiving a coping strategies intervention and control subjects receiving no intervention. *Journal of Otolaryngology, 35,* 88–96. doi:10.2310/7070.2005.5002

61. Zimmermann, T., Heinrichs, N., & Baucom, D.H. (2007). Does one size fit all? Moderators in psychosocial interventions for breast cancer patients: A meta-analysis. *Annals of Behavioral Medicine, 34,* 225–239. doi:10.1007/BF02874548

62. Newell, S.A., Sanson-Fisher, R.W., & Savolainen, N.J. (2002). Systematic review of psychological therapies for cancer patients: Overview and recommendations for future research. *Journal of the National Cancer Institute, 94,* 558–584. doi:10.1093/jnci/94.8.558

63. Walker, J., Sawhney, A., Hansen, C.H., Symeonides, S., Martin, P., Murray, G., & Sharpe, M. (2013). Treatment of depression in people with lung cancer: A systematic review. *Lung Cancer, 79,* 46–53. doi:10.1016/j.lungcan.2012.09.014

64. Barsevick, A.M., Sweeney, C., Haney, E., & Chung, E. (2002). A systematic qualitative analysis of psychoeducational interventions for depression in patients with cancer. *Oncology Nursing Forum, 29,* 73–84. doi:10.1188/02.ONF.73-87

65. Hirai, K., Motooka, H., Ito, N., Wada, N., Yoshizaki, A., Shiozaki, M., ... Akechi, T. (2012). Problem-solving therapy for psychological distress in Japanese early-stage breast cancer patients. *Japanese Journal of Clinical Oncology, 42,* 1168–1174. doi:10.1093/jjco/hys158

66. Hopko, D.R., Armento, M.E., Robertson, S.M., Ryba, M.M., Carvalho, J.P., Colman, L.K., ... Lejuez, C.W. (2011). Brief behavioral activation and

problem-solving therapy for depressed breast cancer patients: Randomized trial. *Journal of Consulting and Clinical Psychology, 79,* 834–849. doi:10.1037/a0025450

67. Hopko, D.R., Robertson, S.M., & Carvalho, J.P. (2009). Sudden gains in depressed cancer patients treated with behavioral activation therapy. *Behavior Therapy, 40,* 346–356. doi:10.1016/j.beth.2008.09.001

68. Lindemalm, C., Mozaffari, F., Choudhury, A., Granstam-Björneklett, H., Lekander, M., Nilsson, B., … Mellstedt, H. (2008). Immune response, depression and fatigue in relation to support intervention in mammary cancer patients. *Supportive Care in Cancer, 16,* 57–65. doi:10.1007/s00520-007-0275-2

69. Ramachandra, P., Booth, S., Pieters, T., Vrotsou, K., & Huppert, F.A. (2009). A brief self-administered psychological intervention to improve well-being in patients with cancer: Results from a feasibility study. *Psycho-Oncology, 18,* 1323–1326. doi:10.1002/pon.1516

70. National Health and Medical Research Council Australia. (2003). Clinical practice guidelines for the psychosocial care of adults with cancer. Retrieved from http://www.nhmrc.gov.au/publications/synopses/cp90syn.htm

71. Goerling, U., Foerg, A., Sander, S., Schramm, N., & Schlag, P.M. (2011). The impact of short-term psycho-oncological interventions on the psychological outcome of cancer patients of a surgical-oncology department: A randomised controlled study. *European Journal of Cancer, 47,* 2009–2014. doi:10.1016/j.ejca.2011.04.031

72. Strong, V., Waters, R., Hibberd, C., Murray, G., Wall, L., Walker, J., … Sharpe, M. (2008). Management of depression for people with cancer (SMaRT oncology 1): A randomised trial. *Lancet, 372,* 40–48. doi:10.1016/S0140-6736(08)60991-5

73. Akechi, T., Okuyama, T., Onishi, J., Morita, T., & Furukawa, T.A. (2008). Psychotherapy for depression among incurable cancer patients. *Cochrane Database of Systematic Reviews, 2008*(2). doi:10.1002/14651858.CD005537.pub2

74. Weber, B.A., Roberts, B.L., Yarandi, H., Mills, T.L., Chumbler, N.R., & Wajsman, Z. (2007). The impact of dyadic social support on self-efficacy and depression after radical prostatectomy. *Journal of Aging and Health, 19,* 630–645. doi:10.1177/0898264307300979

75. Luebbert, K., Dahme, B., & Hasenbring, M. (2001). The effectiveness of relaxation training in reducing treatment related symptoms and improving emotional adjustment in acute and non-surgical cancer treatment: A meta-analytical review. *Psycho-Oncology, 10,* 490–502. doi:10.1002/pon.537

76. Sloman, R. (2002). Relaxation and imagery for anxiety and depression control in community patients with advanced cancer. *Cancer Nursing, 25,* 432–435. doi:10.1097/00002820-200212000-00005

77. Lutgendorf, S.K., Mullen-Houser, E., Russell, D., DeGeest, K., Jacobson, G., Hart, L., … Lubaroff, D.M. (2010). Preservation of immune function in cervical cancer patients during chemoradiation using a novel integrative approach. *Brain, Behavior, and Immunity, 24,* 1231–1240. doi:10.1016/j.bbi.2010.06.014

78. Raison, C.L., Rutherford, R.E., Woolwine, B.J., Shuo, C., Schettler, P., Drake, D.F., … Miller, A.H. (2013). A randomized controlled trial of the tumor necrosis factor antagonist infliximab for treatment-resistant depression: The role of baseline inflammatory biomarkers. *JAMA Psychiatry, 70,* 31–41. doi:10.1001/2013.jamapsychiatry.4

79. Gehring, K., Patwardhan, S.Y., Collins, R., Groves, M.D., Etzel, C.J., Meyers, C.A., & Wefel, J.S. (2012). A randomized trial on the efficacy of methylphenidate and modafinil for improving cognitive functioning and symptoms in patients with a primary brain tumor. *Journal of Neuro-Oncology, 107,* 165–174. doi:10.1007/s11060-011-0723-1

80. Herschbach, P., Berg, P., Waadt, S., Duran, G., Engst-Hastreiter, U., Henrich, G., … Dinkel, A. (2010). Group psychotherapy of dysfunctional fear

of progression in patients with chronic arthritis or cancer. *Psychotherapy and Psychosomatics, 79,* 31–38. doi:10.1159/000254903

81. Vos, P.J., Visser, A.P., Garssen, B., Duivenvoorden, H.J., & de Haes, H.C.J.M. (2007). Effectiveness of group psychotherapy compared to social support groups in patients with primary, non-metastatic breast cancer. *Journal of Psychosocial Oncology, 25*(4), 37–60. doi:10.1300/J077v25n04_03

82. Rajasekaran, M., Edmonds, P.M., & Higginson, I.L. (2005). Systematic review of hypnotherapy for treating symptoms in terminally ill adult cancer patients. *Palliative Medicine, 19,* 418–426. doi:10.1191/0269216305pm1030oa

83. Lloyd-Williams, M., Cobb, M., O'Connor, C., Dunn, L., & Shiels, C. (2012). A pilot randomised controlled trial to reduce suffering and emotional distress in patients with advanced cancer. *Journal of Affective Disorders, 148,* 141–145. doi:10.1016/j.jad.2012.11.013

84. Griffiths, K.M., Calear, A.L., & Banfield, M. (2009). Systematic review on Internet support groups (ISGs) and depression (1): Do ISGs reduce depressive symptoms? *Journal of Medical Internet Research, 11*(3), e40. doi:10.2196/jmir.1270

85. Klemm, P. (2012). Effects of online support group format (moderated vs. peer-led) on depressive symptoms and extent of participation in women with breast cancer. *CIN: Computers, Informatics, Nursing, 30,* 9–18. doi:10.1097/NCN.0b013e3182343efa

86. Deng, G., Chan, Y., Sjoberg, D., Vickers, A., Yeung, K.S., Kris, M., ... Cassileth, B. (2013). Acupuncture for the treatment of post-chemotherapy chronic fatigue: A randomized, blinded, sham-controlled trial. *Supportive Care in Cancer, 21,* 1735–1741. doi:10.1007/s00520-013-1720-z

87. Feng, Y., Wang, X.Y., Li, S.D., Zhang, Y., Wang, H.M., Li, M., ... Zhang, Z. (2011). Clinical research of acupuncture on malignant tumor patients for improving depression and sleep quality. *Journal of Traditional Chinese Medicine, 31,* 199–202. doi:10.1016/S0254-6272(11)60042-3

88. Molassiotis, A., Bardy, J., Finnegan-John, J., Mackereth, P., Ryder, D.W., Filshie, J., ... Richardson, A. (2012). Acupuncture for cancer-related fatigue in patients with breast cancer: A pragmatic randomized controlled trial. *Journal of Clinical Oncology, 30,* 4470–4476. doi:10.1200/JCO.2012.41.6222

89. Molassiotis, A., Bardy, J., Finnegan-John, J., Mackereth, P., Ryder, W.D., Filshie, J., ... Richardson, A. (2013). A randomized, controlled trial of acupuncture self-needling as maintenance therapy for cancer-related fatigue after therapist-delivered acupuncture. *Annals of Oncology, 24,* 1645–1652. doi:10.1093/annonc/mdt034

90. Garcia, M.K., McQuade, J., Haddad, R., Patel, S., Lee, R., Yang, P., ... Cohen, L. (2013). Systematic review of acupuncture in cancer care: A synthesis of the evidence. *Journal of Clinical Oncology, 31,* 952–960. doi:10.1200/JCO.2012.43.5818

91. Yim, V.W.C., Ng, A.K.Y., Tsang, H.W.H., & Leung, A.Y. (2009). A review on the effects of aromatherapy for patients with depressive symptoms. *Journal of Alternative and Complementary Medicine, 15,* 187–195. doi:10.1089/acm.2008.0333

92. Bar-Sela, G., Atid, L., Danos, S., Gabay, N., & Epelbaum, R. (2007). Art therapy improved depression and influenced fatigue levels in cancer patients on chemotherapy. *Psycho-Oncology, 6,* 980–984. doi:10.1002/pon.1175

93. Thyme, K.E., Sundin, E.C., Wiberg, B., Öster, I., Åström, S., & Lindh, J. (2009). Individual brief art therapy can be helpful for women with breast cancer: A randomized controlled clinical study. *Palliative and Supportive Care, 7,* 87–95. doi:10.1017/S147895150900011X

94. Chen, Z., Meng, Z., Milbury, K., Bei, W., Zhang, Y., Thornton, B., ... Cohen, L. (2012). Qigong improves quality of life in women undergoing radiotherapy for breast cancer: Results of a randomized controlled trial. *Cancer, 119,* 1690–1698. doi:10.1002/cncr.27904

95. Liu, C.J., Hsiung, P.-C., Chang, K.-J., Liu, Y.-F., Wang, K.-C., Hsiao, F.-H., ... Chan, C.L.W. (2008). A study on the efficacy of body-mind-spirit group

therapy for patients with breast cancer. *Journal of Clinical Nursing, 17,* 2539–2549. doi:10.1111/j.1365-2702.2008.02296.x

96. Pirl, W.F., Greer, J.A., Traeger, L., Jackson, V., Lennes, I.T., Gallagher, E.R., … Temel, J.S. (2012). Depression and survival in metastatic non-small-cell lung cancer: Effects of early palliative care. *Journal of Clinical Oncology, 30,* 1310–1315. doi:10.1200/JCO.2011.38.3166

97. Berglund, G., Petersson, L.-M., Eriksson, K.C., Wallenius, I., Roshanai, A., Nordin, K.M., … Häggman, M. (2007). "Between men": A psychosocial rehabilitation programme for men with prostate cancer. *Acta Oncologica, 46,* 83–89. doi:10.1080/02841860600857326

98. Brown, J.C., Huedo-Medina, T.B., Pescatello, L.S., Ryan, S.M., Pescatello, S.M., Moker, E., … Johnson, B.T. (2012). The efficacy of exercise in reducing depressive symptoms among cancer survivors: A meta-analysis. *PLOS One, 7*(1), e30955. doi:10.1371/journal.pone.0030955

99. Cantarero-Villanueva, I., Fernández-Lao, C., Cuesta-Vargas, A.I., Del Moral-Avila, R., Fernández-de-las-Peñas, C., & Arroyo-Morales, M. (2013). The effectiveness of a deep water aquatic exercise program in cancer-related fatigue in breast cancer survivors: A randomized controlled trial. *Archives of Physical Medicine and Rehabilitation, 94,* 221–230. doi:10.1016/j.apmr.2012.09.008

100. Eyigor, S., Karapolat, H., Yesil, H., Uslu, R., & Durmaz, B. (2010). Effects of Pilates exercises on functional capacity, flexibility, fatigue, depression and quality of life in female breast cancer patients: A randomized controlled study. *European Journal of Physical and Rehabilitation Medicine, 46,* 481–487. Retrieved from http://www.minervamedica.it/en/journals/europa-medicophysica/article.php?cod=R33Y2010N04A0481

101. Hanna, L.R., Avila, P.F., Meteer, J.D., Nicholas, D.R., & Kaminsky, L.A. (2008). The effects of a comprehensive exercise program on physical function, fatigue, and mood in patients with various types of cancer. *Oncology Nursing Forum, 35,* 461–469. doi:10.1188/08.ONF.461-469

102. Midtgaard, J., Rørth, M., Stelter, R., Tveterås, A., Andersen, C., Quist, M., … Adamsen, L. (2005). The impact of a multidimensional exercise program on self-reported anxiety and depression in cancer patients undergoing chemotherapy: A phase II study. *Palliative and Supportive Care, 3,* 197–208. doi:10.1017/S1478951505050327

103. Payne, J.K., Held, J., Thorpe, J., & Shaw, H. (2008). Effect of exercise on biomarkers, fatigue, sleep disturbances, and depressive symptoms in older women with breast cancer receiving hormonal therapy. *Oncology Nursing Forum, 35,* 635–642. doi:10.1188/08.ONF.635-642

104. Saarto, T., Penttinen, H.M., Sievänen, H., Kellokumpu-Lehtinen, P.L., Hakamies-Blomqvist, L., Nikander, R., … Luoma, M.L. (2012). Effectiveness of a 12-month exercise program on physical performance and quality of life of breast cancer survivors. *Anticancer Research, 32,* 3875–3884.

105. Yang, C.-Y., Tsai, J.-C., Huang, Y.-C., & Lin, C.-C. (2010). Effects of a home-based walking program on perceived symptom and mood status in postoperative breast cancer women receiving adjuvant chemotherapy. *Journal of Advanced Nursing, 67,* 158–168. doi:10.1111/j.1365-2648.2010.05492.x

106. Craft, L.L., Vaniterson, E.H., Helenowski, I.B., Rademaker, A.W., & Courneya, K.S. (2012). Exercise effects on depressive symptoms in cancer survivors: A systematic review and meta-analysis. *Cancer Epidemiology, Biomarkers and Prevention, 21,* 3–19. doi:10.1158/1055-9965.EPI-11-0634

107. da Costa Miranda, V., Trufelli, D.C., Santos, J., Campos, M.P., Nobuo, M., da Costa Miranda, M., … del Giglio, A. (2009). Effectiveness of guaraná (*Paullinia cupana*) for postradiation fatigue and depression: Results of a pilot double-blind randomized study. *Journal of Alternative and Complementary Medicine, 15,* 431–433. doi:10.1089/acm.2008.0324

108. Post-White, J., Kinney, M.E., Savik, K., Gau, J.B., Wilcox, C., & Lerner, I. (2003). Therapeutic massage and healing touch improve symptoms in cancer. *Integrative Cancer Therapies, 2,* 332–344. doi:10.1177/1534735403259064

109. Krohn, M., Listing, M., Tjahjono, G., Reisshauer, A., Peters, E., Klapp, B.F., & Rauchfuss, M. (2011). Depression, mood, stress, and Th1/Th2 immune balance in primary breast cancer patients undergoing classical massage therapy. *Supportive Care in Cancer, 19,* 1303–1311. doi:10.1007/s00520-010-0946-2

110. Zhou, K.N., Li, X.M., Yan, H., Dang, S.N., & Wang, D.L. (2011). Effects of music therapy on depression and duration of hospital stay of breast cancer patients after radical mastectomy. *Chinese Medical Journal, 124,* 2321–2327. Retrieved from http://www.cmj.org/ch/reader/view_abstract.aspx?volume=124&issue=15&start_page=2321

111. Bradt, J., Dileo, C., Grocke, D., & Magill, L. (2011). Music interventions for improving psychological and physical outcomes in cancer patients. *Cochrane Database of Systematic Reviews, 2011*(8). doi:10.1002/14651858.CD006911.pub2

112. Potter, P.J. (2007). Breast biopsy and distress: Feasibility of testing a Reiki intervention. *Journal of Holistic Nursing, 25,* 238–248. doi:10.1177/0898010107301618

113. Nunes, D.F., Rodriguez, A.L., da Silva Hoffmann, F., Luz, C., Braga Filho, A.P., Muller, M.C., & Bauer, M.E. (2007). Relaxation and guided imagery program in patients with breast cancer undergoing radiotherapy is not associated with neuroimmunomodulatory effects. *Journal of Psychosomatic Research, 63,* 647–655. doi:10.1016/j.jpsychores.2007.07.004

114. McMillan, S.C., Small, B.J., & Haley, W.E. (2011). Improving hospice outcomes through systematic assessment. *Cancer Nursing, 34,* 89–97. doi:10.1097/NCC.0b013e3181f70aee

115. Meijer, A., Roseman, M., Milette, K., Coyne, J.C., Stefanek, M.E., Ziegelstein, R.C., ... Thombs, B.D. (2011). Depression screening and patient outcomes in cancer: A systematic review. *PLOS One, 6*(11), e27181. doi:10.1371/journal.pone.0027181

116. Hanssens, S., Luyten, R., Watthy, C., Fontaine, C., Decoster, L., Baillon, C., ... De Grève, J. (2011). Evaluation of a comprehensive rehabilitation program for post-treatment patients with cancer [Online exclusive]. *Oncology Nursing Forum, 38,* E418–E424. doi:10.1188/11.ONF.E418-E424

117. Khan, F., Amatya, B., Pallant, J.F., Rajapaksa, I., & Brand, C. (2012). Multidisciplinary rehabilitation in women following breast cancer treatment: A randomized controlled trial. *Journal of Rehabilitation Medicine, 44,* 788–794. doi:10.2340/16501977-1020

118. Girgis, A., Breen, S., Stacey, F., & Lecathelinais, C. (2009). Impact of two supportive care interventions on anxiety, depression, quality of life, and unmet needs in patients with nonlocalized breast and colorectal cancers. *Journal of Clinical Oncology, 27,* 6180–6190. doi:10.1200/JCO.2009.22.8718

119. Gotay, C.C., Moinpour, C.M., Unger, J.M., Jiang, C.S., Coleman, D., Martino, S., ... Albain, K.S. (2007). Impact of a peer-delivered telephone intervention for women experiencing a breast cancer recurrence. *Journal of Clinical Oncology, 25,* 2093–2099. doi:10.1200/JCO.2006.07.4674

120. Kroenke, K., Theobald, D., Wu, J., Norton, K., Morrison, G., Carpenter, J., & Tu, W. (2010). Effect of telecare management on pain and depression in patients with cancer: A randomized trial. *JAMA, 304,* 163–171. doi:10.1001/jama.2010.944

121. White, V.M., Macvean, M.L., Grogan, S., D'Este, C., Akkerman, D., Ieropoli, S., ... Sanson-Fisher, R. (2012). Can a tailored telephone intervention delivered by volunteers reduce the supportive care needs, anxiety and depression of people with colorectal cancer? A randomised controlled trial. *Psycho-Oncology, 21,* 1053–1062. doi:10.1002/pon.2019

122. D'Souza, V., Blouin, E., Zeitouni, A., Muller, K., & Allison, P.J. (2013). An investigation of the effect of tailored information on symptoms of anxiety and depression in head and neck cancer patients. *Oral Oncology, 49,* 431–437. doi:10.1016/j.oraloncology.2012.12.001

123. Li, W.H., Chung, J.O., & Ho, E.K. (2011). The effectiveness of therapeutic play, using virtual reality computer games, in promoting the psychological

well-being of children hospitalised with cancer. *Journal of Clinical Nursing, 20*, 2135–2143. doi:10.1111/j.1365-2702.2011.03733.x

124. Bower, J.E., Garet, D., Sternlieb, B., Ganz, P.A., Irwin, M.R., Olmstead, R., & Greendale, G. (2012). Yoga for persistent fatigue in breast cancer survivors: A randomized controlled trial. *Cancer, 118*, 3766–3775. doi:10.1002/cncr.26702

125. Dhruva, A., Miaskowski, C., Abrams, D., Acree, M., Cooper, B., Goodman, S., & Hecht, F.M. (2012). Yoga breathing for cancer chemotherapy–associated symptoms and quality of life: Results of a pilot randomized controlled trial. *Journal of Alternative and Complementary Medicine, 18*, 473–479. doi:10.1089/acm.2011.0555

126. D'Silva, S., Poscablo, C., Habousha, R., Kogan, M., & Kligler, B. (2012). Mind-body medicine therapies for a range of depression severity: A systematic review. *Psychosomatics, 53*, 407–423. doi:10.1016/j.psym.2012.04.006

127. Kligler, B., Homel, P., Harrison, L.B., Sackett, E., Levenson, H., Kenney, J., ... Merrell, W. (2011). Impact of the Urban Zen Initiative on patients' experience of admission to an inpatient oncology floor: A mixed-methods analysis. *Journal of Alternative and Complementary Medicine, 17*, 729–734. doi:10.1089/acm.2010.0533

128. Quintard, B., & Lakdja, F. (2008). Assessing the effect of beauty treatments on psychological distress, body image, and coping: A longitudinal study of patients undergoing surgical procedures for breast cancer. *Psycho-Oncology, 17*, 1032–1038. doi:10.1002/pon.1321

129. Jensen-Johansen, M.B., Christensen, S., Valdimarsdottir, H., Zakowski, S., Jensen, A.B., Bovbjerg, D.H., & Zachariae, R. (2012). Effects of an expressive writing intervention on cancer-related distress in Danish breast cancer survivors—Results from a nationwide randomized clinical trial. *Psycho-Oncology, 22*, 1492–1500. doi:10.1002/pon.3193

130. Low, C.A., Stanton, A.L., Dower, J.E., & Gyllenhammer, L. (2010). A randomized controlled trial of emotionally expressive writing for women with metastatic breast cancer. *Health Psychology, 29*, 460–466. doi:10.1037/a0020153

131. Mosher, C.E., Duhamel, K.N., Lam, J., Dickler, M., Li, Y., Massie, M.J., & Norton, L. (2012). Randomised trial of expressive writing for distressed metastatic breast cancer patients. *Psychology and Health, 27*, 88–100. doi:10.1080/08870446.2010.551212

132. Rodríguez Vega, B., Palao, A., Torres, G., Hospital, A., Benito, G., Perez, E., ... Bayon, C. (2011). Combined therapy versus usual care for the treatment of depression in oncologic patients: A randomized controlled trial. *Psycho-Oncology, 20*, 943–952. doi:10.1002/pon.1800

133. Wysocki, W.M., Mituś, J., Komorowski, A.L., & Karolewski, K. (2012). Impact of preoperative information on anxiety and disease-related knowledge in women undergoing mastectomy for breast cancer: A randomized clinical trial. *Acta Chirurgica Belgica, 112*, 111–115.

134. Chan, R.J., Webster, J., & Marquart, L. (2011). Information interventions for orienting patients and their carers to cancer care facilities. *Cochrane Database of Systematic Reviews, 2011*(12). doi:10.1002/14651858. CD008273.pub2

135. Husson, O., Mols, F., & van de Poll-Franse, L.V. (2011). The relation between information provision and health-related quality of life, anxiety and depression among cancer survivors: A systematic review. *Annals of Oncology, 22*, 761–772. doi:10.1093/annonc/mdq413

136. Sharp, D.M., Walker, M.B., Chaturvedi, A., Upadhyay, S., Hamid, A., Walker, A.A., ... Walker, L.G. (2010). A randomized, controlled trial of the psychological effects of reflexology in early breast cancer. *European Journal of Cancer, 46*, 312–322. doi:10.1016/j.ejca.2009.10.006

137. Wyatt, G., Sikorskii, A., Rahbar, M.H., Victorson, D., & You, M. (2012). Health-related quality-of-life outcomes: A reflexology trial with patients with advanced-stage breast cancer. *Oncology Nursing Forum, 39*, 568–577. doi:10.1188/12.ONF.568-577

138. Oncology Nursing Society. (2013, June). Implementing screening for distress: The joint position statement from the American Psychosocial Oncology Society, Association of Oncology Social Work, and Oncology Nursing Society. Retrieved from https://www.ons.org/about-ons/ons-position-statements/nursing-practice/implementing-screening-distress-joint-position

139. Miaskowski, C., Cooper, B.A., Paul, S.M., Dodd, M., Lee, K., Aouizerat, B.E., … Bank, A. (2006). Subgroups of patients with cancer with different symptom experiences and quality-of-life outcomes: A cluster analysis [Online exclusive]. *Oncology Nursing Forum, 33,* E79–E89. doi:10.1188/06.ONF.E79-E89

9

Diarrhea

*Lee Ann Johnson, PhD(c), RN,
and Margaret Irwin, PhD, RN, MN*

Problem and Incidence

Diarrhea is increased stool frequency, liquidity, or volume. Diarrhea can occur as a result of some types of cancer or cancer treatment. This material focuses on chemotherapy-induced diarrhea (CID) and radiation therapy–induced diarrhea (RID). A number of chemotherapy agents are known to cause diarrhea, and CID prevalence varies according to chemotherapy regimen. Incidence of CID has been reported as high as 50%–80% of patients.[1,2] Radiation to the abdomen or pelvis can result in acute or chronic enteritis. Incidence of acute RID has been reported at 30%–90%.[3,5] About 50% of patients overall may have chronic diarrhea.[4] In patients with colorectal cancer, chronic diarrhea has been reported as high as 90%.[6] Patients who are neutropenic may have diarrhea due to gastrointestinal (GI) infection. Incidence of chemotherapy-associated enterocolitis has been reported at 35%.[7] Diarrhea can result in dose reductions and treatment delays or discontinuation. Severe diarrhea often results in higher costs and hospitalization for management and rehydration.[8,9]

Risk Factors and Assessment

Factors that create high risk for diarrhea are
- Chemotherapy, including 5-fluorouracil, irinotecan, capecitabine, taxanes, platinum compounds, epidermal growth factor receptor inhibitors, and tyrosine kinase inhibitors[2]
- Radiation therapy to the abdomen or pelvic area
- Combined chemotherapy and radiation therapy
- Surgery involving radical resection of the GI tract[6]

- Coexisting neutropenia
- GI tract tumors.

Assessment should include the timing, frequency, and severity of diarrhea and accompanying symptoms, such as cramping or blood in the stool. Dehydration should be evaluated by checking the skin, mucous membranes, urine output and color, and orthostatic hypotension. Body temperature should be obtained to assess for potential fever. Stool, blood, and other testing may be needed to assess for infectious or other causes and for electrolyte imbalances.

Assessment tools include
- Diarrhea Assessment Scale
- National Cancer Institute Cancer Therapy Evaluation Program *Common Terminology Criteria for Adverse Events* (open access)[10]
- European Organisation for Research and Treatment of Cancer Quality-of-Life Scale[11]
- Multidimensional symptom distress scales.

What interventions are effective in preventing and managing chemotherapy- and radiation therapy–induced diarrhea in people with cancer?

Evidence retrieved through July 31, 2013

Likely to Be Effective

CID or RID intervention: Loperamide has not been specifically studied for management of treatment-associated diarrhea in cancer, but is recommended in consensus guidelines for low-grade and uncomplicated diarrhea.[1,12]

CID intervention: Octreotide was effective[13-16] and is recommended in professional guidelines.[1,12,17]

RID intervention: **Psyllium fiber** reduced the severity and incidence of diarrhea compared to controls during pelvic radiation.[18]

Benefits Balanced With Harms

CID or RID intervention: **Amifostine** in combination with loperamide reduced the incidence and severity of diarrhea in one small study.[19] Some patients also were given octreotide. The U.S. Food and Drug Administration[20] provided warnings regarding possible interactions of amifostine with cancer treatment, affecting antitumor effects of chemotherapy and radiation therapy.

CID intervention: **Neomycin** showed conflicting results in patients receiving irinotecan.[21,22]

Effectiveness Not Established

CID or RID interventions
- **Glutamine** for CID or RID—One randomized controlled trial showed no effect for CID,[23] and a meta-analysis showed lower diarrhea duration but no difference in severity with glutamine for CID.[24] Results for RID were conflicting.[25,26] Evidence-based guidelines suggest that evidence is inconclusive, but glutamine may be promising in patients with GI tract cancers.[17]
- **Probiotics** have been evaluated for both CID and RID. Mixed results were reported.[4,27-31] Meta-analyses concluded evidence is insufficient to show efficacy in children or adults.[3,32] Varied types of probiotics were used, which may influence findings. Multinational Association of Supportive Care in Cancer guidelines suggest that probiotics might be helpful.[17]

CID interventions
- **AG1004**, a mecamylamine[33]
- **Budesonide**[34]
- **Charcoal/activated charcoal**[35,36]
- **Dietary restrictions of fiber and lactose**[37]

- **Levofloxacin and cholestyramine**[38]
- **Oral alkalization**[35,39]
- **Prophylactic octreotide**[40]—Use of octreotide prophylactically has been recommended for patients with colorectal cancer who experienced diarrhea in a previous chemotherapy cycle in consensus guidelines.[1]

RID interventions
- **Elemental diet supplements** in patients receiving pelvic radiation[5]—Patients randomized to the elemental supplements ingested less than 65% of that prescribed.
- **Vitamin E and C supplements**[41]

Effectiveness Unlikely

RID interventions
- **Octreotide** for RID was examined in two small studies with mixed results[15,42] and had no effect in a large study.[43] A meta-analysis did not show benefit.[40]
- **Pentosan polysulfate** had no effect on RID in one large multisite placebo-controlled trial.[44]

Not Recommended for Practice

RID intervention: Sucralfate was associated with increased fecal incontinence and nausea in one study[45] and was not recommended in evidence-based guidelines.[17]

Expert Opinion

CID or RID interventions: Tincture of opium and paregoric may be beneficial.[12]

A number of dietary practices have been suggested for management of diarrhea.[1,46-48]
- Avoid foods high in fiber and fat.
- Avoid or limit caffeine.
- Avoid alcohol.
- Eat small, frequent meals.

- Avoid insoluble fiber (e.g., raw fruit and vegetables, nuts, popcorn, skins, seeds).
- Add soluble fibers (e.g., pectin-containing foods, canned or cooked fruits and vegetables, bananas, rice, well-cooked eggs, mashed potatoes, applesauce).
- Increase fluid intake (e.g., water, electrolyte replacement drinks, diluted fruit juices).
- Include foods high in potassium to replace electrolyte losses (e.g., bananas, potatoes).

Application to Practice

Nurses should identify those patients who are at risk for development of CID and RID and ensure they are consistently assessed for the development, progression, or resolution of diarrhea. Patients should be educated regarding the potential for diarrhea and the importance of informing the healthcare team of diarrhea symptoms.

Nurses can educate patients regarding dietary interventions from expert opinion that can be employed. Although evidence for dietary restrictions is inconclusive, these may be helpful for some patients.

Nurses can prescribe or advocate use of those interventions that have the best evidence of effectiveness for RID and CID.

Nurses should educate patients regarding symptoms to report, such as lack of resolution despite antidiarrheal medication, dizziness, blood in the stool, fever, or severe abdominal pain or cramping. These symptoms may be indicative of serious acute problems that require action.

Diarrhea Resource Contributors

Topic leader: Deborah M. Thorpe, PhD, APRN, ACHPN
Katherine L. Byar, RN, MSN, APN, BC, Arlene B. Davis, RN, MSN, AOCN®, Jeanne Held-Warmkessel, MSN, RN, AOCN®, ACNS-BC, and Elizabeth S. Kiker, RN, MSN, OCN®

References

1. Maroun, J.A., Anthony, L.B., Blais, N., Burkes, R., Dowden, S.D., Dranitsaris, G., ... Wong, R. (2007). Prevention and management of chemotherapy-induced diarrhea in patients with colorectal cancer: A consensus statement by the Canadian Working Group on Chemotherapy-Induced Diarrhea. *Current Oncology, 14,* 13–20. doi:10.3747/co.2007.96

2. Stein, A., Voigt, W., & Jordan, K. (2010). Chemotherapy-induced diarrhea: Pathophysiology, frequency and guideline-based management. *Therapeutic Advances in Medical Oncology, 2,* 51–63. doi:10.1177/1758834009355164

3. Fuccio, L., Guido, A., Eusebi, L.H., Laterza, L., Grilli, D., Cennamo, V., ... Bazzoli, F. (2009). Effects of probiotics for the prevention and treatment of radiation-induced diarrhea. *Journal of Clinical Gastroenterology, 43,* 506–513. doi:10.1097/MCG.0b013e3181a1f59c

4. Giralt, J., Regadera, J.P., Verges, R., Romero, J., de la Fuente, I., Biete, A., ... Guarner, F. (2008). Effects of probiotic *Lactobacillus casei* DN-114 001 in prevention of radiation-induced diarrhea: Results from multicenter, randomized, placebo-controlled nutritional trial. *International Journal of Radiation Oncology, Biology, Physics, 71,* 1213–1219. doi:10.1016/j.ijrobp.2007.11.009

5. McGough, C., Wedlake, L., Baldwin, C., Hackett, C., Norman, A.R., Blake, P., ... Andreyev, H.J. (2008). Clinical trial: Normal diet vs. partial replacement with oral E028 formula for the prevention of gastrointestinal toxicity in cancer patients undergoing pelvic radiotherapy. *Alimentary Pharmacology and Therapeutics, 27,* 1132–1139. doi:10.1111/j.1365-2036.2008.03665.x

6. Andreyev, H.J.N., Davidson, S.E., Gillespie, G., Allum, W.H., & Swarbrick, E. (2012). Practice guidance on the management of acute and chronic gastrointestinal problems arising as a result of treatment for cancer. *Gut, 61,* 179–192. doi:10.1136/gutjnl-2011-300563

7. Vehreschild, M.J.G.T., Meissner, A.M.K., Cornely, O.A., Maschmeyer, G., Neumann, S., von Lilienfeld-Toal, M., ... Vehreschild, J.J. (2011). Clinically defined chemotherapy-associated bowel syndrome predicts severe complications and death in cancer patients. *Haematologica, 96,* 1855–1860. doi:10.3324/haematol.2011.049627

8. Carlotto, A., Hogsett, V.L., Maiorini, E.M., Razulis, J.G., & Sonis, S.T. (2013). The economic burden of toxicities associated with cancer treatment: Review of the literature and analysis of nausea and vomiting, diarrhoea, oral mucositis and fatigue. *PharmacoEconomics, 31,* 753–766. doi:10.1007/s40273-013-0081-2

9. Dranitsaris, G., Maroun, J., & Shah, A. (2005). Severe chemotherapy-induced diarrhea in patients with colorectal cancer: A cost of illness analysis. *Supportive Care in Cancer, 13,* 318–324. doi:10.1007/s00520-004-0738-7

10. National Cancer Institute Cancer Therapy Evaluation Program. (2010, June 14). *Common terminology criteria for adverse events* [v.4.03]. Retrieved from http://evs.nci.nih.gov/ftp1/CTCAE/CTCAE_4.03_2010-06-14_QuickReference_5x7.pdf

11. European Organisation for Research and Treatment of Cancer. (n.d.). EORTC QLQ-C30. Retrieved from http://groups.eortc.be/qol/eortc-qlq-c30

12. Benson, A.B., III, Ajani, J.A., Catalano, R.B., Engelking, C., Kornblau, S.M., Martenson, J.A., Jr., ... Wadler, S. (2004). Recommended guidelines for the treatment of cancer treatment-induced diarrhea. *Journal of Clinical Oncology, 22,* 2918–2926. doi:10.1200/JCO.2004.04.132

13. Bhattacharya, S., Vijayasekar, C., Worlding, J., & Mathew, G. (2009). Octreotide in chemotherapy induced diarrhoea in colorectal cancer: A review article. *Acta Gastro-Enterologica Belgica, 72,* 289–295.

14. Rosenoff, S.H., Gabrail, N.Y., Conklin, R., Hohneker, J.A., Berg, W.J., Ghulam, M., ... Anthony, L. (2006). A multicenter, randomized trial of long-acting octreotide for the optimum prevention of chemotherapy-induced diarrhea: Results of the STOP trial. *Journal of Supportive Oncology, 4,* 289–294.

15. Topkan, E., & Karaoglu, A. (2006). Octreotide in the management of chemoradiotherapy-induced diarrhea refractory to loperamide in patients with rectal carcinoma. *Oncology, 71,* 354–360. doi:10.1159/000108593

16. Zidan, J., Haim, N., Beny, A., Stein, M., Gez, E., & Kuten, A. (2001). Octreotide in the treatment of severe chemotherapy-induced diarrhea. *Annals of Oncology, 12,* 227–229. doi:10.1023/A:1008372228462

17. Gibson, R.J., Keefe, D.M.K., Lalla, R.V., Bateman, E., Blijlevens, N., Fijlstra, M., ... Bowen, J.M. (2013). Systematic review of agents for the management of gastrointestinal mucositis in cancer patients. *Supportive Care in Cancer, 21,* 313–326. doi:10.1007/s00520-012-1644-z

18. Murphy, J., Stacey, D., Crook, J., Thompson, B., & Panetta, D. (2000). Testing control of radiation-induced diarrhea with a psyllium bulking agent: A pilot study. *Canadian Oncology Nursing Journal, 10,* 96–100. doi:10.5737/1181912x10396100

19. Tsavaris, N., Kosmas, C., Vadiaka, M., Zonios, D., Papalambros, E., Papantoniou, N., ... Koufos, C. (2003). Amifostine, in a reduced dose, protects against severe diarrhea associated with weekly fluorouracil and folinic acid chemotherapy in advanced colorectal cancer: A pilot study. *Journal of Pain and Symptom Management, 26,* 849–854. doi:10.1016/S0885-3924(03)00283-5

20. U.S. Food and Drug Administration. (2013, May). Amifostine. Retrieved from http://www.drugs.com/pro/amifostine.html

21. De Jong, F.A., Kehrer, D.F., Mathijssen, R.H., Creemers, G.J., de Bruijn, P., van Schaik, R.H., ... De Jong, M.J. (2006). Prophylaxis of irinotecan-induced diarrhea with neomycin and potential role for UGT1A1*28 genotype screening: A double-blind, randomized, placebo-controlled study. *Oncologist, 11,* 944–954. doi:10.1634/theoncologist.11-8-944

22. Kehrer, D.F.S., Sparreboom, A., Verweij, J., de Bruijn, P., Nierop, C.A., van de Schraaf, J., ... De Jonge, M.J. (2001). Modulation of irinotecan-induced diarrhea by cotreatment with neomycin in cancer patients. *Clinical Cancer Research, 7,* 1136–1141.

23. Daniele, B., Perrone, F., Gallo, C., Pignata, S., De Martino, S., De Vivo, R., ... D'Agostino, L. (2001). Oral glutamine in the prevention of fluorouracil induced intestinal toxicity: A double blind, placebo controlled, randomised trial. *Gut, 48,* 28–33. doi:10.1136/gut.48.1.28

24. Sun, J., Wang, H., & Hu, H. (2012). Glutamine for chemotherapy induced diarrhea: A meta-analysis. *Asia Pacific Journal of Clinical Nutrition, 21,* 380–385. Retrieved from http://apjcn.nhri.org.tw/server/APJCN/21/3/380.pdf

25. Kozelsky, T.F., Meyers, G.E., Sloan, J.A., Shanahan, T.G., Dick, S.J., Moore, R.L., ... Martenson, J.A. (2003). Phase III double-blind study of glutamine versus placebo for the prevention of acute diarrhea in patients receiving pelvic radiation therapy. *Journal of Clinical Oncology, 21,* 1669–1674. doi:10.1200/JCO.2003.05.060

26. Kucuktulu, E., Guner, A., Kahraman, I., Topbas, M., & Kucuktulu, U. (2013). The protective effects of glutamine on radiation-induced diarrhea. *Supportive Care in Cancer, 21,* 1071–1075. doi:10.1007/s00520-012-1627-0

27. Chitapanarux, I., Chitapanarux, T., Traisathit, P., Kudumpee, S., Tharavichitkul, E., & Lorvidhaya, V. (2010). Randomized controlled trial of live *Lactobacillus acidophilus* plus *Bifidobacterium bifidum* in prophylaxis of diarrhea during radiotherapy in cervical cancer patients. *Radiation Oncology, 5,* 31. doi:10.1186/1748-717X-5-31

28. Österlund, P., Ruotsalainen, T., Korpela, R., Saxelin, M., Ollus, A., Valta, P., ... Joensuu, H. (2007). *Lactobacillus* supplementation for diarrhoea related to chemotherapy of colorectal cancer: A randomised study. *British Journal of Cancer, 97,* 1028–1034. doi:10.1038/sj.bjc.6603990

29. Timko, J. (2010). Probiotics as prevention of radiation-induced diarrhoea. *Journal of Radiotherapy in Practice, 9,* 201–208. doi:10.1017/S1460396910000087

30. Delia, P., Sansotta, G., Donato, V., Frosina, P., Messina, G., De Renzis, C., & Famularo, G. (2007). Use of probiotics for prevention of radiation-induced

diarrhea. *World Journal of Gastroenterology, 13,* 912–915. Retrieved from http://www.wjgnet.com/1007-9327/full/v13/i6/912.htm

31. Urbancsek, H., Kazar, T., Mezes, I., & Neumann, K. (2001). Results of a double-blind, randomized study to evaluate the efficacy and safety of anti-biophilus in patients with radiation-induced diarrhoea. *European Journal of Gastroenterology and Hepatology, 13,* 391–396. doi:10.1097/00042737 -200104000-00015

32. Salari, P., Nikfar, S., & Abdollahi, M. (2012). A meta-analysis and systematic review on the effect of probiotics in acute diarrhea. *Inflammation and Allergy—Drug Targets, 11,* 3–14. doi:10.2174/187152812798889394

33. Coyle, V.M., Lungulescu, D., Toganel, C., Niculescu, A., Pop, S., Ciuleanu, T., ... Wilson, R.H. (2013). A randomised double-blind placebo-controlled phase II study of AGI004 for control of chemotherapy-induced diarrhoea. *British Journal of Cancer, 108,* 1027–1033. doi:10.1038/bjc.2013.35

34. Karthaus, M., Ballo, H., Abenhardt, W., Steinmetz, T., Geer, T., Schimke, J., ... Kleeberg, U. (2005). Prospective, double-blind, placebo-controlled, multicenter, randomized phase III study with orally administered budesonide for prevention of irinotecan (CPT-11)-induced diarrhea in patients with advanced colorectal cancer. *Oncology, 68,* 326–332. doi:10.1159/000086971

35. Maeda, Y., Ohune, T., Nakamura, M., Yamasaki, M., Kiribayashi, Y., & Murakami, T. (2004). Prevention of irinotecan-induced diarrhoea by oral carbonaceous adsorbent (Kremezin) in cancer patients. *Oncology Reports, 12,* 581–585. doi:10.3892/or.12.3.581

36. Michael, M., Brittain, M., Nagai, J., Feld, R., Hedley, D., Oza, A., ... Moore, M.J. (2004). Phase II study of activated charcoal to prevent irinotecan-induced diarrhea. *Journal of Clinical Oncology, 22,* 4410–4417. doi:10.1200/JCO.2004.11.125

37. Pettersson, A., Johansson, B., Persson, C., Berglund, A., & Turesson, I. (2012). Effects of a dietary intervention on acute gastrointestinal side effects and other aspects of health-related quality of life: A randomized controlled trial in prostate cancer patients undergoing radiotherapy. *Radiotherapy and Oncology, 103,* 333–340. doi:10.1016/j.radonc.2012.04.006

38. Flieger, D., Klassert, C., Hainke, S., Keller, R., Kleinschmidt, R., & Fischback, W. (2007). Phase II clinical trial for prevention of delayed diarrhea with cholestyramine/levofloxacin in the second-line treatment with irinotecan biweekly in patients with metastatic colorectal carcinoma. *Oncology, 72,* 10–16. doi:10.1159/000111083

39. Takeda, Y., Kobayashi, K., Akivama, Y., Soma, T., Handa, S., Kudoh, S., & Kudo, K. (2001). Prevention of irinotecan (CPT-11)-induced diarrhea by oral alkalization combined with control of defecation in cancer patients. *International Journal of Cancer, 92,* 269–275. doi:10.1002/1097 -0215(200102)9999:9999<::AID-IJC1179>3.0.CO;2-3

40. Sun, J.X., & Yang, H. (2013). Role of octreotide in post chemotherapy and/or radiotherapy diarrhea: Prophylaxis or therapy? *Asia-Pacific Journal of Clinical Oncology.* Advance online publication. doi:10.1111/ajco.12055

41. Kennedy, M., Bruninga, K., Mutlu, E.A., Losurdo, J., Choudhary, S., & Keshavarzian, A. (2001). Successful and sustained treatment of chronic radiation proctitis with antioxidant vitamins E and C. *American Journal of Gastroenterology, 96,* 1080–1084. doi:10.1111/j.1572-0241.2001 .03742.x

42. Yavuz, M.N., Yavuz, A.A., Aydin, F., Can, G., & Kavgaci, H. (2002). The efficacy of octreotide in the therapy of acute radiation-induced diarrhea: A randomized controlled study. *International Journal of Radiation Oncology, Biology, Physics, 54,* 195–202. doi:10.1016/S0360-3016(02)02870-5

43. Martenson, J.A., Halyard, M.Y., Sloan, J.A., Proulx, G.M., Miller, R.C., Deming, R.L., ... Atherton, P.J. (2008). Phase III, double-blind study of depot octreotide versus placebo in the prevention of acute diarrhea in patients receiving pelvic radiation therapy: Results of North Central Cancer Treatment Group N00CA. *Journal of Clinical Oncology, 26,* 5248–5253. doi:10.1200/JCO.2008.17.1546

44. Pilepich, M.V., Paulus, R., St. Clair, W., Barasacchio, R.A., Rostock, R., & Miller, R.C. (2006). Phase III study of pentosan polysulfate (PPS) in treatment of gastrointestinal tract sequelae of radiotherapy. *American Journal of Clinical Oncology, 29,* 132–137. doi:10.1097/01.coc.0000203758.77490.fd

45. Martenson, J.A., Bollinger, J.W., Sloan, J.A., Novotny, P.J., Urias, R.E., Michalak, J.C., … Levitt, R. (2000). Sucralfate in the prevention of treatment-induced diarrhea in patients receiving pelvic radiation therapy: A North Central Cancer Treatment Group phase III double-blind placebo-controlled trial. *Journal of Clinical Oncology, 18,* 1239–1245. Retrieved from http://jco.ascopubs.org/content/18/6/1239.long

46. American Institute for Cancer Research. (2012). *CancerResource™: Living with cancer.* Retrieved from http://www.aicr.org/assets/docs/pdf/cancerresource/cancerresource-complete.pdf

47. Kornblau, S., Benson, A.B., III, Catalano, R., Champlin, R.E., Engelking, C., Field, M., … Wadler, S. (2000). Management of cancer treatment-related diarrhea: Issues and therapeutic strategies. *Journal of Pain and Symptom Management, 19,* 118–129. doi:10.1016/S0885-3924(99)00149-9

48. McCallum, P., & Polisena, C. (Eds.). (2000). *The clinical guide to oncology nutrition.* Chicago, IL: American Dietetic Association.

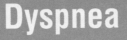

10

Dyspnea

Lee Ann Johnson, PhD(c), RN,
and Angela Adames, RN, BSN, OCN®

Problem and Incidence

Dyspnea is a common symptom among patients with advanced cancer. It is the subjective experience of breathing discomfort, which varies by intensity and quality depending on setting and disease extent.[1] Dyspnea may be acute because of malignant pleural effusion, or a chronic symptom. Malignant pleural effusions are reported to occur in up to 15% of patients with advanced disease.[2] More than 50% of patients with advanced cancer have reported dyspnea at some point throughout their illness.[3] One prospective study involving participants with advanced cancer showed that more than 55% of patients experienced moderate to severe dyspnea and that lung involvement was significantly associated with the presence and intensity of dyspnea.[4] Prevalence and severity of dyspnea increase in the last six months of life regardless of cancer diagnosis.[5]

Risk Factors and Assessment

Dyspnea may be related to disease or treatment or be unrelated to both. Risk factors for dyspnea include
- Progression of disease
- Imminent death
- Underlying lung disease (asthma or chronic obstructive pulmonary disease)
- Tumor involvement in the lung or pleura
- History of smoking
- Lung irradiation
- Anemia
- History of exposure to asbestos, coal dust, cotton dust, or grain dust.

Assessment of dyspnea should include the following.
- Responsive patients: Assess patients using a visual analog scale, a numeric rating scale, or the Borg Dyspnea Scale (open access).[6]
- Nonresponsive patients: Assess tachypnea or distress markers.
- Patients need to be assessed for physiologic causes such as anemia or pleural effusion.

What interventions are effective in managing dyspnea in people with cancer?

Evidence retrieved through July 31, 2013

Optimal treatment of dyspnea includes using specific and appropriate therapies to reverse the causes of dyspnea along with therapies to palliate the irreversible causes of dyspnea. The evidence presented here is palliative.

Recommended for Practice

Immediate-release opioids relieved dyspnea in multiple studies and systematic reviews.[7-18]

Benefits Balanced With Harms

Pleurodesis/pleural catheters relieve symptoms of acute dyspnea related to effusion. Patient preference, costs, and risk for complications should be considered in selection of approach for individual patients.[19-27] A systematic review noted that catheters were complicated by cellulitis, obstruction, and catheter malfunction.[2]

Effectiveness Not Established

A number of interventions for dyspnea have inconsistent results, and for some interventions findings are inconclusive because of small samples or other study limitations. These include the following.

- **Acupuncture**[28]
- **Anxiolytics**[1,17,29-32]—Professional guidelines note there is limited evidence to support use,[1] and systematic reviews have not shown benefit.[8,9,33]
- **Extended- and sustained-release opioids**[12,34]
- **Fan/increasing air flow**[35,36]—A systematic review concluded evidence is insufficient to support effectiveness.[28]
- **Music therapy** with theta music[37]
- **Nebulized furosemide**[9,38-40]
- **Nebulized lidocaine**[41]
- **Nebulized opioids**[9,17,42-46]
- **Progressive muscle relaxation**[47]
- **Psychoeducation/psychoeducational interventions**[16,47-51] —One systematic review concluded the evidence is insufficient to support effectiveness.[28] Another systematic review concluded there is moderate strength of evidence for effects of a nurse-led breathing program.[52] Palliative care guidelines recommend inclusion of psychoeducational interventions.[53]
- **Reflexology**[54]

Not Recommended for Practice

Palliative oxygen (administration in nonhypoxic patients) has consistently been shown not to improve dyspnea in individual studies and systematic reviews.[8,9,13,16,18,29,33,55-64]

Application to Practice

Patients at risk should be assessed for subjective and objective signs of dyspnea as well as severity and intensity of the symptom. Use of patient self-report measurement tools is beneficial in assessment and evaluation of interventions.

Underlying and potentially reversible causes of dyspnea, such as disease progression or anemia, should be identified and treated appropriately.

Nurses should educate patients about and advocate for interventions that are effective for treating dyspnea including the use of immediate-release opioids.

Palliative oxygen use is not shown to be effective. Associated costs and risks are not warranted in patients who do not have hypoxia.

Nurses can have input to selection of pleural catheter versus pleurodesis use. Patients and caregivers need to be assessed for ability to perform catheter care to reduce associated risks such as infection.

Dyspnea Resource Contributors

Topic leader: Margaret M. Joyce, PhD, APRN-BC, AOCN®
Angela Adames, RN, BSN, OCN®, and Brenda K. Shelton, RN, MS,
CCRN, AOCN®

References

1. Parshall, M.B., Schwartzstein, R.M., Adams, L., Banzett, R.B., Manning, H.L., Bourbeau, J., … O'Donnell, D.E. (2012). An official American Thoracic Society statement: Update on the mechanisms, assessment, and management of dyspnea. *American Journal of Respiratory and Critical Care Medicine, 185*, 435–452. doi:10.1164/rccm.201111-2042ST
2. Van Meter, M.E.M., McKee, K.Y., & Kohlwes, R.J. (2011). Efficacy and safety of tunneled pleural catheters in adults with malignant pleural effusions: A systematic review. *Journal of General Internal Medicine, 26*, 70–76. doi:10.1007/s11606-010-1472-0
3. Solano, J., Gomes, B., & Higginson, I. (2006). A comparison of symptom prevalence in far advanced cancer, AIDS, heart disease, chronic obstructive pulmonary disease and renal disease. *Journal of Pain and Symptom Management, 31*, 58–69. doi:10.1016/j.jpainsymman.2005.06.007
4. Bruera, E., Schmitz, B., Pither, J., Neumann, C., & Hanson, J. (2000). The frequency and correlates of dyspnea in patients with advanced cancer. *Journal of Pain and Symptom Management, 19*, 357–362. doi:10.1016/S0885-3924(00)00126-3
5. Currow, D.C., Smith, J., Davidson, P.M., Newton, P.J., Agar, M., & Abernathy, A.P. (2010). Do the trajectories of dyspnea differ in prevalence and intensity by diagnosis at the end of Life? A consecutive cohort study. *Journal Pain and Symptom Management, 39*, 680–690. doi:10.1016/j.jpainsymman.2009.09.017
6. American Academy of Disability Evaluating Physicians. (n.d.). Modified Borg dyspnea scale. Retrieved from http://www.aadep.org/documents/resources/Appendix_G__Modified_Borg_Dyspnea_S_E0BE89914046E.pdf
7. Allard, P., Lamontagne, C., Bernard, P., & Tremblay, C. (1999). How effective are supplementary doses of opioids for dyspnea in terminally ill cancer patients? A randomized continuous sequential clinical trial. *Journal of Pain and Symptom Management, 17*, 256–265. doi:10.1016/S0885-3924(98)00157-2

8. Ben-Aharon, I., Gafter-Gvili, A., Leibovici, I., & Stemmer, S.M. (2012). Interventions for alleviating cancer-related dyspnea: A systematic review and meta-analysis. *Acta Oncologica, 51,* 996–1008. doi:10.3109/028418 6X.2012.709638

9. Ben-Aharon, I., Gafter-Gvili, A., Paul, M., Leibovici, L., & Stemmer, S.M. (2008). Interventions for alleviating cancer-related dyspnea: A systematic review. *Journal of Clinical Oncology, 26,* 2396–2404. doi:10.1200/JCO.2007.15.5796

10. Bruera, E., Macmillan, K., Pither, J., & MacDonald, R.N. (1990). Effects of morphine on the dyspnea of terminal cancer patients. *Journal of Pain and Symptom Management, 5,* 341–344. doi:10.1016/0885-3924(90)90027-H

11. Clemens, K.E., & Klaschik, E. (2007). Symptomatic therapy of dyspnea with strong opioids and its effect on ventilation in palliative care patients. *Journal of Pain and Symptom Management, 33,* 473–481. doi:10.1016/j.jpainsymman.2006.09.015

12. Clemens, K.E., & Klaschik, E. (2008). Effect of hydromorphone on ventilation in palliative care patients with dyspnea. *Supportive Care in Cancer, 16,* 93–99. doi:10.1007/s00520-007-0310-3

13. Clemens, K.E., Quednau, I., & Klaschik, E. (2009). Use of oxygen and opioids in the palliation of dyspnoea in hypoxic and non-hypoxic palliative care patients: A prospective study. *Supportive Care in Cancer, 17,* 367–377. doi:10.1007/s00520-008-0479-0

14. Jennings, A.-L., Davies, A.N., Higgins, J.P.T., Gibbs, J.S.R., & Broadley, K.E. (2002). A systematic review of the use of opioids in the management of dyspnoea. *Thorax, 57,* 939–944. doi:10.1136/thorax.57.11.939

15. Mazzocato, C., Buclin, T., & Rapin, C.-H. (1999). The effects of morphine on dyspnea and ventilatory function in elderly patients with advanced cancer: A randomized double-blind controlled trial. *Annals of Oncology, 10,* 1511–1514. doi:10.1023/A:1008337624200

16. Qaseem, A., Snow, V., Shekelle, P., Casey, D.E., Jr., Cross, J.T., Jr., & Owens, D.K. (2008). Evidence-based interventions to improve the palliative care of pain, dyspnea, and depression at the end of life: A clinical practice guideline from the American College of Physicians. *Annals of Internal Medicine, 148,* 141–146. doi:10.7326/0003-4819-148-2-200801150-00009

17. Viola, R., Kiteley, C., Lloyd, N.S., Mackay, J.A., Wilson, J., Wong, R.K., & Supportive Care Guidelines Group of the Cancer Care Ontario Program in Evidence-Based Care. (2008). The management of dyspnea in cancer patients: A systematic review. *Supportive Care in Cancer, 16,* 329–337. doi:10.1007/s00520-007-0389-6

18. Wiese, C.H., Barrels, U.E., Graf, B.M., & Hanekop, G.G. (2009). Out-of-hospital opioid therapy of palliative care patients with "acute dyspnoea": A retrospective multicenter investigation. *Journal of Opioid Management, 5,* 115–122.

19. Alavi, A.A., Eshraghi, M., Rahim, M.B., Meysami, A.P., Morteza, A., & Hajian, H. (2011). Povidone-iodine and bleomycin in the management of malignant pleural effusion. *Acta Medica Iranica, 49,* 584–587. Retrieved from http://acta.tums.ac.ir/index.php/acta/article/view/4398

20. Davies, H.E., Mishra, E.K., Kahan, B.C., Wrightson, J.M., Stanton, A.E., Guhan, A., ... Rahman, N.M. (2012). Effect of an indwelling pleural catheter vs. chest tube and talc pleurodesis for relieving dyspnea in patients with malignant pleural effusion: The TIME2 randomized controlled trial. *JAMA, 307,* 2383–2389. doi:10.1001/jama.2012.5535

21. Demmy, T.L., Gu, L., Burkhalter, J.E., Toloza, E.M., D'Amico, T.A., Sutherland, S., ... Cancer and Leukemia Group B. (2012). Optimal management of malignant pleural effusions (results of CALGB 30102). *Journal of the National Comprehensive Cancer Network, 10,* 975–982. Retrieved from http://www.jnccn.org/content/10/8/975.long

22. Mohsen, T.A., Zeid, A.A.A., Meshref, M., Tawfeek, N., Redmond, K., Ananiadou, O.G., & Haj-Yahia, S. (2011). Local iodine pleurodesis versus thoracoscopic talc insufflation in recurrent malignant pleural effusion: A

prospective randomized control trial. *European Journal of Cardio-Thoracic Surgery, 40*, 282–286. doi:10.1016/j.ejcts.2010.09.005

23. Musani, A.I., Haas, A.R., Seijo, L., Wilby, M., & Sterman, D.H. (2004). Outpatient management of malignant pleural effusions with small-bore, tunneled pleural catheters. *Respiration, 71*, 559–566. doi:10.1159/000081755

24. Pollak, J.S., Burdge, C.M., Rosenblatt, M., Houston, J.P., Hwu, W.J., & Murren, J. (2001). Treatment of malignant pleural effusions with tunneled long-term drainage catheters. *Journal of Vascular and Interventional Radiology, 12*, 201–208. doi:10.1016/S1051-0443(07)61826-0

25. Schneider, T., Reimer, P., Storz, K., Klopp, M., Pfannschmidt, J., Dienemann, H., & Hoffmann, H. (2009). Recurrent pleural effusion: Who benefits from a tunneled catheter? *Thoracic and Cardiovascular Surgeon, 57*, 42–46. doi:10.1055/s-2008-1039109

26. Suzuki, K., Servais, E.L., Rizk, N.P., Solomon, S.B., Sima, C.S., Park, B.J., … Adusumilli, P.S. (2011). Palliation and pleurodesis in malignant pleural effusion: The role for tunneled pleural catheters. *Journal of Thoracic Oncology, 6*, 762–767. doi:10.1097/JTO.0b013e31820d614f

27. Thornton, R.H., Miller, Z., Covey, A.M., Brody, L., Sofocleous, C.T., Solomon, S.B., & Getrajdman, G.I. (2010). Tunneled pleural catheters for treatment of recurrent malignant pleural effusion following failed pleurodesis. *Journal of Vascular and Interventional Radiology, 21*, 696–700. doi:10.1016/j.jvir.2010.01.021

28. Bausewein, C., Booth, S., Gysels, M., Kühnbach, R., & Higginson, I. (2009). Non-pharmacological interventions for breathlessness in advanced stages of malignant and non-malignant diseases. *Cochrane Database of Systematic Reviews, 2009*(2). doi:10.1002/14651858.CD005623.pub2

29. Booth, S., Moosavi, S.H., & Higginson, I.J. (2008). The etiology and management of intractable breathlessness in patients with advanced cancer: A systematic review of pharmacological therapy. *Nature Clinical Practice Oncology, 5*, 90–100. doi:10.1038/ncponc1034

30. Clemens, K.E., & Klaschik, E. (2011). Dyspnoea associated with anxiety—Symptomatic therapy with opioids in combination with lorazepam and its effect on ventilation in palliative care patients. *Supportive Care in Cancer, 19*, 2027–2033. doi:10.1007/s00520-010-1058-8

31. Navigante, A.H., Castro, M.A., & Cerchietti, L.C. (2010). Morphine versus midazolam as upfront therapy to control dyspnea perception in cancer patients while its underlying cause is sought or treated. *Journal of Pain and Symptom Management, 39*, 820–830. doi:10.1016/j.jpainsymman.2009.10.003

32. Rietjens, J.A.C., van Zuylen, L., van Veluw, H., van der Wijk, L., van der Heide, A., & van der Rijt, C.C.D. (2008). Palliative sedation in a specialized unit for acute palliative care in a cancer hospital: Comparing patients dying with and without palliative sedation. *Journal of Pain and Symptom Management, 36*, 228–234. doi:10.1016/j.jpainsymman.2007.10.014

33. Simon, S.T., Higginson, I.J., Booth, S., Harding, R., & Bausewein, C. (2010). Benzodiazepines for the relief of breathlessness in advanced malignant and non-malignant diseases in adults. *Cochrane Database of Systematic Reviews, 2010*(1). doi:10.1002/14651858.CD007354.pub2

34. Kawabata, M., & Kaneishi, K. (2013). Continuous subcutaneous infusion of compound oxycodone for the relief of dyspnea in patients with terminally ill cancer: A retrospective study. *American Journal of Hospice and Palliative Care, 30*, 305–311. doi:10.1177/1049909112448924

35. Bausewein, C., Booth, S., Gysels, M., Kuhnbach, R., & Higginson, I.J. (2010). Effectiveness of a hand-held fan for breathlessness: A randomised phase II trial. *BMC Palliative Care, 9*, 22. doi:10.1186/1472-684X-9-22

36. Galbraith, S., Fagan, P., Perkins, P., Lynch, A., & Booth, S. (2010). Does the use of a handheld fan improve chronic dyspnea? A randomized, controlled, crossover trial. *Journal of Pain and Symptom Management, 39*, 831–838. doi:10.1016/j.jpainsymman.2009.09.024

37. Lai, W.-S., Chao, C.-S.C., Yang, W.-P., & Chen, C.-H. (2010). Efficacy of guided imagery with theta music for advanced cancer patients with dyspnea: A pilot study. *Biological Research for Nursing, 12,* 188–197. doi:10.1177/1099800409347556

38. Kohara, H., Ueoka, H., Aoe, K., Maeda, T., Takeyama, H., Saito, R., ... Uchitomi, Y. (2003). Effect of nebulized furosemide in terminally ill cancer patients with dyspnea. *Journal of Pain and Symptom Management, 26,* 962–967. doi:10.1016/S0885-3924(03)00322-1

39. Newton, P.J., Davidson, P.M., Macdonald, P., Ollerton, R., & Krum H. (2008). Nebulized furosemide for the management of dyspnea: Does the evidence support its use? *Journal of Pain and Symptom Management, 36,* 424–441. doi:10.1016/j.jpainsymman.2007.10.017

40. Wilcock, A., Walton, A., Manderson, C., Feathers, L., El Khoury, B., Lewis, M., ... Tattersfield, A. (2008). Randomised, placebo controlled trial of nebulised furosemide for breathlessness in patients with cancer. *Thorax, 63,* 872–875. doi:10.1136/thx.2007.091538

41. Wilcock, A., Corcoran, R., & Tattersfield, A.E. (1994). Safety and efficacy of nebulized lignocaine in patients with cancer and breathlessness. *Palliative Medicine, 8,* 35–38. doi:10.1177/026921639400800106

42. Bruera, E., Sala, R., Spruyt, O., Palmer, J.L., Zhang, T., & Willey, J. (2005). Nebulized versus subcutaneous morphine for patients with cancer dyspnea: A preliminary study. *Journal of Pain and Symptom Management, 29,* 613–618. doi:10.1016/j.jpainsymman.2004.08.016

43. Coyne, P.J., Viswanathan, R., & Smith, T.J. (2002). Nebulized fentanyl citrate improves patients' perception of breathing, respiratory rate, and oxygen saturation in dyspnea. *Journal of Pain and Symptom Management, 23,* 157–160. doi:10.1016/S0885-3924(01)00391-8

44. Quigley, C., Joel, S., Patel, N., Baksh, A., & Slevin, M. (2002). A phase I/II study of nebulized morphine-6-glucuronide in patients with cancer-related breathlessness. *Journal of Pain and Symptom Management, 23,* 7–9. doi:10.1016/S0885-3924(01)00381-5

45. Tanaka, K., Shima, Y., Kakinuma, R., Kubota, K., Ohe, Y., Hojo, F., ... Nishiwaki, Y. (1999). Effect of nebulized morphine in cancer patients with dyspnea: A pilot study. *Japanese Journal of Clinical Oncology, 29,* 600–603. doi:10.1093/jjco/29.12.600

46. Zeppetella, G. (1997). Nebulized morphine in the palliation of dyspnoea. *Palliative Medicine, 11,* 267–275. doi:10.1177/026921639701100402

47. Chan, C.W.H., Richardson, A., & Richardson, J. (2011). Managing symptoms in patients with advanced lung cancer during radiotherapy: Results of a psychoeducational randomized controlled trial. *Journal of Pain and Symptom Management, 41,* 347–357. doi:10.1016/j.jpainsymman.2010.04.024

48. Connors, S., Graham, S., & Peel, T. (2007). An evaluation of a physiotherapy led non-pharmacological breathlessness programme for patients with intrathoracic malignancy. *Palliative Medicine, 21,* 285–287. doi:10.1177/0269216307079172

49. Hately, J., Laurence, V., Scott, A., Baker, R., & Thomas, P. (2003). Breathlessness clinics within specialist palliative care settings can improve the quality of life and functional capacity of patients with lung cancer. *Palliative Medicine, 17,* 410–417. doi:10.1191/0269216303pm752oa

50. Yates, P., & Zhao, I. (2012). Update on complex nonpharmacological interventions for breathlessness. *Current Opinion in Supportive and Palliative Care, 6,* 144–152. doi:10.1097/SPC.0b013e3283536413

51. Zhao, I., & Yates, P. (2008). Non-pharmacological interventions for breathlessness management in patients with lung cancer: A systematic review. *Palliative Medicine, 22,* 693–701. doi:10.1177/0269216308095024

52. Rueda, J.-R., Sola, I., Pascual, A., & Casacuberta, M.S. (2012). Non-invasive interventions for improving well-being and quality of life in patients with lung cancer. *Cochrane Database of Systematic Reviews, 2012*(9). doi:10.1002/14651858.CD004282.pub3

53. National Comprehensive Cancer Network. (2013). *NCCN Clinical Practice Guidelines in Oncology: Palliative care* [v.2.2013]. Retrieved from http://www.nccn.org/professionals/physician_gls/pdf/palliative.pdf

54. Wyatt, G., Sikorskii, A., Rahbar, M.H., Victorson, D., & You, M. (2012). Health-related quality-of-life outcomes: A reflexology trial with patients with advanced-stage breast cancer. *Oncology Nursing Forum, 39,* 568–577. doi:10.1188/12.ONF.568-577

55. Abernethy, A.P., McDonald, C.F., Frith, P.A., Clark, K., Herndon, J.E., Marcello, J., … Currow, D.C. (2010). Effect of palliative oxygen versus room air in relief of breathlessness in patients with refractory dyspnoea: A double-blind, randomised controlled trial. *Lancet, 376,* 784–793. doi:10.1016/S0140-6736(10)61115-4

56. Ahmedzai, S.H., Laude, E., Robertson, A., Troy, G., & Vora, V. (2004). A double-blind, randomized, controlled phase II trial of heliox28 gas mixture in lung cancer patients with dyspnoea on exertion. *British Journal of Cancer, 90,* 366–371. doi:10.1038/sj.bjc.6601527

57. Bruera, E., de Stoutz, N., Velasco-Leiva, A., Schoeller, T., & Hanson, J. (1993). Effects of oxygen on dyspnoea in hypoxaemic terminal-cancer patients. *Lancet, 342,* 13–14. doi:10.1016/0140-6736(93)91880-U

58. Bruera, E., Sweeney, C., Willey, J., Palmer, J.L., Strasser, F., Morice, R.C., & Pisters, K. (2003). Randomized controlled trial of supplemental oxygen versus air in cancer patients with dyspnea. *Palliative Medicine, 17,* 659–663. doi:10.1191/0269216303pm826oa

59. Campbell, M.L., Yarandi, H., & Dove-Medows, E. (2013). Oxygen is nonbeneficial for most patients who are near death. *Journal of Pain and Symptom Management, 45,* 517–523. doi:10.1016/j.jpainsymman.2012.02.012

60. Cranston, J.M., Crockett, A., & Currow, D. (2009). Oxygen therapy for dyspnoea in adults. *Cochrane Database of Systematic Reviews, 2009*(3). doi:10.1002/14651858.CD004769.pub2

61. Currow, D.C., Agar, M., Smith, J., & Abernethy, A.P. (2009). Does palliative home oxygen improve dyspnoea? A consecutive cohort study. *Palliative Medicine, 23,* 309–316. doi:10.1177/0269216309104058

62. Philip, J., Gold, M., Milner, A., Di Iulio, J., Miller, B., & Spruyt, O. (2006). A randomized, double-blind, crossover trial of the effect of oxygen on dyspnea in patients with advanced cancer. *Journal of Pain and Symptom Management, 32,* 541–550. doi:10.1016/j.jpainsymman.2006.06.009

63. Uronis, H.E., & Abernethy, A.P. (2008). Oxygen for relief of dyspnea: What is the evidence? *Current Opinion in Supportive and Palliative Care, 2,* 89–94. doi:10.1097/SPC.0b013e3282ff0f5d

64. Uronis, H.E., Currow, D.C., McCrory, D.C., Samsa, G.P., & Abernethy, A.P. (2008). Oxygen for relief of dyspnoea in mildly- or non-hypoxaemic patients with cancer: A systematic review and meta-analysis. *British Journal of Cancer, 98,* 294–299. doi:10.1038/sj.bjc.6604161

11

Fatigue

Margaret Irwin, PhD, RN, MN,
Patricia Poirier, PhD, RN, AOCN®,
and Sandra A. Mitchell, PhD, CRNP, AOCN®

Problem and Incidence

Fatigue is one of the most common and distressing and symptoms reported by adults and children with cancer.[1,2] Fatigue is a multidimensional concept that can be thought of as a continuum from tiredness to exhaustion. Clinical expression of fatigue may include generalized weakness, lack of energy, diminished mental concentration, insomnia or hypersomnia, and emotional reactivity.[3] The prevalence of fatigue during cancer treatment ranges 25%–99% depending on method of measurement used and sample characteristics.[3,4] Fatigue during treatment has been associated with decline in physical and social functioning, emotional and spiritual distress,[5] and reduced employment and lost productivity for both patients and caregivers.[6] Late fatigue, occurring a year or more after completion of cancer treatment, has a significant impact on quality of life and is associated with increased unemployment. Up to 38% of cancer survivors continue to experience fatigue after completion of treatment, and it can persist for many years.[6] Fatigue may be an isolated symptom or can occur as part of a symptom cluster including pain, sleep disturbances, and depression.

Risk Factors and Assessment

Patients receiving multimodality treatment or experiencing multiple symptoms are at highest risk. Patients should be screened for fatigue at regular intervals by asking "How would you rate your fatigue on a scale of 0 to 10 over the past seven days?"[7] Screening for fatigue can be part of general patient distress screening.[8]

Patients with fatigue severity greater than 4 should be further evaluated, including workup to determine whether disease progression or recurrence could be among the causes of fatigue.[7]

Treatable contributing factors[7] need to be addressed.
• Side effects of medications
• Side effects of treatment
• Pain
• Emotional distress
• Sleep disturbances
• Nutritional deficiencies
• Comorbid conditions
• Impaired functional status

One-dimensional and multidimensional measures for fatigue include the following.
• Revised Piper Fatigue Scale
• Brief Fatigue Inventory
• Functional Assessment of Cancer Therapy–Fatigue (FACT-F)
• Numeric or visual analog scale (VAS)
• Patient-Reported Outcomes Measurement Information System (PROMIS®) fatigue short form. (Tools for use with adults and children are available.[9])

What interventions are effective in preventing and managing fatigue in people with cancer?

Evidence retrieved through October 31, 2013

Recommended for Practice

Exercise reduced fatigue in multiple studies.[1,10-31] Systematic reviews and meta-analyses have confirmed efficacy of exercise.[32-44] Exercise is recommended in professional guidelines.[7,45] Studies were done in patients with breast, colon, and prostate cancers; postoperative patients; patients undergoing stem cell transplantation; long-term cancer survivors; and individuals with advanced disease.

Likely to Be Effective

Cognitive behavioral therapy (CBT) for sleep, including stimulus control, sleep restriction, sleep hygiene, and sleep promotion planning, significantly improved fatigue in most studies.[46-56] Interventions were delivered individually, in groups, via telephone, and in multiple types of cancer.

Energy conservation and activity management counseling had a modest positive effect.[57,58] A subsequent study with some design flaws failed to confirm a beneficial effect for fatigue.[46]

Massage showed mixed results in some studies.[1,59-62] However, a post hoc analysis[63] of 1,290 patients demonstrated benefit.

Mindfulness-based stress reduction improved fatigue.[64-67]

Modafinil improved fatigue with minimal toxicity.[68-72]

Psychoeducation reduced fatigue in 16 studies[73-88] and showed no effect in eight studies.[89-96] A systematic review showed positive effects.[3] Guidelines suggest that education and counseling can be helpful.[7,97]

Benefits Balanced With Harms

Erythropoiesis-stimulating agents (ESAs) improved fatigue in patients who were anemic[98-100]; however, these are associated with potential severe adverse effects.[101] The U.S. Food and Drug Administration[102] has issued safety warnings regarding use of ESAs.

Effectiveness Not Established

Structured multidimensional rehabilitation, including multicomponent programs incorporating exercise along with other interventions delivered formally by a multidisciplinary group, had mixed results on fatigue outcomes.[27,79,86,103-115]

Multiple other pharmacologic and nonpharmacologic interventions have been studied for effects on fatigue. Many studies had small samples and employed nonrandomized or open-label study designs. Most interventions showed mixed results.

- **Pharmacologic interventions**
  - **Adenosine triphosphate infusion**[116,117]
  - **Bupropion**[118,119]
  - **Coenzyme Q10**[120]
  - **Dexamphetamine**[121,122]
  - **Donepezil**[101,122]
  - **Methylphenidate**[40,70,122-130]—Use was associated with nervousness, insomnia, and loss of appetite.[122,127,131]
  - **Paroxetine**[101,132-134]
  - **Progestins**[101]
  - **Sertraline**[101,135,136]
  - **Targeted anticytokine therapy with infliximab**[137]
  - **Thalidomide** in combination with megestrol acetate[138]
  - **Thyrotropin-releasing hormone**[139]
  - **Venlafaxine**[140]
- **Biofield and mind-body interventions**
  - **Haptotherapy**[141]
  - **Healing touch**[62,142-144]
  - **Mind-body medicine** combining CBT, yoga, and other complementary therapies[145]
  - **Polarity therapy**[61,146]
  - **Qigong/mind-body-spirit therapy** involving meditation and gentle exercise[147]
  - **Reflexology**[148]
  - **Reiki**[149]
  - **Relaxation and imagery interventions**, including **progressive muscle relaxation**,[150,151] **relaxation breathing**,[152] **guided imagery**,[153,154] and the **combination of relaxation and imagery**[51,155]—A systematic review concluded that effectiveness of these interventions for fatigue could not be determined based on the evidence to date.[156]
  - **Yoga**[157-164]—A systematic review of 18 randomized controlled trials showed that few studies improved fatigue and many were of low quality.[165]

- **Psychosocial Interventions**
  - **CBT** for symptoms, aimed at management of concurrent symptoms[81,156,166-172]
  - **Expressive writing** for emotional disclosure through writing[173,174]
  - **Group psychotherapy**[175,176]
  - **Hypnosis/hypnotherapy** in combination with CBT[171]
- **Dietary interventions and supplements**
  - **Dietary supplements** in varied combinations of protein supplements,[177] antioxidants, omega-3 fatty acids, progestins, vitamins, and other compounds[178-180]
  - **Levocarnitine (L-carnitine)**[122,178,181-185]—Most studies showing positive effects were open-label trials.
  - **Multivitamin supplements**[186]
  - **Vitamin C**[187]
- **Herbal therapies**
  - **Chinese herbal medicine**[188,189]—A systematic review concluded study quality was low, and trials had limited safety assessments.[190]
  - **Ginseng**[191]
  - **Guarana**, a plant extract[192,193]
  - **Mistletoe extract**[194,195]
  - **PG2**, a botanical root extract[196]
  - **Valerian**[197]
- **Other complementary and alternative interventions**
  - **Acupuncture**,[198-206] **acustimulation** with transcutaneous electrical stimulation,[207] and **acupressure**.[208] Systematic reviews[209-211] and a meta-analysis[212] concluded that more studies are needed before drawing conclusions about efficacy.
  - **Animal-assisted therapy**[213]
  - **Art making/art therapy**[214]
  - **Cranial stimulation**, providing low electrical brain stimulation with electrodes placed on the earlobes[215]
  - **Electroencephalography neurofeedback**, a biofeedback approach via display of brain electrical activity provided to the patient in visual or audio form[216]
  - **Light therapy** involving patient exposure to bright light delivered via a light box[217]
  - **Music/music therapy**[218-221]—A systematic review concluded music showed no significant effects on fatigue.[222]
  - **Virtual reality**[223-227]

Application to Practice

Nurses can work with patients to incorporate physical activity into daily routines. The approach to activity that is most acceptable to the patient can be encouraged, such as participation in group programs, individual training with a therapist or exercise physiologist, or self-directed exercise at home. Home use of videos, television programs, and software may be helpful. Some health insurance programs include coverage for gym memberships or provide a discount for membership.

It may seem counterintuitive to plan to exercise when feeling fatigued. Patients may need ongoing education and encouragement to be physically active.

Fatigue may be part of a symptom cluster. Effective management of the full range of patient symptoms is essential to successful fatigue management.

Nurses can educate and counsel patients regarding symptoms of fatigue and those interventions recommended or likely to be effective and assist patients in determining which interventions are most appealing to them.

Nurses may incorporate CBT for sleep into education and counseling and consider referrals to clinicians skilled in CBT and mindfulness-based stress reduction.

Although effectiveness for some interventions (e.g., relaxation therapies, acupuncture) is currently not established because of insufficient strength of the evidence, these may be helpful to select patients.

Fatigue Resource Contributors

*Topic leader: Sandra A. Mitchell, PhD, CRNP, AOCN®
Jane C. Clark, PhD, RN, AOCN®, GNP-C, Regina M. DeGennaro,
DNP, RN, AOCN®, CNL, Amy J. Hoffman, BSN, MSN, PhD,
Patricia Poirier, PhD, RN, AOCN®, Carolene B. Robinson, RN,
MA, AOCN®, CBCN®, Karen Stilwell, RN, MSN, CNS, OCN®, and
Breanna Weisbrod, RN, OCN®*

References

1. Chang, C.-W., Mu, P.-F., Jou, S.-T., Wong, T.-T., & Chen, Y.-C. (2013). Systematic review and meta-analysis of nonpharmacological interventions for fatigue in children and adolescents with cancer. *Worldviews on Evidence-Based Nursing, 10,* 208–217. doi:10.1111/wvn.12007

2. Dhillon, H.M., van der Ploeg, H.P., Bell, M.L., Boyer, M., Clarke, S., & Vardy, J. (2012). The impact of physical activity on fatigue and quality of life in lung cancer patients: A randomised controlled trial protocol. *BMC Cancer, 12,* 572. doi:10.1186/1471-2407-12-572

3. Goedendorp, M.M., Gielissen, M.F.M., Verhagen, C.A., & Bleijenberg, G. (2009). Psychosocial interventions for reducing fatigue during cancer treatment in adults. *Cochrane Database of Systematic Reviews, 2009*(1). doi:10.1002/14651858.CD006953.pub2

4. Kim, J.-E.E., Dodd, M.J., Aouizerat, B.E., Jahan, T., & Miaskowski, C. (2009). A review of the prevalence and impact of multiple symptoms in oncology patients. *Journal of Pain and Symptom Management, 37,* 715–736. doi:10.1016/j.jpainsymman.2008.04.018.

5. Mitchell, S.A. (2010). Cancer-related fatigue: State of the science. *PM&R, 2,* 364–383. doi:10.1016/j.pmrj.2010.03.024

6. Carlotto, A., Hogsett, V.L., Maiorini, E.M., Razulis, J.G., & Sonis, S.T. (2013). The economic burden of toxicities associated with cancer treatment: Review of the literature and analysis of nausea and vomiting, diarrhoea, oral mucositis and fatigue. *PharmacoEconomics, 31,* 753–766. doi:10.1007/s40273-013-0081-2

7. National Comprehensive Cancer Network. (2014). *NCCN Clinical Practice Guidelines in Oncology: Cancer-related fatigue* [v.1.2014]. Retrieved from http://www.nccn.org/professionals/physician_gls/pdf/fatigue.pdf

8. National Comprehensive Cancer Network. (2012). *NCCN Clinical Practice Guidelines in Oncology: Distress management* [v.2.2013]. Retrieved from http://www.nccn.org/professionals/physician_gls/pdf/distress.pdf

9. Assessment Center. (n.d.). What is Assessment Center? Retrieved from http://www.assessmentcenter.net

10. Andersen, C., Rorth, M., Ejlertsen, B., Stage, M., Moller, T., Midtgaard, J., ... Adamsen, L. (2013). The effects of a six-week supervised multimodal exercise intervention during chemotherapy on cancer-related fatigue. *European Journal of Oncology Nursing, 17,* 331–339. doi:10.1016/j.ejon.2012.09.003

11. Bourke, L., Thompson, G., Gibson, D.J., Daley, A., Crank, H., Adam, I., ... Saxton, J. (2011). Pragmatic lifestyle intervention in patients recovering from colon cancer: A randomized controlled pilot study. *Archives of Physical Medicine and Rehabilitation, 92,* 749–755. doi:10.1016/j.apmr.2010.12.020

12. Buss, T., de Walden-Gałuszko, K., Modlińska, A., Osowicka, M., Lichodziejewska-Niemierko, M., & Janiszewska, J. (2010). Kinesitherapy alleviates fatigue in terminal hospice cancer patients—An experimental, controlled study. *Supportive Care in Cancer, 18,* 743–749. doi:10.1007/s00520-009-0709-0

13. Cantarero-Villanueva, I., Fernández-Lao, C., Cuesta-Vargas, A.I., Del Moral-Avila, R., Fernández-de-las-Peñas, C., & Arroyo-Morales, M. (2013). The effectiveness of a deep water aquatic exercise program in cancer-related fatigue in breast cancer survivors: A randomized controlled trial. *Archives of Physical Medicine and Rehabilitation, 94,* 221–230. doi:10.1016/j.apmr.2012.09.008

14. Carayol, M., Bernard, P., Boiché, J., Riou, F., Mercier, B., Cousson-Gélie, F., ... Ninot, G. (2013). Psychological effect of exercise in women with breast cancer receiving adjuvant therapy: What is the optimal dose needed? *Annals of Oncology, 24,* 291–300. doi:10.1093/annonc/mds342

15. Cheville, A.L., Kollasch, J., Vandenberg, J., Shen, T., Grothey, A., Gamble, G., & Basford, J.R. (2013). A home-based exercise program to improve

function, fatigue, and sleep quality in patients with stage IV lung and colorectal cancer: A randomized controlled trial. *Journal of Pain and Symptom Management, 45,* 811–821. doi:10.1016/j.jpainsymman.2012.05.006

16. Coleman, E.A., Goodwin, J.A., Kennedy, R., Coon, S.K., Richards, K., Enderlin, C., … Anaissie, E.J. (2012). Effects of exercise on fatigue, sleep, and performance: A randomized trial. *Oncology Nursing Forum, 39,* 468–477. doi:10.1188/12.ONF.468-477

17. Eyigor, S., Karapolat, H., Yesil, H., Uslu, R., & Durmaz, B. (2010). Effects of Pilates exercises on functional capacity, flexibility, fatigue, depression and quality of life in female breast cancer patients: A randomized controlled study. *European Journal of Physical and Rehabilitation Medicine, 46,* 481–487. Retrieved from http://www.minervamedica.it/en/journals/europa-medicophysica/article.php?cod=R33Y2010N04A0481

18. Hayes, S.C., Rye, S., DiSipio, T., Yates, P., Bashford, J., Pyke, C., … Eakin, E. (2013). Exercise for health: A randomized, controlled trial evaluating the impact of a pragmatic, translational exercise intervention on the quality of life, function and treatment-related side effects following breast cancer. *Breast Cancer Research and Treatment, 137,* 175–186. doi:10.1007/s10549-012-2331-y

19. Hoffman, A.J., Brintnall, R.A., Brown, J.K., von Eye, A., Jones, L.W., Alderink, G., … VanOtteren, G.M. (2013). Too sick not to exercise: Using a 6-week, home-based exercise intervention for cancer-related fatigue self-management for postsurgical non-small cell lung cancer patients. *Cancer Nursing, 36,* 175–188. doi:10.1097/NCC.0b013e31826c7763

20. Hoffman, A.J., Brintnall, R.A., Brown, J.K., von Eye, A., Jones, L.W., Alderink, G., … VanOtteren, G.M. (2013). Virtual reality bringing a new reality to postthoracotomy lung cancer patients via a home-based exercise intervention targeting fatigue while undergoing adjuvant treatment. *Cancer Nursing, 37,* 23–33. doi:10.1097/NCC.0b013e318278d52f

21. Hsieh, C.C., Sprod, L.K., Hydock, D.S., Carter, S.D., Hayward, R., & Schneider, C.M. (2008). Effects of a supervised exercise intervention on recovery from treatment regimens in breast cancer survivors. *Oncology Nursing Forum, 35,* 909–915. doi:10.1188/08.ONF.909-915

22. Litterini, A.J., & Fieler, V.K. (2008). The change in fatigue, strength, and quality of life following a physical therapist prescribed exercise program for cancer survivors. *Rehabilitation Oncology, 26,* 11–17.

23. Oldervoll, L.M., Loge, J.H., Lydersen, S., Paltiel, H., Asp, M.B., Nygaard, U.V., … Kaasa, S. (2011). Physical exercise for cancer patients with advanced disease: A randomized controlled trial. *Oncologist, 16,* 1649–1657. doi:10.1634/theoncologist.2011-0133

24. Rajotte, E.J., Jean, C.Y., Baker, K.S., Gregerson, L., Leiserowitz, A., & Syrjala, K.L. (2012). Community-based exercise program effectiveness and safety for cancer survivors. *Journal of Cancer Survivorship, 6,* 219–228. doi:10.1007/s11764-011-0213-7

25. Saarto, T., Penttinen, H.M., Sievänen, H., Kellokumpu-Lehtinen, P.L., Hakamies-Blomqvist, L., Nikander, R., … Luoma, M.L. (2012). Effectiveness of a 12-month exercise program on physical performance and quality of life of breast cancer survivors. *Anticancer Research, 32,* 3875–3884. Retrieved from http://ar.iiarjournals.org/content/32/9/3875.long

26. Schmidt, T., Weisser, B., Jonat, W., Baumann, F.T., & Mundhenke, C. (2012). Gentle strength training in rehabilitation of breast cancer patients compared to conventional therapy. *Anticancer Research, 32,* 3229–3233. Retrieved from http://ar.iiarjournals.org/content/32/8/3229.long

27. Wang, Y.-J., Boehmke, M., Wu, Y.-W., Dickerson, S.S., & Fisher, N. (2011). Effects of a 6-week walking program on Taiwanese women newly diagnosed with early-stage breast cancer. *Cancer Nursing, 34*(2), E1–E13. doi:10.1097/NCC.0b013e3181e4588d

28. Wenzel, J.A., Griffith, K.A., Shang, J., Thompson, C.B., Hedlin, H., Stewart, K.J., … Mock, V. (2013). Impact of a home-based walking intervention on outcomes of sleep quality, emotional distress, and fatigue in patients un-

dergoing treatment for solid tumors. *Oncologist, 18*, 476–484. doi:10.1634/theoncologist.2012-0278

29. Yang, C.Y., Tsai, J.C., Huang, Y.C., & Lin, C.C. (2010). Effects of a home-based walking program on perceived symptom and mood status in postoperative breast cancer women receiving adjuvant chemotherapy. *Journal of Advanced Nursing, 67*, 158–168. doi:10.1111/j.1365-2648.2010.05492.x

30. Yeh, C.H., Man Wai, J.P., Lin, U.-S., & Chiang, Y.-C. (2011). A pilot study to examine the feasibility and effects of a home-based aerobic program on reducing fatigue in children with acute lymphoblastic leukemia. *Cancer Nursing, 34*, 3–12. doi:10.1097/NCC.0b013e3181e4553c

31. Yeo, T.P., Burrell, S.A., Sauter, P.K., Kennedy, E.P., Lavu, H., Leiby, B.E., & Yeo, C.J. (2012). A progressive postresection walking program significantly improves fatigue and health-related quality of life in pancreas and periampullary cancer patients. *Journal of the American College of Surgeons, 214*, 463–475. doi:10.1016/j.jamcollsurg.2011.12.017

32. Arnold, M., & Taylor, N.F. (2010). Does exercise reduce cancer-related fatigue in hospitalised oncology patients? A systematic review. *Onkologie, 33*, 625–630. doi:10.1159/000321145

33. Bradt, J., Goodill, S.W., & Dileo, C. (2011). Dance/movement therapy for improving psychological and physical outcomes in cancer patients. *Cochrane Database of Systematic Reviews, 2011*(10). doi:10.1002/14651858.CD007103.pub2

34. Brown, J.C., Huedo-Medina, T.B., Pescatello, L.S., Pescatello, S.M., Ferrer, R.A., & Johnson, B.T. (2011). Efficacy of exercise interventions in modulating cancer-related fatigue among adult cancer survivors: A meta-analysis. *Cancer Epidemiology, Biomarkers and Prevention, 20*, 123–133. doi:10.1158/1055-9965.EPI-10-0988

35. Cramp, F., & Byron-Daniel, J. (2012). Exercise for the management of cancer-related fatigue in adults. *Cochrane Database of Systematic Reviews, 2012*(11). doi:10.1002/14651858.CD006145.pub3

36. Keogh, J.W.L., & Macleod, R.D. (2011). Body composition, physical fitness, functional performance, quality of life, and fatigue benefits of exercise for prostate cancer patients: A systematic review. *Journal of Pain and Symptom Management, 43*, 96–110. doi:10.1016/j.jpainsymman.2011.03.006

37. Kuchinski, A., Reading, M., & Lash, A.A. (2009). Treatment-related fatigue and exercise in patients with cancer: A systematic review. *MEDSURG Nursing, 18*, 174–180.

38. McMillan, E.M., & Newhouse, I.J. (2011). Exercise is an effective treatment modality for reducing cancer-related fatigue and improving physical capacity in cancer patients and survivors: A meta-analysis. *Applied Physiology, Nutrition, and Metabolism, 36*, 892–903. doi:10.1139/h11-082

39. Mishra, S.I., Scherer, R.W., Geigle, P.M., Berlanstein, D.R., Topaloglu, O., Gotay, C.C., & Snyder, C. (2012). Exercise interventions on health-related quality of life for cancer survivors. *Cochrane Database of Systematic Reviews, 2012*(8). doi:10.1002/14651858.CD007566.pub2

40. Payne, C., Wiffen, P.J., & Martin, S. (2012). Interventions for fatigue and weight loss in adults with advanced progressive illness. *Cochrane Database of Systematic Reviews, 2012*(1). doi:10.1002/14651858.CD008427.pub2

41. Puetz, T.W., & Herring, M.P. (2012). Differential effects of exercise on cancer-related fatigue during and following treatment: A meta-analysis. *American Journal of Preventive Medicine, 43*(2), e1–e24. doi:10.1016/j.amepre.2012.04.027

42. van Haren, I.E.M., Timmerman, H., Potting, C.M., Blijlevens, N.M., Staal, J.B., & Nijhuis-van der Sanden, M.W. (2013). Physical exercise for patients undergoing hematopoietic stem cell transplantation: Systematic review and meta-analyses of randomized controlled trials. *Physical Therapy, 93*, 514–528. doi:10.2522/ptj.20120181

43. Velthuis, M.J., Agasi-Idenburg, S.C., Aufdemkampe, G., & Wittink, H.M. (2010). The effect of physical exercise on cancer-related fatigue during

cancer treatment: A meta-analysis of randomised controlled trials. *Clinical Oncology, 22*, 208–221. doi:10.1016/j.clon.2009.12.005

44. Wanchai, A., Armer, J.M., & Stewart, B.R. (2011). Nonpharmacologic supportive strategies to promote quality of life in patients experiencing cancer-related fatigue: A systematic review. *Clinical Journal of Oncology Nursing, 15*, 203–214. doi:10.1188/11.CJON.203-214

45. Schmitz, K.H., Courneya, K.S., Matthews, C., Demark-Wahnefried, W., Galvão, D.A., Pinto, B.M., … Schwartz, A. (2010). American College of Sports Medicine roundtable on exercise guidelines for cancer survivors. *Medicine and Science in Sports and Exercise, 42*, 1409–1426. doi:10.1249/MSS.0b013e3181e0c112

46. Barsevick, A., Beck, S.L., Dudley, W.N., Wong, B., Berger, A.M., Whitmer, K., … Stewart, K. (2010). Efficacy of an intervention for fatigue and sleep disturbance during cancer chemotherapy. *Journal of Pain and Symptom Management, 40*, 200–216. doi:10.1016/j.jpainsymman.2009.12.020

47. Berger, A.M., Kuhn, B.R., Farr, L.A., Lynch, J.C., Agrawal, S., Chamberlain, J., & Von Essen, S. (2009). Behavioral therapy intervention trial to improve sleep quality and cancer-related fatigue. *Psycho-Oncology, 18*, 634–646. doi:10.1002/pon.1438

48. Berger, A.M., Kuhn, B.R., Farr, L.A., Von Essen, S., Chamberlain, J., Lynch, J.C., & Agrawal, S. (2009). One-year outcomes of a behavioral intervention trial on sleep quality and cancer-related fatigue. *Journal of Clinical Oncology, 27*, 6033–6040. doi:10.1200/JCO.2008.20.8306

49. Berger, A.M., VonEssen, S., Kuhn, B.R., Piper, B.F., Farr, L., Agrawal, S., … Higginbotham, P. (2002). Feasibility of a sleep intervention during adjuvant breast cancer chemotherapy. *Oncology Nursing Forum, 29*, 1431–1441. doi:10.1188/02.ONF.1431-1441

50. Berger, A.M., VonEssen, S., Kuhn, B.R., Piper, B.F., Agrawal, S., Lynch, J.C., & Higginbotham, P. (2003). Adherence, sleep, and fatigue outcomes after adjuvant breast cancer chemotherapy: Results of a feasibility intervention study. *Oncology Nursing Forum, 30*, 513–522. doi:10.1188/03.ONF.513-522

51. Cohen, M., & Fried, G. (2007). Comparing relaxation training and cognitive-behavioral group therapy for women with breast cancer. *Research on Social Work Practice, 17*, 313–323. doi:10.1177/1049731506293741

52. Dirksen, S.R., & Epstein, D.R. (2008). Efficacy of an insomnia intervention on fatigue, mood and quality of life in breast cancer survivors. *Journal of Advanced Nursing, 61*, 664–675. doi:10.1111/j.1365-2648.2007.04560.x

53. Espie, C.A., Fleming, L., Cassidy, J., Samuel, L., Taylor, L.M., White, C.A., … Paul, J. (2008). Randomized controlled clinical effectiveness trial of cognitive behavior therapy compared with treatment as usual for persistent insomnia in patients with cancer. *Journal of Clinical Oncology, 26*, 4651–4658. doi:10.1200/JCO.2007.13.9006

54. Prinsen, H., Bleijenberg, G., Heijmen, L., Zwarts, M.J., Leer, J.W., Heerschap, A., … van Laarhoven, H.W.M. (2013). The role of physical activity and physical fitness in postcancer fatigue: A randomized controlled trial. *Supportive Care in Cancer, 21*, 2279–2288. doi:10.1007/s00520-013-1784-9

55. Quesnel, C., Savard, J., Simard, S., Ivers, H., & Morin, C.M. (2003). Efficacy of cognitive-behavioral therapy for insomnia in women treated for nonmetastatic breast cancer. *Journal of Consulting and Clinical Psychology, 71*, 189–200. doi:10.1037/0022-006X.71.1.189

56. Savard, J., Simard, S., Ivers, H., & Morin, C.M. (2005). Randomized study on the efficacy of cognitive-behavioral therapy for insomnia secondary to breast cancer, part I: Sleep and psychological effects. *Journal of Clinical Oncology, 23*, 6083–6096. doi:10.1200/JCO.2005.09.548

57. Barsevick, A.M., Dudley, W., Beck, S., Sweeney, C., Whitmer, K., & Nail, L. (2004). A randomized clinical trial of energy conservation for patients with cancer-related fatigue. *Cancer, 100*, 1302–1310. doi:10.1002/cncr.20111

58. Barsevick, A.M., Whitmer, K., Sweeney, C., & Nail, L.M. (2002). A pilot study examining energy conservation for cancer treatment-related fatigue. *Cancer Nursing, 25*, 333–341. doi:10.1097/00002820-200210000-00001

59. Ahles, T.A., Tope, D.M., Pinkson, B., Walch, S., Hann, D., Whedon, M., ... Silberfarb, P.M. (1999). Massage therapy for patients undergoing autologous bone marrow transplantation. *Journal of Pain and Symptom Management, 18*, 157–163. doi:10.1016/S0885-3924(99)00061-5

60. Currin, J., & Meister, E.A. (2008). A hospital-based intervention using massage to reduce distress among oncology patients. *Cancer Nursing, 31*, 214–221. doi:10.1097/01.NCC.0000305725.65345.f3

61. Mustian, K.M., Roscoe, J.A., Palesh, O.G., Sprod, L.K., Heckler, C.E., Peppone, L.J., ... Morrow, G.R. (2011). Polarity therapy for cancer-related fatigue in patients with breast cancer receiving radiation therapy: A randomized controlled pilot study. *Integrative Cancer Therapies, 10*, 27–37. doi:10.1177/1534735410397044

62. Post-White, J., Kinney, M.E., Savik, K., Gau, J.B., Wilcox, C., & Lerner, I. (2003). Therapeutic massage and healing touch improve symptoms in cancer. *Integrative Cancer Therapies, 2*, 332–344. doi:10.1177/1534735403259064

63. Cassileth, B.R., & Vickers, A.J. (2004). Massage therapy for symptom control: Outcome study at a major cancer center. *Journal of Pain and Symptom Management, 28*, 244–249. doi:10.1016/j.jpainsymman.2003.12.016

64. Garland, S.N., Tamagawa, R., Todd, S.C., Speca, M., & Carlson, L.E. (2013). Increased mindfulness is related to improved stress and mood following participation in a mindfulness-based stress reduction program in individuals with cancer. *Integrative Cancer Therapies, 12*, 31–40. doi:10.1177/1534735412442370

65. Hoffman, C.J., Ersser, S.J., Hopkinson, J.B., Nicholls, P.G., Harrington, J.E., & Thomas, P.W. (2012). Effectiveness of mindfulness-based stress reduction in mood, breast- and endocrine-related quality of life, and well-being in stage 0 to III breast cancer: A randomized, controlled trial. *Journal of Clinical Oncology, 30*, 1335–1342. doi:10.1200/JCO.2010.34.0331

66. Lengacher, C.A., Reich, R.R., Post-White, J., Moscoso, M., Shelton, M.M., Barta, M., ... Budhrani, P. (2012). Mindfulness based stress reduction in post-treatment breast cancer patients: An examination of symptoms and symptom clusters. *Journal of Behavioral Medicine, 35*, 86–94. doi:10.1007/s10865-011-9346-4

67. van der Lee, M.L., & Garssen, B. (2012). Mindfulness-based cognitive therapy reduces chronic cancer-related fatigue: A treatment study. *Psycho-Oncology, 21*, 264–272. doi:10.1002/pon.1890

68. Blackhall, L., Petroni, G., Shu, J., Baum, L., & Farace, E. (2009). A pilot study evaluating the safety and efficacy of modafinil for cancer-related fatigue. *Journal of Palliative Medicine, 12*, 433–439. doi:10.1089/jpm.2008.0230

69. Cooper, M.R., Bird, H.M., & Steinberg, M. (2009). Efficacy and safety of modafinil in the treatment of cancer-related fatigue. *Annals of Pharmacotherapy, 43*, 721–725. doi:10.1345/aph.1L532

70. Gehring, K., Patwardhan, S.Y., Collins, R., Groves, M.D., Etzel, C.J., Meyers, C.A., & Wefel, J.S. (2012). A randomized trial on the efficacy of methylphenidate and modafinil for improving cognitive functioning and symptoms in patients with a primary brain tumor. *Journal of Neuro-Oncology, 107*, 165–174. doi:10.1007/s11060-011-0723-1

71. Jean-Pierre, P., Morrow, G.R., Roscoe, J.A., Heckler, C., Mohile, S., Janelsins, M., ... Hopkins, J.O. (2010). A phase 3 randomized, placebo-controlled, double-blind, clinical trial of the effect of modafinil on cancer-related fatigue among 631 patients receiving chemotherapy: A University of Rochester Cancer Center Community Clinical Oncology Program Research Base study. *Cancer, 116*, 3513–3520. doi:10.1002/cncr.25083

72. Spathis, A., Dhillan, R., Booden, D., Forbes, K., Vrotsou, K., & Fife, K. (2009). Modafinil for the treatment of fatigue in lung cancer: A pilot study. *Palliative Medicine, 23*, 325–331. doi:10.1177/0269216309102614

73. Allison, P.J., Edgar, L., Nicolau, B., Archer, J., Black, M., & Hier, M. (2004). Results of a feasibility study for a psycho-educational intervention in head and neck cancer. *Psycho-Oncology, 13*, 482–485. doi:10.1002/pon.816

74. Arving, C., Sjödén, P.O., Bergh, J., Hellbom, M., Johansson, B., Glimelius, B., & Brandberg, Y. (2007). Individual psychosocial support for breast cancer patients: A randomized study of nurse versus psychologist interventions and standard care. *Cancer Nursing, 30*(3), E10–E19. doi:10.1097/01.NCC.0000270709.64790.05

75. Chan, C.W., Richardson, A., & Richardson, J. (2011). Managing symptoms in patients with advanced lung cancer during radiotherapy: Results of a psychoeducational randomized controlled trial. *Journal of Pain and Symptom Management, 41,* 347–357. doi:10.1016/j.jpainsymman.2010.04.024

76. Fillion, L., Gagnon, P., Leblond, F., Gelinas, C., Sayard, J., Dupuis, R., ... Larochelle, M. (2008). A brief intervention for fatigue management in breast cancer survivors. *Cancer Nursing, 31,* 145–159. doi:10.1097/01.NCC.0000305698.97625.95

77. Gaston-Johansson, F., Fall-Dickson, J.M., Nanda, J., Ohly, K.V., Stillman, S., Krumm, S., ... Kennedy, M.J. (2000). The effectiveness of the comprehensive coping strategy program on clinical outcomes in breast cancer autologous bone marrow transplantation. *Cancer Nursing, 23,* 277–285. doi:10.1097/00002820-200008000-00004

78. Genc, R.E., & Conk, Z. (2008). Impact of effective nursing interventions to the fatigue syndrome in children who receive chemotherapy. *Cancer Nursing, 31,* 312–317. doi:10.1097/01.NCC.0000305740.18711.c6

79. Gjerset, G.M., Fosså, S.D., Dahl, A.A., Loge, J.H., Ensby, T., & Thorsen, L. (2011). Effects of a 1-week inpatient course including information, physical activity, and group sessions for prostate cancer patients. *Journal of Cancer Education, 26,* 754–760. doi:10.1007/s13187-011-0245-8

80. Godino, C., Jodar, L., Durán, Á., Martinez, I., & Schiaffino, A. (2006). Nursing education as an intervention to decrease fatigue perception in oncology patients. *European Journal of Oncology Nursing, 10,* 150–155. doi:10.1016/j.ejon.2005.03.004

81. Kwekkeboom, K.L., Abbott-Anderson, K., Cherwin, C., Roiland, R., Serlin, R.C., & Ward, S.E. (2012). Pilot randomized controlled trial of a patient-controlled cognitive-behavioral intervention for the pain, fatigue, and sleep disturbance symptom cluster in cancer. *Journal of Pain and Symptom Management, 44,* 810–822. doi:10.1016/j.jpainsymman.2011.12.281

82. Lindemalm, C., Strang, P., & Lekander, M. (2005). Support group for cancer patients: Does it improve their physical and psychological wellbeing? A pilot study. *Supportive Care in Cancer, 13,* 652–657. doi:10.1007/s00520-005-0785-8

83. Ream, E., Richardson, A., & Alexander-Dann, C. (2006). Supportive intervention for fatigue in patients undergoing chemotherapy: A randomized controlled trial. *Journal of Pain and Symptom Management, 31,* 148–161. doi:10.1016/j.jpainsymman.2005.07.003

84. Reif, K., de Vries, U., Petermann, F., & Görres, S. (2013). A patient education program is effective in reducing cancer-related fatigue: A multi-centre randomised two-group waiting-list controlled intervention trial. *European Journal of Oncology Nursing, 17,* 204–213. doi:10.1016/j.ejon.2012.07.002

85. Vilela, L.D., Nicolau, B., Mahmud, S., Edgar, L., Hier, M., Black, M., ... Allison, P.J. (2006). Comparison of psychosocial outcomes in head and neck cancer patients receiving a coping strategies intervention and control subjects receiving no intervention. *Journal of Otolaryngology, 35,* 88–96. doi:10.2310/7070.2005.5002

86. Yates, P., Aranda, S., Hargraves, M., Mirolo, B., Clavarino, A., McLachlan, S., & Skerman, H. (2005). Randomized controlled trial of an educational intervention for managing fatigue in women receiving adjuvant chemotherapy for early-stage breast cancer. *Journal of Clinical Oncology, 23,* 6027–6036. doi:10.1200/JCO.2005.01.271

87. Yesilbalkan, O.U., Karadakovan, A., & Göker, E. (2009). The effectiveness of nursing education as an intervention to decrease fatigue in Turkish patients receiving chemotherapy [Online exclusive]. *Oncology Nursing Forum, 36,* E215–E222. doi:10.1188/09.ONF.E215-E222

88. Yun, Y.H., Lee, K.S., Kim, Y.-W., Park, S.Y., Lee, E.S., Noh, D.-Y., ... Park, S. (2012). Web-based tailored education program for disease-free cancer survivors with cancer-related fatigue: A randomized controlled trial. *Journal of Clinical Oncology, 30,* 1296–1303. doi:10.1200/JCO.2011.37.2979

89. Berglund, G., Petersson, L.-M., Eriksson, K.C., Wallenius, I., Roshanai, A., Nordin, K.M., ... Häggman, M. (2007). "Between Men": A psychosocial rehabilitation programme for men with prostate cancer. *Acta Oncologica, 46,* 83–89. doi:10.1080/02841860600857326

90. Bjorneklett, H.G., Lindemalm, C., Ojutkangas, M.L., Berglund, A., Letocha, H., Strang, P., & Bergkvist, L. (2012). A randomized controlled trial of a support group intervention on the quality of life and fatigue in women after primary treatment for early breast cancer. *Supportive Care in Cancer, 20,* 3325–3334. doi:10.1007/s00520-012-1480-1

91. Brown, P., Clark, M.M., Atherton, P., Huschka, M., Sloan, J.A., Gamble, G., ... Rummans, T.A. (2006). Will improvement in quality of life (QOL) impact fatigue in patients receiving radiation therapy for advanced cancer? *American Journal of Clinical Oncology, 29,* 52–58. doi:10.1097/01.coc.0000190459.14841.55

92. Bruera, E., Yennurajalingam, S., Palmer, J.L., Perez-Cruz, P.E., Frisbee-Hume, S., Allo, J.A., ... Cohen, M.Z. (2013). Methylphenidate and/or a nursing telephone intervention for fatigue in patients with advanced cancer: A randomized, placebo-controlled, phase II trial. *Journal of Clinical Oncology, 31,* 2421–2427. doi:10.1200/JCO.2012.45.3696

93. Kearney, N., Miller, M., Maguire, R., Dolan, S., MacDonald, R., McLeod, J., ... Wengström, Y. (2008). WISECARE+: Results of a European study of a nursing intervention for the management of chemotherapy-related symptoms. *European Journal of Oncology Nursing, 12,* 443–448. doi:10.1016/j.ejon.2008.07.005

94. Purcell, A., Fleming, J., Burmeister, B., Bennett, S., & Haines, T. (2011). Is education an effective management strategy for reducing cancer-related fatigue? *Supportive Care in Cancer, 19,* 1429–1439. doi:10.1007/s00520-010-0970-2

95. Williams, S.A., & Schreier, A.M. (2005). The role of education in managing fatigue, anxiety, and sleep disorders in women undergoing chemotherapy for breast cancer. *Applied Nursing Research, 18,* 138–147. doi:10.1016/j.apnr.2004.08.005

96. Windsor, P.M., Potter, J., McAdam, K., & McCowan, C. (2009). Evaluation of a fatigue initiative: Information on exercise for patients receiving cancer treatment. *Clinical Oncology, 21,* 473–482. doi:10.1016/j.clon.2009.01.009

97. Howell, D., Keller-Olaman, S., Oliver, T.K., Hack, T.F., Broadfield, L., Biggs, K., ... Olson, K. (2013). A pan-Canadian practice guideline and algorithm: Screening, assessment, and supportive care of adults with cancer-related fatigue. *Current Oncology, 20*(3), e233–e246. doi:10.3747/co.20.1302

98. Auerbach, M., Silberstein, P.T., Webb, R.T., Averyanova, S., Ciuleanu, T.E., Shao, J., & Bridges, K. (2010). Darbepoetin alfa 300 or 500 μg once every 3 weeks with or without intravenous iron in patients with chemotherapy-induced anemia. *American Journal of Hematology, 85,* 655–663. doi:10.1002/ajh.21779

99. Hoskin, P.J., Robinson, M., Slevin, N., Morgan, D., Harrington, K., & Gaffney, C. (2009). Effect of epoetin alfa on survival and cancer treatment-related anemia and fatigue in patients receiving radical radiotherapy with curative intent for head and neck cancer. *Journal of Clinical Oncology, 27,* 5751–5756. doi:10.1200/JCO.2009.22.3693

100. Pronzato, P., Cortesi, E., van der Rijt, C.C., Bols, A., Moreno-Nogueira, J.A., de Oliveira, C.F., ... Rosso, R. (2010). Epoetin alfa improves anemia and anemia-related, patient-reported outcomes in patients with breast cancer receiving myelotoxic chemotherapy: Results of a European, multicenter, randomized, controlled trial. *Oncologist, 15,* 935–943. doi:10.1634/theoncologist.2009-0279

101. Minton, O., Richardson, A., Sharpe, M., Hotopf, M., & Stone, P. (2010). Drug therapy for the management of cancer-related fatigue. *Cochrane Database of Systematic Reviews, 2010*(7). doi:10.1002/14651858.CD006704 .pub3

102. U.S. Food and Drug Administration. (2009, March 27). Erythropoiesis stimulating agents (ESA) safety alert. Retrieved from http://www.fda .gov/forconsumers/byaudience/forpatientadvocates/hivandaidsactivities/ ucm124422.htm

103. Cheville, A.L., Girardi, J., Clark, M.M., Rummans, T.A., Pittelkow, T., Brown, P., ... Gamble, G. (2010). Therapeutic exercise during outpatient radiation therapy for advanced cancer: Feasibility and impact on physical well-being. *American Journal of Physical Medicine and Rehabilitation, 89,* 611–619. doi:10.1097/PHM.0b013e3181d3e782

104. Culos-Reed, S.N., Robinson, J.W., Lau, H., Stephenson, L., Keats, M., Norris, S., ... Faris, P. (2010). Physical activity for men receiving androgen deprivation therapy for prostate cancer: Benefits from a 16-week intervention. *Supportive Care in Cancer, 18,* 591–599. doi:10.1007/s00520-009-0694-3

105. de Nijs, E., Ros, W., & Grijpdonck, M.H. (2008). Nursing intervention for fatigue during the treatment for cancer. *Cancer Nursing, 31,* 191–206. doi:10.1097/01.NCC.0000305721.98518.7c

106. Dodd, M.J., Cho, M.H., Miaskowski, C., Painter, P.L., Paul, S.M., Cooper, B.A., ... Bank, K.A. (2010). A randomized controlled trial of home-based exercise for cancer-related fatigue in women during and after chemotherapy with or without radiation therapy. *Cancer Nursing, 33,* 245–257. doi:10.1097/ NCC.0b013e3181ddc58c

107. Hanna, L.R., Avila, P.F., Meteer, J.D., Nicholas, D.R., & Kaminsky, L.A. (2008). The effects of a comprehensive exercise program on physical function, fatigue, and mood in patients with various types of cancer. *Oncology Nursing Forum, 35,* 461–469. doi:10.1188/08.ONF.461-469

108. Hanssens, S., Luyten, R., Watthy, C., Fontaine, C., Decoster, L., Baillon, C., ... De Grève, J. (2011). Evaluation of a comprehensive rehabilitation program for post-treatment patients with cancer [Online exclusive]. *Oncology Nursing Forum, 38,* E418–E424. doi:10.1188/11.ONF.E418-E424

109. Heim, M.E., v.d Malsburg, M.L., & Niklas, A. (2007). Randomized controlled trial of a structured training program in breast cancer patients with tumor-related chronic fatigue. *Onkologie, 30,* 429–434. doi:10.1159/000104097

110. Korstjens, I., Mesters, I., van der Peet, E., Gijsen, B., & van den Borne, B. (2006). Quality of life of cancer survivors after physical and psychosocial rehabilitation. *European Journal of Cancer Prevention, 15,* 541–547. doi:10.1097/01.cej.0000220625.77857.95

111. Pinto, B.M., Papandonatos, G.D., Goldstein, M.G., Marcus, B.H., & Farrell, N. (2013). Home-based physical activity intervention for colorectal cancer survivors. *Psycho-Oncology, 22,* 54–64. doi:10.1002/pon.2047

112. Rabin, C., Pinto, B., Dunsiger, S., Nash, J., & Trask, P. (2009). Exercise and relaxation intervention for breast cancer survivors: Feasibility, acceptability and effects. *Psycho-Oncology, 18,* 258–266. doi:10.1002/pon.1341

113. Strauss-Blasche, G., Gnad, E., Ekmekcioglu, C., Hladschik, B., & Marktl, W. (2005). Combined inpatient rehabilitation and spa therapy for breast cancer patients: Effects on quality of life and CA15-3. *Cancer Nursing, 28,* 390–398. doi:10.1097/00002820-200509000-00009

114. van Weert, E., Hoekstra-Weebers, J., Otter, R., Postema, K., Sanderman, R., & van der Schans, C. (2006). Cancer-related fatigue: Predictors and effects of rehabilitation. *Oncologist, 11,* 184–196. doi:10.1634/theoncologist .11-2-184

115. van Weert, E., May, A.M., Korstjens, I., Post, W.J., van der Schans, C.P., van den Borne, B., ... Hoekstra-Weebers, J.E. (2010). Cancer-related fatigue and rehabilitation: A randomized controlled multicenter trial comparing physical training combined with cognitive-behavioral therapy with physical training only and with no intervention. *Physical Therapy, 90,* 1413–1425. doi:10.2522/ptj.20090212

116. Agteresch, H.J., Dagnelie, P.C., van der Gaast, A., Stijnen, T., & Wilson, J.H.P. (2000). Randomized clinical trial of adenosine 5'-triphosphate in patients with advanced non-small-cell lung cancer. *Journal of the National Cancer Institute, 92,* 321–328. doi:10.1093/jnci/92.4.321

117. Beijer, S., I lupperets, P.S., van den Borne, B.E., Wijckmans, N.E., Spreeu-wenberg, C., van den Brandt, P.A., & Dagnelie, P.C. (2010). Randomized clinical trial on the effects of adenosine 5'-triphosphate infusions on quality of life, functional status, and fatigue in preterminal cancer patients. *Journal of Pain and Symptom Management, 40,* 520–530. doi:10.1016/j.jpainsymman.2010.01.023

118. Cullum, J.L., Wojciechowski, A.E., Pelletier, G., & Simpson, J.S. (2004). Bupropion sustained release treatment reduces fatigue in cancer patients. *Canadian Journal of Psychiatry, 49,* 139–144. Retrieved from https://ww1.cpa-apc.org/Publications/Archives/CJP/2004/february/simpson.pdf

119. Moss, E.L., Simpson, J.S.A., Pelletier, G., & Forsyth, P. (2006). An open-label study of the effects of bupropion SR on fatigue, depression and quality of life of mixed-site cancer patients and their partners. *Psycho-Oncology, 15,* 259–267. doi:10.1002/pon.952

120. Lesser, G.J., Case, D., Stark, N., Williford, S., Giguere, J., Garino, L.A., … Shaw, E.G. (2013). A randomized, double-blind, placebo-controlled study of oral coenzyme Q_{10} to relieve self-reported treatment-related fatigue in newly diagnosed patients with breast cancer. *Journal of Supportive Oncology, 11,* 31–42. doi:10.1016/j.suponc.2012.03.003

121. Auret, K.A., Schug, S.A., Bremner, A.P., & Bulsara, M. (2009). A randomized, double-blind, placebo-controlled trial assessing the impact of dexamphetamine on fatigue in patients with advanced cancer. *Journal of Pain and Symptom Management, 37,* 613–621. doi:10.1016/j.jpainsymman.2008.03.016

122. Peuckmann-Post, V., Elsner, F., Krumm, N., Trottenberg, P., & Radbruch, L. (2010). Pharmacological treatments for fatigue associated with palliative care. *Cochrane Database of Systematic Reviews, 2010*(11). doi:10.1002/14651858.CD006788.pub2

123. Johnson, R.L., Block, I., Gold, M.A., Markwell, S., & Zupancic, M. (2010). Effect of methylphenidate on fatigue in women with recurrent gynecologic cancer. *Psycho-Oncology, 19,* 955–958. doi:10.1002/pon.1646

124. Lower, E.E., Fleishman, S., Cooper, A., Zeldis, J., Faleck, H., Yu, Z., & Manning, D. (2009). Efficacy of dexmethylphenidate for the treatment of fatigue after cancer chemotherapy: A randomized clinical trial. *Journal of Pain and Symptom Management, 38,* 650–662. doi:10.1016/j.jpainsymman.2009.03.011

125. Mar Fan, H., Clemons, M., Xu, W., Chemerynsky, I., Breunis, H., Braganza, S., & Tannock, I.F. (2008). A randomised, placebo-controlled, double-blind trial of the effects of d-methylphenidate on fatigue and cognitive dysfunction in women undergoing adjuvant chemotherapy for breast cancer. *Supportive Care in Cancer, 16,* 577–583. doi:10.1007/s00520-007-0341-9

126. Minton, O., Richardson, A., Sharpe, M., Hotopf, M., & Stone, P.C. (2011). Psychostimulants for the management of cancer-related fatigue: A systematic review and meta-analysis. *Journal of Pain and Symptom Management, 41,* 761–767. doi:10.1016/j.jpainsymman.2010.06.020

127. Roth, A.J., Nelson, C., Rosenfeld, B., Scher, H., Slovin, S., Morris, M., … Breitbart, W. (2010). Methylphenidate for fatigue in ambulatory men with prostate cancer. *Cancer, 116,* 5102–5110. doi:10.1002/cncr.25424

128. Sarhill, N., Walsh, D., Nelson, K.A., Homsi, J., LeGrand, S., & Davis, M.P. (2001). Methylphenidate for fatigue in advanced cancer: A prospective open-label pilot study. *American Journal of Hospice and Palliative Care, 18,* 187–192. doi:10.1177/104990910101800310

129. Schwartz, A.L., Thompson, J.A., & Masood, N. (2002). Interferon-induced fatigue in patients with melanoma: A pilot study of exercise and methylphenidate [Online exclusive]. *Oncology Nursing Forum, 29,* E85–E90. doi:10.1188/02.ONF.E85-E90

130. Sugawara, Y., Akechi, T., Shima, Y., Okuyana, T., Akizuki, N., Nakano, T., & Uchitomi, Y. (2002). Efficacy of methylphenidate for fatigue in advanced cancer patients: A preliminary study. *Palliative Medicine, 16,* 261–263. doi:10.1191/0269216302pm547xx

131. Moraska, A.R., Sood, A., Dakhil, S.R., Sloan, J.A., Barton, D., Atherton, P.J., ... Loprinzi, C.L. (2010). Phase III, randomized, double-blind, placebo-controlled study of long-acting methylphenidate for cancer-related fatigue: North Central Cancer Treatment Group NCCTG-N05C7 trial. *Journal of Clinical Oncology, 28,* 3673–3679. doi:10.1200/JCO.2010.28.1444

132. Capuron, L., Gumnick, J.F., Musselman, D.L., Lawson, D.H., Reemsnyder, A., Nemeroff, C.B., & Miller, A.H. (2002). Neurobehavioral effects of interferon-α in cancer patients: Phenomenology and paroxetine responsiveness of symptom dimensions. *Neuropsychopharmacology, 26,* 643–652. doi:10.1016/S0893-133X(01)00407-9

133. Morrow, G.R., Hickok, J.T., Roscoe, J.A., Raubertas, R.F., Andrews, P.L.R., Flynn, P.J., ... King, D.K. (2003). Differential effects of paroxetine on fatigue and depression: A randomized, double-blind trial from the University of Rochester Cancer Center Community Clinical Oncology Program. *Journal of Clinical Oncology, 21,* 4635–4641. doi:10.1200/JCO.2003.04.070

134. Roscoe, J.A., Morrow, G.R., Hickok, J.T., Mustian, K.M., Griggs, J.J., Matteson, S.E., ... Smith, D. (2005). Effect of paroxetine hydrochloride (Paxil) on fatigue and depression in breast cancer patients receiving chemotherapy. *Breast Cancer Research and Treatment, 89,* 243–249. doi:10.1007/s10549-004-2175-1

135. Stockler, M.R., O'Connell, R., Nowak, A.K., Goldstein, D., Turner, J., Wilcken, N.R.C., ... Simes, R.J. (2007). Effect of sertraline on symptoms and survival in patients with advanced cancer, but without major depression: A placebo-controlled double-blind randomised trial. *Lancet Oncology, 8,* 603–612. doi:10.1016/S1470-2045(07)70148-1

136. Torta, R., Siri, I., & Caldera, P. (2008). Sertraline effectiveness and safety in depressed oncological patients. *Supportive Care in Cancer, 16,* 83–91. doi:10.1007/s00520-007-0269-0

137. Tookman, A.J., Jones, C.L., DeWitte, M., & Lodge, P.J. (2008). Fatigue in patients with advanced cancer: A pilot study of an intervention with infliximab. *Supportive Care in Cancer, 16,* 1131–1140. doi:10.1007/s00520-008-0429-x

138. Wen, H.-S., Li, X., Cao, Y.-Z., Zhang, C.-C., Yang, F., Shi, Y.-M., & Peng, L.-M. (2012). Clinical studies on the treatment of cancer cachexia with megestrol acetate plus thalidomide. *Chemotherapy, 58,* 461–467. doi:10.1159/000346446

139. Kamath, J., Feinn, R., & Winokur, A. (2012). Thyrotropin-releasing hormone as a treatment for cancer-related fatigue: A randomized controlled study. *Supportive Care in Cancer, 20,* 1745–1753. doi:10.1007/s00520-011-1268-8

140. Carpenter, J.S., Storniolo, A.M., Johns, S., Monahan, P.O., Azzouz, F., Elam, J.L., ... Shelton, R.C. (2007). Randomized, double-blind, placebo-controlled crossover trials of venlafaxine for hot flashes after breast cancer. *Oncologist, 12,* 124–135. doi:10.1634/theoncologist.12-1-124

141. van den Berg, M., Visser, A., Schoolmeesters, A., Edelman, P., & van den Borne, B. (2006). Evaluation of haptotherapy for patients with cancer treated with chemotherapy at a day clinic. *Patient Education and Counseling, 60,* 336–343. doi:10.1016/j.pec.2005.10.012

142. Aghabati, N., Mohammadi, E., & Esmaiel, Z.P. (2010). The effect of therapeutic touch on pain and fatigue of cancer patients undergoing chemotherapy. *Evidence-Based Complementary and Alternative Medicine, 7,* 375–381. doi:10.1093/ecam/nen006

143. Danhauer, S.C., Tooze, J.A., Holder, P., Miller, C., & Jesse, M.T. (2008). Healing touch as a supportive intervention for adult acute leukemia patients:

A pilot investigation of effects on distress and symptoms. *Journal of the Society for Integrative Oncology, 6,* 89–97. Retrieved from http://www.ncbi.nlm.nih.gov/pmc/articles/PMC3891375

144. Jain, S., Pavlik, D., Distefan, J., Bruyere, R.L., Acer, J., Garcia, R., ... Mills, P.J. (2012). Complementary medicine for fatigue and cortisol variability in breast cancer survivors: A randomized controlled trial. *Cancer, 118,* 777–787. doi:10.1002/cncr.26345

145. Appling, S.E., Scarvalone, S., MacDonald, R., McBeth, M., & Helzlsouer, K.J. (2012). Fatigue in breast cancer survivors: The impact of a mind-body medicine intervention. *Oncology Nursing Forum, 39,* 278–286. doi:10.1188/12.ONF.278-286

146. Roscoe, J.A., Matteson, S.E., Mustian, K.M., Padmanaban, D., & Morrow, G.R. (2005). Treatment of radiotherapy-induced fatigue through a nonpharmacological approach. *Integrative Cancer Therapies, 4,* 8–13. doi:10.1177/1534735404273726

147. Chen, Z., Meng, Z., Milbury, K., Bei, W., Zhang, Y., Thornton, B., ... Cohen, L. (2013). Qigong improves quality of life in women undergoing radiotherapy for breast cancer: Results of a randomized controlled trial. *Cancer, 119,* 1690–1698. doi:10.1002/cncr.27904

148. Wyatt, G., Sikorskii, A., Rahbar, M.H., Victorson, D., & You, M. (2012). Health-related quality-of-life outcomes: A reflexology trial with patients with advanced-stage breast cancer. *Oncology Nursing Forum, 39,* 568–577. doi:10.1188/12.ONF.568-577

149. Tsang, K.L., Carlson, L.E., & Olson, K. (2007). Pilot crossover trial of Reiki versus rest for treating cancer-related fatigue. *Integrative Cancer Therapies, 6,* 25–35. doi:10.1177/1534735406298986

150. Decker, T.W., Cline-Elsen, J., & Gallagher, M. (1992). Relaxation therapy as an adjunct in radiation oncology. *Journal of Clinical Psychology, 48,* 388–393. doi:10.1002/1097-4679(199205)48:3<388::AID-JCLP2270480318>3.0.CO;2-O

151. Demiralp, M., Oflaz, F., & Komurcu, S. (2010). Effects of relaxation training on sleep quality and fatigue in patients with breast cancer undergoing adjuvant chemotherapy. *Journal of Clinical Nursing, 19,* 1073–1083. doi:10.1111/j.1365-2702.2009.03037.x

152. Hayama, Y., & Inoue, T. (2012). The effects of deep breathing on 'tension-anxiety' and fatigue in cancer patients undergoing adjuvant chemotherapy. *Complementary Therapies in Clinical Practice, 18,* 94–98. doi:10.1016/j.ctcp.2011.10.001

153. Menzies, V., & Jallo, N. (2011). Guided imagery as a treatment option for fatigue: A literature review. *Journal of Holistic Nursing, 29,* 279–286. doi:10.1177/0898010111412187

154. Serra, D., Parris, C.R., Carper, E., Homel, P., Fleishman, S.B., Harrison, L.B., & Chadha, M. (2012). Outcomes of guided imagery in patients receiving radiation therapy for breast cancer. *Clinical Journal of Oncology Nursing, 16,* 617–623. doi:10.1188/12.CJON.617-623

155. Kwekkeboom, K.L., Abbott-Anderson, K., & Wanta, B. (2010). Feasibility of a patient-controlled cognitive-behavioral intervention for pain, fatigue, and sleep disturbance in cancer [Online exclusive]. *Oncology Nursing Forum, 37,* E151–E159. doi:10.1188/10.ONF.E151-E159

156. Kwekkeboom, K.L., Cherwin, C.H., Lee, J.W., & Wanta, B. (2010). Mind-body treatments for the pain-fatigue-sleep disturbance symptom cluster in persons with cancer. *Journal of Pain and Symptom Management, 39,* 126–138. doi:10.1016/j.jpainsymman.2009.05.022

157. Bower, J.E., Garet, D., Sternlieb, B., Ganz, P.A., Irwin, M.R., Olmstead, R., & Greendale, G. (2012). Yoga for persistent fatigue in breast cancer survivors: A randomized controlled trial. *Cancer, 118,* 3766–3775. doi:10.1002/cncr.26702

158. Buffart, L.M., van Uffelen, J.G.Z., Riphagen, I.I., Brug, J., van Mechelen, W., Brown, W.J., & Chinapaw, M.J. (2012). Physical and psychosocial benefits of yoga in cancer patients and survivors, a systematic review

and meta-analysis of randomized controlled trials. *BMC Cancer, 12*, 559. doi:10.1186/1471-2407-12-559

159. Carson, J.W., Carson, K.M., Porter, L.S., Keefe, F.J., Shaw, H., & Miller, J.M. (2007). Yoga for women with metastatic breast cancer: Results from a pilot study. *Journal of Pain and Symptom Management, 33*, 331–341. doi:10.1016/j.jpainsymman.2006.08.009

160. Carson, J.W., Carson, K.M., Porter, L.S., Keefe, F.J., & Seewaldt, V.L. (2009). Yoga of Awareness program for menopausal symptoms in breast cancer survivors: Results from a randomized trial. *Supportive Care in Cancer, 17*, 1301–1309. doi:10.1007/s00520-009-0587-5

161. Cohen, L., Warneke, C., Fouladi, R.T., Rodriguez, M.A., & Chaoul-Reich, A. (2004). Psychological adjustment and sleep quality in a randomized trial of the effects of a Tibetan yoga intervention in patients with lymphoma. *Cancer, 100*, 2253–2260. doi:10.1002/cncr.20236

162. Dhruva, A., Miaskowski, C., Abrams, D., Acree, M., Cooper, B., Goodman, S., & Hecht, F.M. (2012). Yoga breathing for cancer chemotherapy-associated symptoms and quality of life: Results of a pilot randomized controlled trial. *Journal of Alternative and Complementary Medicine, 18*, 473–479. doi:10.1089/acm.2011.0555

163. Moadel, A.B., Shah, C., Wylie-Rosett, J., Harris, M.S., Patel, S.R., Hall, C.B., & Sparano, J.A. (2007). Randomized controlled trial of yoga among a multiethnic sample of breast cancer patients: Effects on quality of life. *Journal of Clinical Oncology, 25*, 4387–4395. doi:10.1200/JCO.2006.06.6027

164. Zhang, J., Yang, K.-H., Tian, J.-H., & Wang, C.-M. (2012). Effects of yoga on psychologic function and quality of life in women with breast cancer: A meta-analysis of randomized controlled trials. *Journal of Alternative and Complementary Medicine, 18*, 994–1002. doi:10.1089/acm.2011.0514

165. Harder, H., Parlour, L., & Jenkins, V. (2012). Randomised controlled trials of yoga interventions for women with breast cancer: A systematic literature review. *Supportive Care in Cancer, 20*, 3055–3064. doi:10.1007/s00520-012-1611-8

166. Armes, J., Chalder, T., Addington-Hall, J., Richardson, A., & Hotopf, M. (2007). A randomized controlled trial to evaluate the effectiveness of a brief, behaviorally oriented intervention for cancer-related fatigue. *Cancer, 110*, 1385–1395. doi:10.1002/cncr.22923

167. Dalton, J.A., Keefe, F.J., Carlson, J., & Youngblood, R. (2004). Tailoring cognitive behavioral treatment for cancer pain. *Pain Management Nursing, 5*, 3–18. doi:10.1016/S1524-9042(03)00027-4

168. Gielissen, M.F.M., Verhagen, S., Witjes, F., & Bleijenberg, G. (2006). Effects of cognitive behavior therapy in severely fatigued disease-free cancer patients compared with patients waiting for cognitive behavior therapy: A randomized controlled trial. *Journal of Clinical Oncology, 24*, 4882–4887. doi:10.1200/JCO.2006.06.8270

169. Goedendorp, M.M., Peters, M.E.W.J., Gielissen, M.F.M., Witjes, J.A., Leer, J.W., Verhagen, C.A.H.H.V.M., & Bleijenberg, G. (2010). Is increasing physical activity necessary to diminish fatigue during cancer treatment? Comparing cognitive behavior therapy and a brief nursing intervention with usual care in a multicenter randomized controlled trial. *Oncologist, 15*, 1122–1132. doi:10.1634/theoncologist.2010-0092

170. Lee, H., Lim, Y., Yoo, M.-S., & Kim, Y. (2011). Effects of a nurse-led cognitive-behavior therapy on fatigue and quality of life of patients with breast cancer undergoing radiotherapy: An exploratory study. *Cancer Nursing, 34*(6), E22–E30. doi:10.1097/NCC.0b013e31820d1734

171. Montgomery, G.H., Kangas, M., David, D., Hallquist, M.N., Green, S., Bovbjerg, D.H., & Schnur, J.B. (2009). Fatigue during breast cancer radiotherapy: An initial randomized study of cognitive-behavioral therapy plus hypnosis. *Health Psychology, 28*, 317–322. doi:10.1037/a0013582

172. Strong, V., Waters, R., Hibberd, C., Murray, G., Wall, L., Walker, J., … Sharpe, M. (2008). Management of depression for people with cancer

(SMaRT oncology 1), a randomised trial. *Lancet, 372,* 40–48. doi:10.1016/S0140-6736(08)60991-5

173. Lu, Q., Zheng, D., Young, L., Kagawa-Singer, M., & Loh, A. (2012). A pilot study of expressive writing intervention among Chinese-speaking breast cancer survivors. *Health Psychology, 31,* 548–551. doi:10.1037/a0026834

174. Mosher, C.E., Duhamel, K.N., Lam, J., Dickler, M., Li, Y., Massie, M.J., & Norton, L. (2012). Randomised trial of expressive writing for distressed metastatic breast cancer patients. *Psychology and Health, 27,* 88–100. doi:10.1080/08870446.2010.551212

175. Boesen, E.H., Ross, L., Frederiksen, K., Thomsen, B.L., Dahlstrøm, K., Schmidt, G., … Johansen, C. (2005). Psychoeducational intervention for patients with cutaneous malignant melanoma: A replication study. *Journal of Clinical Oncology, 23,* 1270–1277. doi:10.1200/JCO.2005.05.193

176. Courneya, K.S., Friedenreich, C.M., Sela, R.A., Quinney, H.A., Rhodes, R.E., & Handman, M.T. (2003). The group psychotherapy and home-based physical exercise (group-hope) trial in cancer survivors: Physical fitness and quality of life outcomes. *Psycho-Oncology, 12,* 357–374. doi:10.1002/pon.658

177. Jensen, M.B., & Hessov, I. (1997). Randomization to nutritional intervention at home did not improve postoperative function, fatigue or well-being. *British Journal of Surgery, 84,* 113–118. doi:10.1046/j.1365-2168.1997.02457.x

178. Mantovani, G., Macciò, A., Madeddu, C., Gramignano, G., Serpe, R., Massa, E., … Floris, C. (2008). Randomized phase III clinical trial of five different arms of treatment for patients with cancer cachexia: Interim results. *Nutrition, 24,* 305–313. doi:10.1016/j.nut.2007.12.010

179. Cerchietti, L.C.A., Navigante, A.H., Peluffo, G.D., Diament, M.J., Stillitani, I., Klein, S.A., & Cabalar, M.E. (2004). Effects of celecoxib, medroxyprogesterone, and dietary intervention on systemic syndromes in patients with advanced lung adenocarcinoma: A pilot study. *Journal of Pain and Symptom Management, 27,* 85–95. doi:10.1016/j.jpainsymman.2003.05.010

180. Mantovani, G., Macciò, A., Madeddu, C., Gramignano, G., Lusso, M.R., Serpe, R., … Deiana, L. (2006). A phase II study with antioxidants, both in the diet and supplemented, pharmaconutritional support, progestogen, and anti-cyclooxygenase-2 showing efficacy and safety in patients with cancer-related anorexia/cachexia and oxidative stress. *Cancer Epidemiology, Biomarkers and Prevention, 15,* 1030–1034. doi:10.1158/1055-9965.EPI-05-0538

181. Cruciani, R.A., Dvorkin, E., Homel, P., Culliney, B., Malamud, S., Shaiova, L., … Esteban-Cruciani, N. (2004). L-carnitine supplementation for the treatment of fatigue and depressed mood in cancer patients with carnitine deficiency: A preliminary analysis. *Annals of the New York Academy of Sciences, 1033,* 168–176. doi:10.1196/annals.1320.016

182. Cruciani, R.A., Dvorkin, E., Homel, P., Malamud, S., Culliney, B., Lapin, J., … Esteban-Cruciani, N. (2006). Safety, tolerability and symptom outcomes associated with L-carnitine supplementation in patients with cancer, fatigue, and carnitine deficiency: A phase I/II study. *Journal of Pain and Symptom Management, 32,* 551–559. doi:10.1016/j.jpainsymman.2006.09.001

183. Cruciani, R.A., Zhang, J.J., Manola, J., Cella, D., Ansari, B., & Fisch, M.J. (2012). L-carnitine supplementation for the management of fatigue in patients with cancer: An Eastern Cooperative Oncology Group phase III, randomized, double-blind, placebo-controlled trial. *Journal of Clinical Oncology, 30,* 3864–3869. doi:10.1200/JCO.2011.40.2180

184. Gramignano, G., Lusso, M.R., Madeddu, C., Massa, E., Serpe, R., Deiana, L., … Mantovani, G. (2006). Efficacy of l-carnitine administration on fatigue, nutritional status, oxidative stress, and related quality of life in 12 advanced cancer patients undergoing anticancer therapy. *Nutrition, 22,* 136–145. doi:10.1016/j.nut.2005.06.003

185. Graziano, F., Bisonni, R., Catalano, V., Silva, R., Rovidati, S., Mencarini, E., … Lai, V. (2002). Potential role of levocarnitine supplementation for the

treatment of chemotherapy-induced fatigue in non-anaemic cancer patients. *British Journal of Cancer, 86,* 1854–1857. doi:10.1038/sj.bjc.6600413

186. de Souza Fêde, Â.B., Bensi, C.G., Trufelli, D.C., de Oliveira Campos, M.P., Pecoroni, P.G., Ranzatti, R.P., ... del Glio, A. (2007). Multivitamins do not improve radiation therapy-related fatigue: Results of a double-blind randomized crossover trial. *American Journal of Clinical Oncology, 30,* 432–436. doi:10.1097/COC.0b013e31804b40d9

187. Yeom, C.H., Jung, G.C., & Song, K.J. (2007). Changes of terminal cancer patients' health-related quality of life after high dose vitamin C administration. *Journal of Korean Medical Science, 22,* 7–11. doi:10.3346/jkms.2007.22.1.7

188. Jeong, J.S., Ryu, B.H., Kim, J.S., Park, J.W., Choi, W.C., & Yoon, S.W. (2010). Bojungikki-tang for cancer-related fatigue: A pilot randomized clinical trial. *Integrative Cancer Therapies, 9,* 331–338. doi:10.1177/1534735410383170

189. Zhao, H., Zhang, Q., Zhao, L., Huang, X., Wang, J., & Kang, X. (2012). Spore powder of *Ganoderma lucidum* improves cancer-related fatigue in breast cancer patients undergoing endocrine therapy: A pilot clinical trial. *Evidence-Based Complementary and Alternative Medicine, 2012,* 809614. doi:10.1155/2012/809614

190. Zhang, M., Liu, X., Li, J., He, L., & Tripathy, D. (2009). Chinese medicinal herbs to treat the side-effects of chemotherapy in breast cancer patients. *Cochrane Database of Systematic Reviews, 2009*(1). doi:10.1002/14651858.CD004921.pub2

191. Barton, D.L., Soori, G.S., Bauer, B.A., Sloan, J.A., Johnson, P.A., Figueras, C., ... Loprinzi, C.L. (2010). Pilot study of *Panax quinquefolius* (American ginseng) to improve cancer-related fatigue: A randomized, double-blind, dose-finding evaluation: NCCTG trial N03CA. *Supportive Care in Cancer, 18,* 179–187. doi:10.1007/s00520-009-0642-2

192. da Costa Miranda, V., Trufelli, D.C., Santos, J., Campos, M.P., Nobuo, M., da Costa Miranda, M., ... del Glio, A. (2009). Effectiveness of guaraná (*Paullinia cupana*) for postradiation fatigue and depression: Results of a pilot double-blind randomized study. *Journal of Alternative and Complementary Medicine, 15,* 431–433. doi:10.1089/acm.2008.0324

193. de Oliveira Campos, M.P., Riechelmann, R., Martins, L.C., Hassan, B.J., Casa, F.B., & Del Glio, A. (2011). Guarana (*Paullinia cupana*) improves fatigue in breast cancer patients undergoing systemic chemotherapy. *Journal of Alternative and Complementary Medicine, 17,* 505–512. doi:10.1089/acm.2010.0571

194. Beuth, J., Schneider, B., & Schierholz, J.M. (2008). Impact of complementary treatment of breast cancer patients with standardized mistletoe extract during aftercare: A controlled multicontor comparative epidemiological cohort study. *Anticancer Research, 28,* 523–527. Retrieved from http://ar.iiarjournals.org/content/28/1B/523.long

195. Schumacher, K., Schneider, B., Reich, G., Stiefel, T., Stoll, G., Bock, P.R., ... Beuth, J. (2003). Influence of postoperative complementary treatment with lectin-standardized mistletoe extract on breast cancer patients. A controlled epidemiological multicentric retrolective cohort study. *Anticancer Research, 23,* 5081–5087.

196. Chen, H.-W., Lin, I.-H., Chen, Y.-J., Chang, K.-H., Wu, M.-H., Su, W.-H., ... Lai, Y.-L. (2012). A novel infusible botanically-derived drug, PG2, for cancer-related fatigue: A phase II double-blind, randomized placebo-controlled study. *Clinical and Investigative Medicine, 35,* E1–E11. Retrieved from http://cimonline.ca/index.php/cim/article/view/16100/13111

197. Barton, D.L., Atherton, P.J., Bauer, B.A., Moore, D.F., Jr., Mattar, B.I., Lavasseur, B.I., ... Loprinzi, C.L. (2011). The use of *Valeriana officinalis* (valerian) in improving sleep in patients who are undergoing treatment for cancer: A phase III randomized, placebo-controlled, double-blind study (NCCTG Trial, N01C5). *Journal of Supportive Oncology, 9,* 24–31. doi:10.1016/j.suponc.2010.12.008

198. Balk, J., Day, R., Rosenzweig, M., & Beriwal, S. (2009). Pilot, randomized, modified, double-blind, placebo-controlled trial of acupuncture for

cancer-related fatigue. *Journal of the Society for Integrative Oncology, 7,* 4–11. Retrieved from https://www.integrativeonc.org/index.php/component/dropbox/?view=dropbox&id=7

199. Deng, G., Chan, Y., Sjoberg, D., Vickers, A., Yeung, K.S., Kris, M., ... Cassileth, B. (2013). Acupuncture for the treatment of post-chemotherapy chronic fatigue: A randomized, blinded, sham-controlled trial. *Supportive Care in Cancer, 21,* 1735–1741. doi:10.1007/s00520-013-1720-z

200. Johnston, M.F., Hays, R.D., Subramanian, S.K., Elashoff, R.M., Axe, E.K., Li, J.J., ... Hui, K.K. (2011). Patient education integrated with acupuncture for relief of cancer-related fatigue randomized controlled feasibility study. *BMC Complementary and Alternative Medicine, 11,* 49. doi:10.1186/1472-6882-11-49

201. Molassiotis, A., Bardy, J., Finnegan-John, J., Mackereth, P., Ryder, D.W., Filshie, J., ... Richardson, A. (2012). Acupuncture for cancer-related fatigue in patients with breast cancer: A pragmatic randomized controlled trial. *Journal of Clinical Oncology, 30,* 4470–4476. doi:10.1200/JCO.2012.41.6222

202. Molassiotis, A., Sylt, P., & Diggins, H. (2007). The management of cancer-related fatigue after chemotherapy with acupuncture and acupressure: A randomised controlled trial. *Complementary Therapies in Medicine, 15,* 228–237. doi:10.1016/j.ctim.2006.09.009

203. Molassiotis, A., Bardy, J., Finnegan-John, J., Mackereth, P., Ryder, W.D., Filshie, J., ... Richardson, A. (2013). A randomized, controlled trial of acupuncture self-needling as maintenance therapy for cancer-related fatigue after therapist-delivered acupuncture. *Annals of Oncology, 24,* 1645–1652. doi:10.1093/annonc/mdt034

204. Robertshawe, P. (2008). Cancer-related fatigue managed with acupuncture and acupressure. *Journal of the Australian Traditional-Medicine Society, 14,* 229. Retrieved from http://www.highbeam.com/doc/1G1-222679405.html

205. Smith, C., Carmady, B., Thornton, C., Perz, J., & Ussher, J.M. (2013). The effect of acupuncture on post-cancer fatigue and well-being for women recovering from breast cancer: A pilot randomised controlled trial. *Acupuncture in Medicine, 31,* 9–15. doi:10.1136/acupmed-2012-010228

206. Vickers, A.J., Straus, D.J., Fearon, B., & Cassileth, B.R. (2004). Acupuncture for postchemotherapy fatigue: A phase II study. *Journal of Clinical Oncology, 22,* 1731–1735. doi:10.1200/JCO.2004.04.102

207. Gadsby, J.G., Franks, A., Jarvis, P., & Dewhurst, F. (1997). Acupuncture-like transcutaneous electrical nerve stimulation in palliative care: A pilot study. *Complementary Therapies in Medicine, 5,* 13–18. doi:10.1016/S0965-2299(97)80084-2

208. Lee, E.J., & Frazier, S.K. (2011). The efficacy of acupressure for symptom management: A systematic review. *Journal of Pain and Symptom Management, 42,* 589–603. doi:10.1016/j.jpainsymman.2011.01.007

209. Finnegan-John, J., Molassiotis, A., Richardson, A., & Ream, E. (2013). A systematic review of complementary and alternative medicine interventions for the management of cancer-related fatigue. *Integrative Cancer Therapies, 12,* 276–290. doi:10.1177/1534735413485816

210. Garcia, M.K., McQuade, J., Haddad, R., Patel, S., Lee, R., Yang, P., ... Cohen, L. (2013). Systematic review of acupuncture in cancer care: A synthesis of the evidence. *Journal of Clinical Oncology, 31,* 952–960. doi:10.1200/JCO.2012.43.5818

211. Posadzki, P., Moon, T.-W., Choi, T.-Y., Park, T.-Y., Lee, M.S., & Ernst, E. (2013). Acupuncture for cancer-related fatigue: A systematic review of randomized clinical trials. *Supportive Care in Cancer, 21,* 2067–2073. doi:10.1007/s00520-013-1765-z

212. He, X.R., Wang, Q., & Li, P.P. (2013). Acupuncture and moxibustion for cancer-related fatigue: A systematic review and meta-analysis. *Asian Pacific Journal of Cancer Prevention, 14,* 3067–3074. doi:10.7314/APJCP.2013.14.5.3067

213. Johnson, R.A., Meadows, R.L., Haubner, J.S., & Sevedge, K. (2008). Animal-assisted activity among patients with cancer: Effects on mood,

fatigue, self-perceived health, and sense of coherence. *Oncology Nursing Forum, 35,* 225–232. doi:10.1188/08.ONF.225-232

214. Bar-Sela, G., Atid, L., Danos, S., Gabay, N., & Epelbaum, R. (2007). Art therapy improved depression and influenced fatigue levels in cancer patients on chemotherapy. *Psycho-Oncology, 16,* 980–984. doi:10.1002/pon.1175

215. Lyon, D.E., Schubert, C., & Taylor, A.G. (2010). Pilot study of cranial stimulation for symptom management in breast cancer. *Oncology Nursing Forum, 37,* 476–483. doi:10.1188/10.ONF.476-483

216. Alvarez, J., Meyer, F.L., Granoff, D.L., & Lundy, A. (2013). The effect of EEG biofeedback on reducing postcancer cognitive impairment. *Integrative Cancer Therapies, 12,* 475–487. doi:10.1177/1534735413477192

217. Ancoli-Israel, S., Rissling, M., Neikrug, A., Trofimenko, V., Natarajan, L., Parker, B.A., … Liu, L. (2012). Light treatment prevents fatigue in women undergoing chemotherapy for breast cancer. *Supportive Care in Cancer, 20,* 1211–1219. doi:10.1007/s00520-011-1203-z

218. Bozcuk, H., Artac, M., Kara, A., Ozdogan, M., Sualp, Y., Topcu, Z., … Savas, B. (2006). Does music exposure during chemotherapy improve quality of life in early breast cancer patients? A pilot study. *Medical Science Monitor, 12,* 200–205. Retrieved from http://www.medscimonit.com/download/index/idArt/450288

219. Burns, D.S., Azzouz, F., Sledge, R., Rutledge, C., Hincher, K., Monahan, P.O., & Cripe, L.D. (2008). Music imagery for adults with acute leukemia in protective environments: A feasibility study. *Supportive Care in Cancer, 16,* 507–513. doi:10.1007/s00520-007-0330-z

220. Chuang, C.-Y., Han, W.-R., Li, P.-C., & Young, S.-T. (2010). Effects of music therapy on subjective sensations and heart rate variability in treated cancer survivors: A pilot study. *Complementary Therapies in Medicine, 18,* 224–226. doi:10.1016/j.ctim.2010.08.003

221. Clark, M., Isaacks-Downton, G., Wells, N., Redlin-Grazier, S., Eck, C., Hepworth, J.T., & Chakravarthy, B. (2006). Use of preferred music to reduce emotional distress and symptom activity during radiation therapy. *Journal of Music Therapy, 43,* 247–265. doi:10.1093/jmt/43.3.247

222. Bradt, J., Dileo, C., Grocke, D., & Magill, L. (2011). Music interventions for improving psychological and physical outcomes in cancer patients. *Cochrane Database of Systematic Reviews, 2011*(8). doi:10.1002/14651858.CD006911.pub2

223. Oyama, H., Kaneda, M., Katsumata, N., Akechi, T., & Ohsuga, M. (2000). Using the bedside wellness system during chemotherapy decreases fatigue and emesis in cancer patients. *Journal of Medical Systems, 24,* 173–182. doi:10.1023/A:1005591626518

224. Oyama, H., Ohsuga, M., Tatsuno, Y., & Katsumata, H. (1999). Evaluation of the psycho-oncological effectiveness of the bedside wellness system. *CyberPsychology and Behavior, 2,* 81–84. doi:10.1089/cpb.1999.2.81

225. Schneider, S.M., Ellis, M., Coombs, W.T., Shonkwiler, E.L., & Folsom, L.C. (2003). Virtual reality intervention for older women with breast cancer. *CyberPsychology and Behavior, 6,* 301–307. doi:10.1089/109493103322011605

226. Schneider, S.M., & Hood, L.E. (2007). Virtual reality: A distraction intervention for chemotherapy. *Oncology Nursing Forum, 34,* 39–46. doi:10.1188/07.ONF.39-46

227. Schneider, S.M., Prince-Paul, M., Allen, M.J., Silverman, P., & Talaba, D. (2004). Virtual reality as a distraction intervention for women receiving chemotherapy. *Oncology Nursing Forum, 31,* 81–88. doi:10.1188/04.ONF.81-88

12

Hot Flashes

Lee Ann Johnson, PhD(c), RN,
Dale Grimmer, RN, MS, AOCN®, CCRC,
and Maria Paz Fernandez-Ortega, PhD(c), RN

Problem and Incidence

Hot flashes are intense heat sensations, flushing, and diaphoresis that generally involve the face and trunk.[1] Hot flashes and night sweats have been reported in 65%–80% of breast cancer survivors[2,3] and in 34%–80% of men with prostate cancer who have received androgen deprivation or ablation therapy.[4] Many men have reported hot flashes as the most troublesome adverse treatment effect.[4]

Chemotherapy and endocrine treatments can induce or exacerbate these symptoms in breast cancer survivors, who report more frequent and severe symptoms than menopausal women without cancer.[5] Symptoms may be problematic enough to lead patients with breast cancer to discontinue endocrine therapy, despite its role in reducing the risk of cancer recurrence.[6]

Hot flashes can range from mild to severe, with skin color changes from pink to deep red. Some patients may experience multiple hot flashes daily, with significant negative effects on social functioning and quality of life. Hot flashes can occur as part of a symptom cluster including fatigue and sleep disturbances.[3,7]

Risk Factors and Assessment

Individuals with cancer at highest risk for hot flashes include
- Women with breast cancer receiving aromatase inhibitors or tamoxifen

- Men with prostate cancer receiving androgen deprivation or ablation treatment
- Women with treatment-induced ovarian disruption or damage.

Assessment includes frequency, duration, and intensity of hot flash symptoms and associated sleep disruption and fatigue. The perceived degree of hot flash interference with daily life is an important and useful component of assessment.[8]

Assessment tools include
- National Cancer Institute Cancer Therapy Evaluation Program *Common Terminology Criteria for Adverse Events* hot flash scale (open access)[9]
- Hot flash diary
- Hot Flash Related Daily Interference Scale.[10]

What interventions are effective in managing hot flashes in people with cancer?

Evidence retrieved through May 31, 2013

Likely to Be Effective

Gabapentin reduced hot flashes in men with prostate cancer[4,11,12] and women with breast cancer.[13-17]

Venlafaxine reduced hot flashes in women with breast cancer.[14,18-23]

Benefits Balanced With Harms

Paroxetine[24,25]—This is a strong CYP2D6 inhibitor and should be used with caution in women with breast cancer who are taking tamoxifen, a drug metabolized to its active form through the CYP2D6 enzyme system.[26]

Effectiveness Not Established

Several medical, pharmacologic, and nonpharmacologic interventions have been studied for hot flashes. The strength of this evidence is limited because of small samples, other study design limitations, or mixed findings regarding effectiveness.

- Pharmacologic and medical interventions
  - Clonidine[4,17,21,23,27-29]
  - Cyproterone acetate in men[4,20]
  - Estrogen replacement in men on hormonal therapy[30]
  - Fluoxetine[31]
  - Magnesium[32]
  - Mirtazapine[33]
  - Progestins, megestrol and medroxyprogesterone, in men with prostate cancer and women with breast cancer[4,20,34-36]—There are concerns about the potential effects of progestins in women with a history of breast cancer.
  - Sertraline[37,38]
  - Stellate ganglion block[39,40]—Hot flashes returned over time.[39]
  - Testosterone replacement after treatment for prostate cancer[41]
  - Zolpidem with venlafaxine and selective serotonin reuptake inhibitors[42]
- Nonpharmacologic and complementary and alternative interventions
  - Acupuncture[43-55]—A meta-analysis did not show an effect, and it was noted that all studies had high risk of bias.[56]
  - Black cohosh[57-60]
  - Cognitive behavioral interventions[61-63]
  - Hypnosis/hypnotherapy[64-66]
  - Peer counseling[67]
  - Relaxation therapy[68]
  - *Salvia officinalis* (sage)[69]
  - Vitamin E[13,70]—A systematic review concluded vitamin E supplements were not effective.[17]
  - Yoga[71]

Effectiveness Unlikely

Homeopathic interventions showed no consistent benefit, and studies had multiple limitations.[72-74]

Soy did not affect hot flashes in women with breast cancer[75-78] or men with prostate cancer.[79]

Not Recommended for Practice

Tibolone did not show consistent benefit for breast cancer survivors.[80,81] It has been reported to increase the risk of breast cancer recurrence.[82]

Expert Opinion

Some lifestyle behaviors may reduce symptoms.[83]
- Triggers for hot flashes may include caffeine, smoking, and alcohol. Reducing use of these triggers may be of benefit.
- Dressing in layers, use of cotton clothing and bedding, strategic placement of electric fans, and drinking cold beverages may reduce symptoms.
- Reusable cooling bandanas soaked in cold water for 10–30 minutes and tied around the neck may be beneficial.
- Stress reduction behaviors may be helpful.

Application to Practice

Patients at risk should be assessed for hot flashes. Hot flash interference can be a practical way to determine symptom severity.

Nurses can advocate for the use of pharmacologic interventions with demonstrated efficacy in appropriate patients.

Nurses can assist patients to identify triggers or factors that may affect the experience of hot flashes and educate patients regarding behavior changes that might be helpful.

Hot Flashes Resource Contributors

Topic leader: Janet Carpenter, PhD, RN, FAAN
Elizabeth Abernathy, RN, MSN, AOCNS®, Maria Paz Fernandez-Ortega, PhD(c), RN, Jacqueline Foster, RN, OCN®, MPH, and Dale Grimmer, RN, MS, AOCN®, CCRC
Reviewer: Marcelle Kaplan, RN, MS, AOCN®, CBCN®

References

1. Jones, J.M., Kohli, M., & Loprinzi, C.L. (2012). Androgen deprivation therapy-associated vasomotor symptoms. *Asian Journal of Andrology, 14,* 193–197. doi:10.1038/aja.2011.101

2. Kontos, M., Agbaje, O.F., Rymer, J., & Fentiman, I.S. (2010). What can be done about hot flushes after treatment for breast cancer? *Climacteric, 13,* 4–21. doi:10.3109/13697130903291058

3. Mann, E., Smith, M., Hellier, J., & Hunter, M. (2011). A randomised controlled trial of a cognitive behavioural intervention for women who have menopausal symptoms following breast cancer treatment (MENOS 1): Trial protocol. *BMC Cancer, 11,* 44. doi:10.1186/1471-2407-11-44

4. Frisk, J. (2010). Managing hot flushes in men after prostate cancer—A systematic review. *Maturitas, 65,* 15–22. doi:10.1016/j.maturitas.2009.10.017

5. Carpenter, J.S., Wu, M.J., Burns, D.S., & Yu, M. (2012). Perceived control and hot flashes in treatment-seeking breast cancer survivors and menopausal women. *Cancer Nursing, 35,* 195–202. doi:10.1097/NCC.0b013e31822e78eb

6. Hickey, M., Emery, L.I., Gregson, J., Doherty, D.A., & Saunders, C.M. (2010). The multidisciplinary management of menopausal symptoms after breast cancer: A unique model of care. *Menopause, 17,* 727–733. doi:10.1097/gme.0b013e3181d672f6

7. Balabanovic, J., Ayers, B., & Hunter, M.S. (2012). Women's experiences of group cognitive behaviour therapy for hot flushes and night sweats following breast cancer treatment: An interpretative phenomenological analysis. *Maturitas, 72,* 236–242. doi:10.1016/j.maturitas.2012.03.013

8. Rand, K.L., Otte, J.L., Flockhart, D., Hayes, D., Storniolo, A.M., Stearns, V., ... Carpenter, J.S. (2011). Modeling hot flushes and quality of life in breast cancer survivors. *Climacteric, 14,* 171–180. doi:10.3109/13697131003717070

9. National Cancer Institute Cancer Therapy Evaluation Program. (2010, June 14). *Common terminology ctiteria for adverse events* [v.4.03]. Retrieved from http://evs.nci.nih.gov/ftp1/CTCAE/CTCAE_4.03_2010-06-14_QuickReference_5x7.pdf

10. Carpenter, J.S. (2001). The Hot Flash Related Daily Interference Scale: A tool for assessing the impact of hot flashes on quality of life following breast cancer. *Journal of Pain and Symptom Management, 22,* 979–989. doi:10.1016/S0885-3924(01)00353-0

11. Loprinzi, C.L., Sloan, J., Stearns, V., Slack, R., Iyengar, M., Diekmann, B., ... Novotny, P. (2009). Newer antidepressants and gabapentin for hot

flashes: An individual patient pooled analysis. *Journal of Clinical Oncology, 27*, 2831–2837. doi:10.1200/JCO.2008.19.6253

12. Moraska, A.R., Atherton, P.J., Szydlo, D.W., Barton, D.L., Stella, P.J., Rowland, K.M., Jr., ... Loprinzi, C.L. (2010). Gabapentin for the management of hot flashes in prostate cancer survivors: A longitudinal continuation study—NCCTG Trial N00CB. *Journal of Supportive Oncology, 8*, 128–132. Retrieved from http://www.ncbi.nlm.nih.gov/pmc/articles/PMC3075822

13. Biglia, N., Sgandurra, P., Peano, E., Marenco, D., Moggio, G., Bounous, V., ... Sismondi, P. (2009). Non-hormonal treatment of hot flushes in breast cancer survivors: Gabapentin vs. vitamin E. *Climacteric, 12*, 310–318. doi:10.1080/13697130902736921

14. Bordeleau, L., Pritchard, K.I., Loprinzi, C.L., Ennis, M., Jugovic, O., Warr, D., ... Goodwin, P.J. (2010). Multicenter, randomized, cross-over clinical trial of venlafaxine versus gabapentin for the management of hot flashes in breast cancer survivors. *Journal of Clinical Oncology, 28*, 5147–5152. doi:10.1200/JCO.2010.29.9230

15. Loprinzi, C.L., Kugler, J.W., Barton, D.L., Dueck, A.C., Tschetter, L.K., Nelimark, R.A., ... Jaslowski, A.J. (2007). Phase III trial of gabapentin alone or in conjunction with an antidepressant in the management of hot flashes in women who have inadequate control with an antidepressant alone. *Journal of Clinical Oncology, 25*, 308–312. doi:10.1200/JCO.2006.07.5390

16. Pandya, K.J., Morrow, G.R., Roscoe, J.A., Zhao, H., Hickok, J.T., Pajon, E., ... Flynn, P.J. (2005). Gabapentin for hot flashes in 420 women with breast cancer: A randomised double-blind placebo-controlled trial. *Lancet, 366*, 818–824. doi:10.1016/S0140-6736(05)67215-7

17. Rada, G., Capurro, D., Pantoja, T., Corbalán, J., Moreno, G., Letelier, L.M., & Vera, C. (2010). Non-hormonal interventions for hot flushes in women with a history of breast cancer. *Cochrane Database of Systematic Reviews, 2010*(9). doi:10.1002/14651858.CD004923.pub2

18. Biglia, N., Torta, R., Roagna, R., Maggiorotto, F., Cacciari, F., Ponzone, R., ... Sismondi, P. (2005). Evaluation of low-dose venlafaxine hydrochloride for the therapy of hot flushes in breast cancer survivors. *Maturitas, 52*, 78–85. doi:10.1016/j.maturitas.2005.01.001

19. Carpenter, J.S., Storniolo, A.M., Johns, S., Monahan, P.O., Azzouz, F., Elam, J.L., ... Shelton, R.C. (2007). Randomized, double-blind, placebo-controlled crossover trials of venlafaxine for hot flashes after breast cancer. *Oncologist, 12*, 124–135. doi:10.1634/theoncologist.12-1-124

20. Irani, J., Salomon, L., Oba, R., Bouchard, P., & Mottet, N. (2010). Efficacy of venlafaxine, medroxyprogesterone acetate, and cyproterone acetate for the treatment of vasomotor hot flushes in men taking gonadotropin-releasing hormone analogues for prostate cancer: A double-blind, randomised trial. *Lancet Oncology, 11*, 147–154. doi:10.1016/S1470-2045(09)70338-9

21. Loibl, S., Schwedler, K., von Minckwitz, G., Strohmeier, R., Mehta, K.M., & Kaufmann, M. (2007). Venlafaxine is superior to clonidine as treatment of hot flashes in breast cancer patients—A double-blind, randomized study. *Annals of Oncology, 18*, 689–693. doi:10.1093/annonc/mdl478

22. Loprinzi, C.L., Kugler, J.W., Sloan, J.A., Mailliard, J.A., LaVasseur, B.I., Barton, D.L., ... Christensen, B.J. (2000). Venlafaxine in management of hot flashes in survivors of breast cancer: A randomised controlled trial. *Lancet, 356*, 2059–2063. doi:10.1016/S0140-6736(00)03403-6

23. Boekhout, A.H., Vincent, A.D., Dalesio, O.B., van den Bosch, J., Foekema-Tons, J.H., Adriaansz, S., ... Schellens, J.H. (2011). Management of hot flashes in patients who have breast cancer with venlafaxine and clonidine: A randomized, double-blind, placebo-controlled trial. *Journal of Clinical Oncology, 29*, 3862–3868. doi:10.1200/JCO.2010.33.1298

24. Kelly, C.M., Juurlink, D.N., Gomes, T., Duong-Hua, M., Pritchard, K., Austin, P., & Paszat, L. (2010). Selective serotonin reuptake inhibitors and breast cancer mortality in women receiving tamoxifen: A population based cohort study. *BMJ, 340*, c693. doi:10.1136/bmj.c693

25. Stearns, V., Slack, R., Greep, N., Henry-Tilman, R., Osborne, M., Bunnoll, C., … Isaacs, C. (2005). Paroxetine is an effective treatment for hot flashes: Results from a prospective randomized clinical trial. *Journal of Clinical Oncology, 23,* 6919–6930. doi:10.1200/JCO.2005.10.081

26. National Comprehensive Cancer Network. (2013). *NCCN Clinical Practice Guidelines in Oncology: Breast cancer* [v.3.2013]. Retrieved from http://www.nccn.org/professionals/physician_gls/pdf/breast.pdf

27. Buijs, C., Mom, C.H., Willemse, P.H., Marike Boezen, H., Maurer, J.M., Wymenga, A.N., … Mourits, M.J. (2009). Venlafaxine versus clonidine for the treatment of hot flashes in breast cancer patients: A double-blind, randomized cross-over study. *Breast Cancer Research and Treatment, 115,* 573–580. doi:10.1007/s10549-008-0138-7

28. Goldberg, R.M., Loprinzi, C.L., O'Fallon, J.R., Veeder, M.H., Miser, A.W., Mailliard, J.A., … Burnham, N.L. (1994). Transdermal clonidine for ameliorating tamoxifen-induced hot flashes. *Journal of Clinical Oncology, 12,* 155–158. Retrieved from http://jco.ascopubs.org/content/12/1/155.long

29. Pandya, K.J., Raubertas, R.F., Flynn, P.J., Hynes, H.E., Rosenbluth, R.J., Kirshner, J., … Morrow, G.R. (2000). Oral clonidine in postmenopausal patients with breast cancer experiencing tamoxifen-induced hot flashes: A University of Rochester Cancer Center Community Clinical Oncology Program study. *Annals of Internal Medicine, 132,* 788–793. doi:10.7326/0003-4819-132-10-200005160-00004

30. Gerber, G.S., Zagaja, G.P., Ray, P.S., & Rukstalis, D.B. (2000). Transdermal estrogen in the treatment of hot flushes in men with prostate cancer. *Urology, 55,* 97–101. doi:10.1016/S0090-4295(99)00370-2

31. Loprinzi, C.L., Sloan, J.A., Perez, E.A., Quella, S.K., Stella, P.J., Mailliard, J.A., … Rummans, T.A. (2002). Phase III evaluation of fluoxetine for treatment of hot flashes. *Journal of Clinical Oncology, 20,* 1578–1583. doi:10.1200/JCO.20.6.1578

32. Park, H., Parker, G.L., Boardman, C.H., Morris, M.M., & Smith, T.J. (2011). A pilot phase II trial of magnesium supplements to reduce menopausal hot flashes in breast cancer patients. *Supportive Care in Cancer, 19,* 859–863. doi:10.1007/s00520-011-1099-7

33. Biglia, N., Kubatzki, F., Sgandurra, P., Ponzone, R., Marenco, D., Peano, E., & Sismondi, P. (2007). Mirtazapine for the treatment of hot flushes in breast cancer survivors: A prospective pilot trial. *Breast Journal, 13,* 490–495. doi:10.1111/j.1524-4741.2007.00470.x

34. Bertelli, G., Venturini, M., Del Mastro, L., Bergaglio, M., Sismondi, P., Biglia, N., … Rosso, R. (2002). Intramuscular depot medroxyprogesterone versus oral megestrol for the control of postmenopausal hot flashes in breast cancer patients: A randomized study. *Annals of Oncology, 13,* 883–888. doi:10.1093/annonc/mdf151

35. Goodwin, J.W., Green, S.J., Moinpour, C.M., Bearden, J.D., III, Giguere, J.K., Jiang, C.S., … Albain, K.S. (2008). Phase III randomized placebo-controlled trial of two doses of megestrol acetate as treatment for menopausal symptoms in women with breast cancer: Southwest Oncology Group Study 9626. *Journal of Clinical Oncology, 26,* 1650–1656. doi:10.1200/JCO.2006.10.6179

36. Loprinzi, C.L., Michalak, J.C., Quella, S.K., O'Fallon, J.R., Hatfield, A.K., Nelimark, R.A., … Oesterling, J.E. (1994). Megestrol acetate for the prevention of hot flashes. *New England Journal of Medicine, 331,* 347–352. doi:10.1056/NEJM199408113310602

37. Kimmick, G.G., Lovato, J., McQuellon, R., Robinson, E., & Hyman, B.M. (2006). Randomized double-blind, placebo-controlled, crossover study of sertraline (Zoloft) for the treatment of hot flashes in women with early stage breast cancer taking tamoxifen. *Breast Journal, 12,* 114–122. doi:10.1111/j.1075-122X.2006.00218.x

38. Wu, M.F., Hilsenbeck, S.G., Tham, Y.L., Kramer, R., Elledge, R.M., Chang, J.C., & Friedman, L.C. (2009). The efficacy of sertraline for controlling hot flashes in women with or at high risk of developing breast cancer.

Breast Cancer Research and Treatment, 118, 369–375. doi:10.1007/
s10549-009-0425-y

39. Haest, K., Kumar, A., Van Calster, B., Leunen, K., Smeets, A., Amant, F.,
... Neven, P. (2012). Stellate ganglion block for the management of hot
flashes and sleep disturbances in breast cancer survivors: An uncontrolled
experimental study with 24 weeks of follow-up. *Annals of Oncology, 23,*
1449–1454. doi:10.1093/annonc/mdr478

40. Lipov, E.G., Joshi, J.R., Sanders, S., Wilcox, K., Lipov, S., Xie, H., ...
Slavin, K. (2008). Effects of stellate-ganglion block on hot flushes and night
awakenings in survivors of breast cancer: A pilot study. *Lancet Oncology,
9,* 523–532. doi:10.1016/S1470-2045(08)70131-1

41. Agarwal, P.K., & Oefelein, M.G. (2005). Testosterone replacement therapy after primary treatment for prostate cancer. *Journal of Urology, 173,*
533–536. doi:10.1097/01.ju.0000143942.55896.64

42. Joffe, H., Partridge, A., Giobbie-Hurder, A., Li, X., Habin, K., Goss, P., ...
Garber, J. (2010). Augmentation of venlafaxine and selective serotonin
reuptake inhibitors with zolpidem improves sleep and quality of life in breast
cancer patients with hot flushes: A randomized, double-blind, placebo-
controlled trial. *Menopause, 17,* 908–916. doi:10.1097/gme.0b013e3181dbee1b

43. Ashamalla, H., Jiang, M.L., Guirguis, A., Peluso, F., & Ashamalla, M. (2011).
Acupuncture for the alleviation of hot flashes in men treated with androgen
ablation therapy. *International Journal of Radiation Oncology, Biology,
Physics, 79,* 1358–1363. doi:10.1016/j.ijrobp.2010.01.025

44. Beer, T.M., Benavides, M., Emmons, S.L., Hayes, M., Liu, G., Garzotto, M.,
... Eilers, K. (2010). Acupuncture for hot flashes in patients with prostate
cancer. *Urology, 76,* 1182–1188. doi:10.1016/j.urology.2010.03.033

45. de Valois, B.A., Young, T.E., Robinson, N., McCourt, C., & Maher, E.J.
(2010). Using traditional acupuncture for breast cancer-related hot flashes
and night sweats. *Journal of Alternative and Complementary Medicine, 16,*
1047–1057. doi:10.1089/acm.2009.0472

46. Deng, G., Vickers, A., Yeung, S., D'Andrea, G.M., Xiao, H., Heerdt, A.S.,
... Cassileth, B. (2007). Randomized, controlled trial of acupuncture for
the treatment of hot flashes in breast cancer patients. *Journal of Clinical
Oncology, 25,* 5584–5590. doi:10.1200/JCO.2007.12.0774

47. Filshie, J., Bolton, T., Browne, D., & Ashley, S. (2005). Acupuncture and
self acupuncture for long-term treatment of vasomotor symptoms in cancer
patients—Audit and treatment algorithm. *Acupuncture in Medicine, 23,*
171–180. doi:10.1136/aim.23.4.171

48. Frisk, J., Carlhall, S., Kallstrom, A.C., Lindh-Astrand, L., Malmstrom, A.,
& Hammar, M. (2008). Long-term follow-up of acupuncture and hormone
therapy on hot flushes in women with breast cancer: A prospective,
randomized, controlled multicenter trial. *Climacteric, 11,* 166–174.
doi:10.1080/13697130801958709

49. Frisk, J., Kallstrom, A.C., Wall, N., Fredrikson, M., & Hammar, M. (2012).
Acupuncture improves health-related quality-of-life (HRQoL) and sleep in
women with breast cancer and hot flushes. *Supportive Care in Cancer, 20,*
715–724. doi:10.1007/s00520-011-1134-8

50. Hammar, M., Frisk, J., Grimås, O., Höök, M., Spetz, A.C., & Wyon, Y. (1999).
Acupuncture treatment of vasomotor symptoms in men with prostatic
carcinoma: A pilot study. *Journal of Urology, 161,* 853–856. doi:10.1016/
S0022-5347(01)61789-0

51. Harding, C., Harris, A., & Chadwick, D. (2008). Auricular acupuncture: A novel
treatment for vasomotor symptoms associated with luteinizing-hormone
releasing hormone agonist treatment for prostate cancer. *BJU International,
103,* 186–190. doi:10.1111/j.1464-410X.2008.07884.x

52. Hervik, J., & Mjåland, J. (2009). Acupuncture for the treatment of hot flashes
in breast cancer patients, a randomized, controlled trial. *Breast Cancer
Research and Treatment, 116,* 311–316. doi:10.1007/s10549-008-0210-3

53. Liljegren, A., Gunnarsson, P., Landgren, B.M., Robeus, N., Johansson, H.,
& Rotstein, S. (2012). Reducing vasomotor symptoms with acupuncture

in breast cancer patients treated with adjuvant tamoxifen: A randomized controlled trial. *Breast Cancer Research and Treatment, 135*, 791–798. doi:10.1007/s10549-010-1283-3

54. Otte, J.L., Carpenter, J.S., Zhong, X., & Johnstone, P.A. (2011). Feasibility study of acupuncture for reducing sleep disturbances and hot flashes in postmenopausal breast cancer survivors. *Clinical Nurse Specialist, 25*, 228–236. doi:10.1097/NUR.0b013e318229950b

55. Walker, E.M., Rodriguez, A.I., Kohn, B., Ball, R.M., Pegg, J., Pocock, J.R., ... Levine, R.A. (2010). Acupuncture versus venlafaxine for the management of vasomotor symptoms in patients with hormone receptor-positive breast cancer: A randomized controlled trial. *Journal of Clinical Oncology, 28*, 634–640. doi:10.1200/JCO.2009.23.5150

56. Garcia, M.K., McQuade, J., Haddad, R., Patel, S., Lee, R., Yang, P., ... Cohen, L. (2013). Systematic review of acupuncture in cancer care: A synthesis of the evidence. *Journal of Clinical Oncology, 31*, 952–960. doi:10.1200/JCO.2012.43.5818

57. Hernández Muñoz, G., & Pluchino, S. (2003). *Cimicifuga racemosa* for the treatment of hot flushes in women surviving breast cancer. *Maturitas, 44*(Suppl. 1), S59–S65. doi:10.1016/S0378-5122(02)00349-3

58. Jacobson, J.S., Troxel, A.B., Evans, J., Klaus, L., Vahdat, L., Kinne, D., ... Grann, V.R. (2001). Randomized trial of black cohosh for the treatment of hot flashes among women with a history of breast cancer. *Journal of Clinical Oncology, 19*, 2739–2745. Retrieved from http://jco.ascopubs.org/content/19/10/2739.long

59. Pockaj, B.A., Gallagher, J.G., Loprinzi, C.L., Stella, P.J., Barton, D.L., Sloan, J.A., ... Fauq, A.H. (2006). Phase III double-blind, randomized, placebo-controlled crossover trial of black cohosh in the management of hot flashes: NCCTG trial N01CC1. *Journal of Clinical Oncology, 24*, 2836–2841. doi:10.1200/JCO.2005.05.4296

60. Rostock, M., Fischer, J., Mumm, A., Stammwitz, U., Saller, R., & Bartsch, H.H. (2011). Black cohosh (*Cimicifuga racemosa*) in tamoxifen-treated breast cancer patients with climacteric complaints—A prospective observational study. *Gynecological Endocrinology, 27*, 844–848. doi:10.3109/09513590.2010.538097

61. Ganz, P.A., Greendale, G.A., Petersen, L., Zibecchi, L., Kahn, B., & Berlin, T.R. (2000). Managing menopausal symptoms in breast cancer survivors: Results of a randomized controlled trial. *Journal of the National Cancer Institute, 92*, 1054–1064. doi:10.1093/jnci/92.13.1054

62. Hunter, M.S., Coventry, S., Hamed, H., Fentiman, I., & Grunfeld, E.A. (2009). Evaluation of a group cognitive behavioural intervention for women suffering from menopausal symptoms following breast cancer treatment. *Psycho-Oncology, 18*, 560–563. doi:10.1002/pon.1414

63. Mann, E., Smith, M.J., Hellier, J., Balabanovic, J.A., Hamed, H., Grunfeld, E.A., & Hunter, M.S. (2012). Cognitive behavioural treatment for women who have menopausal symptoms after breast cancer treatment (MENOS 1): A randomised controlled trial. *Lancet Oncology, 13*, 309–318. doi:10.1016/S1470-2045(11)70364-3

64. Elkins, G., Marcus, J., Stearns, V., Perfect, M., Rajab, M.H., Ruud, C., ... Keith, T. (2008). Randomized trial of a hypnosis intervention for treatment of hot flashes among breast cancer survivors. *Journal of Clinical Oncology, 26*, 5022–5026. doi:10.1200/JCO.2008.16.6389

65. Elkins, G., Marcus, J., Stearns, V., & Rajab, M.H. (2007). Pilot evaluation of hypnosis for the treatment of hot flashes in breast cancer survivors. *Psycho-Oncology, 16*, 487–492. doi:10.1002/pon.1096

66. Younus, J., Simpson, I., Collins, A., & Wang, X. (2003). Mind control of menopause. *Women's Health Issues, 13*, 74–78. doi:10.1016/S1049-3867(02)00196-2

67. Schover, L.R., Jenkins, R., Sui, D., Adams, J.H., Marion, M.S., & Jackson, K.E. (2006). Randomized trial of peer counseling on reproductive health in African American breast cancer survivors. *Journal of Clinical Oncology, 24*, 1620–1626. doi:10.1200/JCO.2005.04.7159

68. Fenlon, D.R., Corner, J.L., & Haviland, J.S. (2008). A randomized controlled trial of relaxation training to reduce hot flashes in women with primary breast cancer. *Journal of Pain and Symptom Management, 35,* 397–405. doi:10.1016/j.jpainsymman.2007.05.014

69. Vandecasteele, K., Ost, P., Oosterlinck, W., Fonteyne, V., De Neve, W., & De Meerleer, G. (2012). Evaluation of the efficacy and safety of *Salvia officinalis* in controlling hot flashes in prostate cancer patients treated with androgen deprivation. *Phytotherapy Research, 26,* 208–213. doi:10.1002/ptr.3528

70. Barton, D.L., Loprinzi, C.L., Quella, S.K., Sloan, J.A., Veeder, M.H., Egner, J.R., ... Novotny, P. (1998). Prospective evaluation of vitamin E for hot flashes in breast cancer survivors. *Journal of Clinical Oncology, 16,* 495–500. Retrieved from http://jco.ascopubs.org/content/16/2/495.long

71. Carson, J.W., Carson, K.M., Porter, L.S., Keefe, F.J., & Seewaldt, V.L. (2009). Yoga of Awareness program for menopausal symptoms in breast cancer survivors: Results from a randomized trial. *Supportive Care in Cancer, 17,* 1301–1309. doi:10.1007/s00520-009-0587-5

72. Clover, A., & Ratsey, D. (2002). Homeopathic treatment of hot flushes: A pilot study. *Homeopathy, 91,* 75–79. doi:10.1054/homp.2002.0004

73. Jacobs, J., Herman, P., Heron, K., Olsen, S., & Vaughters, L. (2005). Homeopathy for menopausal symptoms in breast cancer survivors: A preliminary randomized controlled trial. *Journal of Alternative and Complementary Medicine, 11,* 21–27. doi:10.1089/acm.2005.11.21

74. Thompson, E.A., & Reilly, D. (2003). The homeopathic approach to the treatment of symptoms of oestrogen withdrawal in breast cancer patients: A prospective observational study. *Homeopathy, 92,* 131–134. doi:10.1016/S1475-4916(03)00035-3

75. MacGregor, C.A., Canney, P.A., Patterson, G., McDonald, R., & Paul, J. (2005). A randomised double-blind controlled trial of oral soy supplements versus placebo for treatment of menopausal symptoms in patients with early breast cancer. *European Journal of Cancer, 41,* 708–714. doi:10.1016/j.ejca.2005.01.005

76. Nikander, E., Metsä-Heikkilä, M., Ylikorkala, O., & Tiitinen, A. (2004). Effects of phytoestrogens on bone turnover in postmenopausal women with a history of breast cancer. *Journal of Clinical Endocrinology and Metabolism, 89,* 1207–1212. doi:10.1210/jc.2003-031166

77. Quella, S.K., Loprinzi, C.L., Barton, D.L., Knost, J.A., Sloan, J.A., LaVasseur, B.I., ... Novotny, P.J. (2000). Evaluation of soy phytoestrogens for the treatment of hot flashes in breast cancer survivors: A North Central Cancer Treatment Group trial. *Journal of Clinical Oncology, 18,* 1068–1074. Retrieved from http://jco.ascopubs.org/content/18/5/1068.long

78. Van Patten, C.L. (2002). Effect of soy phytoestrogens on hot flashes in postmenopausal women with breast cancer: A randomized, controlled clinical trial. *Journal of Clinical Oncology, 20,* 1449–1455. doi:10.1200/JCO.20.6.1449

79. Sharma, P., Wisniewski, A., Braga-Basaria, M., Xu, X., Yep, M., Denmeade, S., ... Basaria, S. (2009). Lack of an effect of high dose isoflavones in men with prostate cancer undergoing androgen deprivation therapy. *Journal of Urology, 182,* 2265–2272. doi:10.1016/j.juro.2009.07.030

80. Kroiss, R., Fentiman, I.S., Helmond, F.A., Rymer, J., Foidart, J.M., Bundred, N., ... Kubista, E. (2005). The effect of tibolone in postmenopausal women receiving tamoxifen after surgery for breast cancer: A randomised, double-blind, placebo-controlled trial. *BJOG: An International Journal of Obstetrics and Gynaecology, 112,* 228–233. doi:10.1111/j.1471-0528.2004.00309.x

81. Sismondi, P., Kimmig, R., Kubista, E., Biglia, N., Egberts, J., Mulder, R., ... Kenemans, P. (2011). Effects of tibolone on climacteric symptoms and quality of life in breast cancer patients—Data from LIBERATE trial. *Maturitas, 70,* 365–372. doi:10.1016/j.maturitas.2011.09.003

82. Beral, V., Danks, E., Reeves, G., & Bull, D. (2003). Breast cancer and hormone-replacement therapy: The Million Women Study. *Lancet, 362,* 1330–1331. doi:10.1016/S0140-6736(03)14596-5

83. Kligman, K., & Younus, J. (2010). Nursing management of hot flashes in women with breast cancer. *Current Oncology, 17,* 81–86. doi:10.3747/co.v17i1.473

Lymphedema

Lee Ann Johnson, PhD(c), RN,
Jie Deng, PhD, RN, OCN®,
and Marcia Beck, RN, ACNS-BC, CLT-LANA

Problem and Incidence

Lymphedema is a persistent swelling of an affected body part caused by an obstruction and subsequent accumulation of lymphatic fluid in the lymph system. In patients with cancer, lymphedema is most often caused by radiation therapy and lymph node dissection and can affect one or more upper or lower extremities, the head and neck, breasts, and genitalia.[1] Upper-extremity lymphedema is most often reported in women who have undergone treatment for breast cancer and affects 12%–26% of survivors.[2] Other types of cancer are also associated with lymphedema, and incidence has been reported as follows: melanoma (16%), gynecologic cancers (20%), genitourinary cancers (10%),[4,5] and head and neck cancers (75%).[6]

Risk Factors and Assessment

Factors that place patients at high risk for lymphedema include
- Inherited abnormalities of the lymphatic system
- Surgical removal of lymph nodes
- Radiation therapy to specific lymphatic territories
- Infection or parasites
- Recurrence or new malignancy.

Factors that place patients at low to moderate risk for lymphedema include
- Obesity
- Trauma resulting in damage to the lymphatic system.

Assessment related to lymphedema should include
- Physical exam of affected body parts
- Measurements of affected body parts
- Identification of patient-perceived changes in affected body parts.

Assessment tools include
- National Cancer Institute Cancer Therapy Evaluation Program *Common Terminology Criteria for Adverse Events* lymphedema scale (open access)[7]
- Stages of lymphedema (Földi's Scale)[8,9]
- International Society of Lymphedema Stages of Lymphedema[10]
- Standard, objective, and reproducible limb volume measurements
- Photographs of affected body parts.

What interventions are effective in preventing and managing lymphedema in people with cancer?

Evidence retrieved through August 31, 2013

Recommended for Practice

Complete decongestive therapy, the gold standard for lymphedema therapy, consists of manual lymphatic drainage, compression bandaging, lymphatic exercise, and skin care. It reduced arm volume[1,11-24] and lower-limb volume.[25,26]

Compression garments and bandages reduced volume in upper limbs[27-36] and lower limbs.[37-38]

Likely to Be Effective

Exercise benefitted women with breast cancer and did not exacerbate symptoms or increase limb volume.[1,17,34,39-60]

Orientation and information provision to breast cancer survivors reduced symptoms and risky behaviors.[61]

Prevention and early intervention protocols with consistent surveillance reduced arm volume in women with breast cancer.[28,62]

Weight management was associated with reduced swelling in one study[63] and is recommended in guidelines.[1]

Benefits Balanced With Harms

Activity restriction did not improve outcomes in a large multisite randomized controlled trial,[64] and inactivity can adversely affect function.

Kinesio® tape bandage improved limb circumference and water volume and was more acceptable to patients than bandages but led to significantly more wounds.[35]

Effectiveness Not Established

Multiple other interventions have been studied for effects on lymphedema. Some studies were small, nonrandomized, and open-label designs.

- **Compression interventions**
  - **Manual lymph drainage**[3,11,19,32,36,65-70]
  - **Pneumatic compression**[1,15,32,69,71-79]
- **Mind-body interventions**
  - **Acupuncture**[80]
  - **Massage and aromatherapy massage**[81,82]
- **Physical activity interventions**
  - **Aquatherapy**[83]
  - **Avoidance of lifting weight**[84-90]
  - **Mechanical exercise**[91-93]—Exercise increased arm volume when performed without a compression garment.[94]
- **Surgical interventions**
  - **Axillary reverse mapping**[95]
  - **Liposuction**[96]
  - **Lymphatic venous anastomosis**[97-99]

- **Stromal and stem cell transplantation**[98,100-102]
  - **Surgical techniques** such as lymph node transfer, various microsurgical techniques, and use of fibrin sealant.[98,102-104]
- **Other interventions**
  - **Hyperbaric oxygen**[105,106]
  - **Low-intensity electrostatic stimulation**[107,108]
  - **Low-level laser therapy**[109-114]—Systematic reviews suggested benefits; however, studies had different lymphedema definitions and varied dosing, and co-interventions were often not described.[69,115]

Expert Opinion

Compression garments when flying are recommended by experts.[116,117]

Skin and hygiene care are recommended as part of lymphedema management.[1,12]

Application to Practice

Nurses can advocate for complete decongestive therapy provided by a certified lymphedema therapist followed by home self-management.

Individuals with severe lymphedema need to use properly fitted home compression bandaging, including custom garments, and should wear compression at night. Nurses can educate and counsel patients regarding these needs.

Individuals with lymphedema can be encouraged to carry out proper exercise. While lifting some weight has been shown to be safe, patients should be initially trained and supervised in exercise with weights by appropriate professionals.

Nurses can educate patients and caregivers on the importance of skin and nail care, signs and symptoms of cellulitis, the importance of maintaining a healthy weight, and the benefits of exercise and that lifting moderate weight as part of daily activities does not need to be avoided.

Nurses can educate at-risk patients about the risks of lymphedema occurrence and self-monitoring. Evidence shows that surveillance and early intervention are beneficial.

Lymphedema Resource Contributors

Topic leader: Jane M. Armer, RN, PhD, FAAN
Marcia Beck, RN, ACNS-BC, CLT-LANA, Jie Deng, PhD, RN, OCN®,
Mei R. Fu, PhD, RN, ACNS-BC, FAAN,
and Karen A. Giammicchio, MSN, APN, AOCNS®

References

1. Lymphoedema Framework. (2006). *Best practice for the management of lymphoedema.* London, UK: Medical Education Partnership.
2. DiSipio, T., Rye, S., Newman, B., & Hayes, S. (2013). Incidence of unilateral arm lymphoedema after breast cancer: A systematic review and meta-analysis. *Lancet Oncology, 14,* 500–515. doi:10.1016/S1470-2045(13)70076-7
3. Huang, T.-W., Tseng, S.-H., Lin, C.-C., Bai, C.-H., Chen, C.-S., Hung, C.-S., ... Tam, K.-W. (2013). Effects of manual lymphatic drainage on breast cancer-related lymphedema: A systematic review and meta-analysis of randomized controlled trials. *World Journal of Surgical Oncology, 11,* 15. doi:10.1186/1477-7819-11-15
4. Cormier, J.N., Askew, R.L., Mungovan, K.S., Xing, Y., Ross, M.I., & Armer, J.M. (2010). Lymphedema beyond breast cancer: A systematic review and meta-analysis of cancer-related secondary lymphedema. *Cancer, 116,* 5138–5149. doi:10.1002/cncr.25458
5. Fu, M.R., Ridner, S.H., Hu, S.H., Stewart, B.R., Cormier, J.N., & Armer, J.M. (2013). Psychosocial impact of lymphedema: A systematic review of literature from 2004 to 2011. *Psycho-Oncology, 22,* 1466–1484. doi:10.1002/pon.3201
6. Deng, J., Ridner, S.H., Dietrich, M.S., Wells, N., & Murphy, B.A. (2013). Assessment of external lymphedema in patients with head and neck cancer: A comparison of four scales. *Oncology Nursing Forum, 40,* 501–506. doi:10.1188/13.ONF.501-506
7. National Cancer Institute Cancer Therapy Evaluation Program. (2010, June 14). *Common terminology criteria for adverse events* [v.4.03]. Retrieved from http://evs.nci.nih.gov/ftp1/CTCAE/CTCAE_4.03_2010-06-14_QuickReference_5x7.pdf
8. Földi, M., Földi, E., & Kubik, S. (2003). *Textbook of lymphology for physicians and lymphedema therapists.* Munich, Germany: Urban and Fischer.
9. Földi, M.D., Földi, E., Strössenreuther, R.H.K., & Kubik, S. (Eds.). (2007). *Földi's textbook of lymphology: For physicians and lymphedema therapists* (2nd ed.). Munich, Germany: Urban and Fischer.
10. OncoLink. (2006, August 13). Staging system for lymphedema. Retrieved from https://www.oncolink.org/experts/article.cfm?id=2293
11. Beck, M., Wanchai, A., Stewart, B.R., Cormier, J.N., & Armer, J.M. (2012). Palliative care for cancer-related lymphedema: A systematic review. *Journal of Palliative Medicine, 15,* 821–827. doi:10.1089/jpm.2011.0494
12. Browning, C. (1997). *Lymphoedema: Prevalence, risk factors and management: A review of research.* Retrieved from http://canceraustralia.gov.au/sites/default/files/publications/lym-lymphoedema-prevalence-risk-factors-and-management-a-review-of-research_504af02f48fff.pdf

13. da Silva Leal, N.F.B., Angotti Carrara, H.H., Vieira, K.F., & Jorge Ferreira, C.H. (2009). Physiotherapy treatments for breast cancer–related lymphedema: A literature review. *Revista Latino-Americana De Enfermagem, 17,* 730–736. doi:10.1590/S0104-11692009000500021

14. Didem, K., Ufuk, Y.S., Serdar, S., & Zumre, A. (2005). The comparison of two different physiotherapy methods in treatment of lymphedema after breast surgery. *Breast Cancer Research and Treatment, 93,* 49–54. doi:10.1007/s10549-005-3781-2

15. Haghighat, S., Lotfi-Tokaldany, M., Yunesian, M., Akbari, M.E., Nazemi, F., & Weiss, J. (2010). Comparing two treatment methods for post mastectomy lymphedema: Complex decongestive therapy alone and in combination with intermittent pneumatic compression. *Lymphology, 43,* 25–33.

16. Hamner, J.B., & Fleming, M.D. (2007). Lymphedema therapy reduces the volume of edema and pain in patients with breast cancer. *Annals of Surgical Oncology, 14,* 1904–1908. doi:10.1245/s10434-006-9332-1

17. International Society of Lymphology. (2009). The diagnosis and treatment of peripheral lymphedema: 2009 consensus document of the International Society of Lymphology. *Lymphology, 42,* 51–60. Retrieved from http://www.u.arizona.edu/~witte/contents/2009.42.2.consensus.pdf

18. Karadibak, D., Yavuzsen, T., & Saydam, S. (2008). Prospective trial of intensive decongestive physiotherapy for upper extremity lymphedema. *Journal of Surgical Oncology, 97,* 572–577. doi:10.1002/jso.21035

19. Koul, R., Dufan, T., Russell, C., Guenther, W., Nugent, Z., Sun, X., & Cooke, A.L. (2007). Efficacy of complete decongestive therapy and manual lymphatic drainage on treatment-related lymphedema in breast cancer. *International Journal of Radiation Oncology, Biology, Physics, 67,* 841–846. doi:10.1016/j.ijrobp.2006.09.024

20. Lasinski, B.B., Thrift, K.M., Squire, D., Austin, M.K., Smith, K.M., Wanchai, A., ... Armer, J.M. (2012). A systematic review of the evidence for complete decongestive therapy in the treatment of lymphedema from 2004 to 2011. *PM&R, 4,* 580–601. doi:10.1016/j.pmrj.2012.05.003

21. Liao, S.-F., Li, S.-H., Huang, H.-Y., Chen, S.-T., Kuo, S.-J., Chen, D.-R., & Wei, T.-S. (2013). The efficacy of complex decongestive physiotherapy (CDP) and predictive factors of lymphedema severity and response to CDP in breast cancer–related lymphedema (BCRL). *Breast, 22,* 703–706. doi:10.1016/j.breast.2012.12.018

22. Pereira de Godoy, J.M., & Guerreiro Godoy, M.D. (2013). Evaluation of a new approach to the treatment of lymphedema resulting from breast cancer therapy. *European Journal of Internal Medicine, 24,* 59–62. doi:10.1016/j.ejim.2012.08.008

23. Randheer, S., Kadambari, D., Srinivasan, K., Bhuvaneswari, V., Bhanumathy, M., & Salaja, R. (2011). Comprehensive decongestive therapy in postmastectomy lymphedema: An Indian perspective. *Indian Journal of Cancer, 48,* 397–402. doi:10.4103/0019-509X.92250

24. Ridner, S.H., Murphy, B., Deng, J., Kidd, N., Galford, E., Bonner, C., ... Dietrich, M.S. (2012). A randomized clinical trial comparing advanced pneumatic truncal, chest, and arm treatment to arm treatment only in self-care of arm lymphedema. *Breast Cancer Research and Treatment, 131,* 147–158. doi:10.1007/s10549-011-1795-5

25. Carmeli, E., & Bartoletti, R. (2011). Retrospective trial of complete decongestive physical therapy for lower extremity secondary lymphedema in melanoma patients. *Supportive Care in Cancer, 19,* 141–147. doi:10.1007/s00520-009-0803-3

26. Liao, S.-F., Li, S.-H., & Huang, H.-Y. (2012). The efficacy of complex decongestive physiotherapy (CDP) and predictive factors of response to CDP in lower limb lymphedema (LLL) after pelvic cancer treatment. *Gynecologic Oncology, 125,* 712–715. doi:10.1016/j.ygyno.2012.03.017

27. Damstra, R.J., & Partsch, H. (2009). Compression therapy in breast cancer-related lymphedema: A randomized, controlled comparative study of relation between volume and interface pressure changes.

Journal of Vascular Surgery, 49, 1256–1263. doi:10.1016/j.jvs.2008.12.018

28. Gergich, N.L.S., Pfalzer, L.A., McGarvey, C., Springer, B., Gerber, L.H., & Soballe, P. (2008). Preoperative assessment enables the early diagnosis and successful treatment of lymphedema. *Cancer, 112,* 2809–2819. doi:10.1002/cncr.23494

29. Harris, S.R., Schmitz, K.H., Campbell, K.L., & McNeely, M.L. (2012). Clinical practice guidelines for breast cancer rehabilitation: Syntheses of guideline recommendations and qualitative appraisals. *Cancer, 118*(Suppl. 8), 2312–2324. doi:10.1002/cncr.27461

30. Jeffs, E. (2006). Treating breast cancer–related lymphoedema at the London Haven: Clinical audit results. *European Journal of Oncology Nursing, 10,* 71–79. doi:10.1016/j.ejon.2005.02.005

31. Kasseroller, R.G., & Brenner, E. (2010). A prospective randomised study of alginate-drenched low stretch bandages as an alternative to conventional lymphologic compression bandaging. *Supportive Care in Cancer, 18,* 343–350. doi:10.1007/s00520-009-0658-7

32. McNeely, M.L., Peddle, C.J., Yurick, J.L., Dayes, I.S., & Mackey, J.R. (2011). Conservative and dietary interventions for cancer-related lymphedema: A systematic review and meta-analysis. *Cancer, 117,* 1136–1148. doi:10.1002/cncr.25513

33. Partsch, H., Flour, M., & Smith, P.C. (2008). Indications for compression therapy in venous and lymphatic disease consensus based on experimental data and scientific evidence. Under the auspices of the IUP. *International Angiology, 27,* 193–219. Retrieved from http://www.minervamedica.it/en/journals/international-angiology/article.php?cod=R34Y2008N03A0193&acquista=1

34. Preston, N.J., Seers, K., & Mortimer, P.S. (2008). Physical therapies for reducing and controlling lymphoedema of the limbs. *Cochrane Database of Systematic Reviews, 2008*(4). doi:10.1002/14651858.CD003141.pub2

35. Tsai, H.-J., Hung, H.-C., Yang, J.-L., Huang, C.-S., & Tsauo, J.-Y. (2009). Could Kinesio tape replace the bandage in decongestive lymphatic therapy for breast-cancer–related lymphedema? A pilot study. *Supportive Care in Cancer, 17,* 1353–1360. doi:10.1007/s00520-009-0592-8

36. Vignes, S., Porcher, R., Arrault, M., & Dupuy, A. (2011). Factors influencing breast cancer–related lymphedema volume after intensive decongestive physiotherapy. *Supportive Care in Cancer, 19,* 935–940. doi:10.1007/s00520-010-0906-x

37. Damstra, R.J., Brouwer, E.R., & Partsch, H. (2008). Controlled, comparative study of relation between volume changes and interface pressure under short-stretch bandages in leg lymphedema patients. *Dermatologic Surgery, 34,* 773–779. doi:10.1111/j.1524-4725.2008.34145.x

38. Sawan, S., Mugnai, R., Lopes Ade, B., Hughes, A., & Edmondson, R.J. (2009). Lower-limb lymphedema and vulval cancer: Feasibility of prophylactic compression garments and validation of leg volume measurement. *International Journal of Gynecological Cancer, 19,* 1649–1654. doi:10.1111/IGC.0b013e3181a8446a

39. Anderson, R.T., Kimmick, G.G., McCoy, T.P., Hopkins, J., Levine, E., Miller, G., … Mihalko, S.L. (2012). A randomized trial of exercise on well-being and function following breast cancer surgery: The RESTORE trial. *Journal of Cancer Survivorship: Research and Practice, 6,* 172–181. doi:10.1007/s11764-011-0208-4

40. Bicego, D., Brown, K., Ruddick, M., Storey, D., Wong, C., & Harris, S.R. (2006). Exercise for women with or at risk for breast cancer–related lymphedema. *Physical Therapy, 86,* 1398–1405. doi:10.2522/ptj.20050328

41. Box, R.C., Reul-Hirsch, H.M., Bullock-Saxton, J.E., & Furnival, C.M. (2002). Physiotherapy after breast cancer surgery: Results of a randomized controlled study to minimise lymphoedema. *Breast Cancer Research and Treatment, 75,* 51–64. doi:10.1023/A:1016591121762

42. Chan, D.N., Lui, L.Y., & So, W.K. (2010). Effectiveness of exercise programmes on shoulder mobility and lymphoedema after axillary lymph node dissection for breast cancer: Systematic review. *Journal of Advanced Nursing, 66,* 1902–1914. doi:10.1111/j.1365-2648.2010.05374.x

43. Cheema, B., Gaul, C.A., Lane, K., & Singh, M.A.F. (2008). Progressive resistance training in breast cancer: A systematic review of clinical trials. *Breast Cancer Research and Treatment, 109,* 9–26. doi:10.1007/s10549 -007-9638-0

44. Cinar, N., Seckin, Ü., Keskin, D., Bodur, H., Bozkurt, B., & Cengiz, Ö. (2008). The effectiveness of early rehabilitation in patients with modified radical mastectomy. *Cancer Nursing, 31,* 160–165. doi:10.1097/01 .NCC.0000305696.12873.0e

45. de Rezende, L.F., Franco, R.L., de Rezende, M.F., Beletti, P.O., Morais, S.S., & Gurgel, M.S. (2006). Two exercise schemes in postoperative breast cancer: Comparison of effects on shoulder movement and lymphatic disturbance. *Tumori, 92,* 55–61. doi:10.1700/230.2687

46. Gautam, A.P., Maiya, A.G., & Vidyasagar, M.S. (2011). Effect of home-based exercise program on lymphedema and quality of life in female postmastectomy patients: Pre-post intervention study. *Journal of Rehabilitation Research and Development, 48,* 1261–1268. doi:10.1682/JRRD.2010.05.0089

47. Hayes, S.C., Reul-Hirche, H., & Turner, J. (2009). Exercise and secondary lymphedema: Safety, potential benefits, and research issues. *Medicine and Science in Sports and Exercise, 41,* 483–489. doi:10.1249/ MSS.0b013e31818b98fb

48. Johansson, K., Hayes, S., Speck, R.M., & Schmitz, K.H. (2013). Water-based exercise for patients with chronic arm lymphedema: A randomized controlled pilot trial. *American Journal of Physical Medicine and Rehabilitation, 92,* 312–319. doi:10.1097/PHM.0b013e318278b0e8

49. Johansson, K., Tibe, K., Weibull, A., & Newton, R.C. (2005). Low intensity resistance exercise for breast cancer patients with arm lymphedema with or without compression sleeve. *Lymphology, 38,* 167–180.

50. Jonsson, C., & Johansson, K. (2009). Pole walking for patients with breast cancer–related arm lymphedema. *Physiotherapy Theory and Practice, 25,* 165–173. doi:10.1080/09593980902776621

51. Kilgour, R., Jones, D., & Keyserlink, J. (2008). Effectiveness of a self-administered, home-based exercise rehabilitation program for women following a modified radical mastectomy and axillary node dissection: A preliminary study. *Breast Cancer Research and Treatment, 109,* 285–295. doi:10.1007/s10549-007-9649-x

52. Kim, D.S., Sim, Y.-J., Jeong, H.J., & Kim, G.C. (2010). Effect of active resistive exercise on breast cancer–related lymphedema: A randomized controlled trial. *Archives of Physical Medicine and Rehabilitation, 91,* 1844–1848. doi:10.1016/j.apmr.2010.09.008

53. Kwan, M.L., Cohn, J.C., Armer, J.M., Stewart, B.R., & Cormier, J.N. (2011). Exercise in patients with lymphedema: A systematic review of the contemporary literature. *Journal of Cancer Survivorship: Research and Practice, 5,* 320–336. doi:10.1007/s11764-011-0203-9

54. Malicka, I., Stefańska, M., Rudziak, M., Jarmoluk, P., Pawłowska, K., Szczepańska-Gieracha, J., & Woźniewski, M. (2011). The influence of Nordic walking exercise on upper extremity strength and the volume of lymphoedema in women following breast cancer treatment. *Isokinetics and Exercise Science, 19,* 295–304. doi:10.3233/IES-2011-0430

55. McClure, M.K., McClure, R.J., Day, R., & Brufsky, A.M. (2010). Randomized controlled trial of the Breast Cancer Recovery Program for women with breast cancer-related lymphedema. *American Journal of Occupational Therapy, 64,* 59–72. doi:10.5014/ajot.64.1.59

56. McNeely, M.L., Campbell, K., Ospina, M., Rowe, B.H., Dabbs, K., Klassen, T.P., ... Courneya, K. (2010). Exercise interventions for upper-limb dysfunction due to breast cancer treatment. *Cochrane Database of Systematic Reviews, 2010*(6). doi:10.1002/14651858.CD005211.pub2

57. Schmitz, K.H., Courneya, K.S., Matthews, C., Demark-Wahnefried, W., Galvão, D.A., Pinto, B.M., ... Schwartz, A.L. (2010). American College of Sports Medicine roundtable on exercise guidelines for cancer survivors. *Medicine and Science in Sports and Exercise, 42,* 1409–1426. doi:10.1249/MSS.0b013e3181e0c112

58. Sisman, H., Sahin, B., Duman, B.B., & Tanriverdi, G. (2012). Nurse-assisted education and exercise decrease the prevalence and morbidity of lymphedema following breast cancer surgery. *Journal of B.U.ON., 17,* 565–569.

59. Torres Lacomba, M., Yuste Sánchez, M.J., Zapico Goñi, Á., Prieto Merino, D., Mayoral del Moral, O., Cerezo Téllez, E., & Minayo Mogollón, E. (2010). Effectiveness of early physiotherapy to prevent lymphoedema after surgery for breast cancer: Randomised, single blinded, clinical trial. *BMJ, 340,* b5396. doi:10.1136/bmj.b5396

60. Young-McCaughan, S., & Arzola, S.M. (2007). Exercise intervention research for patients with cancer on treatment. *Seminars in Oncology Nursing, 23,* 264–274. doi:10.1016/j.soncn.2007.08.004

61. Fu, M.R., Axelrod, D., & Haber, J. (2008). Breast-cancer-related lymphedema: Information, symptoms, and risk-reduction behaviors. *Journal of Nursing Scholarship, 40,* 341–348. doi:10.1111/j.1547-5069.2008.00248.x

62. Boccardo, F.M., Ansaldi, F., Bellini, C., Accogli, S., Taddei, G., Murdaca, G., ... Campisi, C. (2009). Prospective evaluation of a prevention protocol for lymphedema following surgery for breast cancer. *Lymphology, 42,* 1–9.

63. Shaw, C., Mortimer, P., & Judd, P.A. (2007). Randomized controlled trial comparing a low-fat diet with a weight-reduction diet in breast cancer-related lymphedema. *Cancer, 109,* 1949–1956. doi:10.1002/cncr.22638

64. Sagen, A., Karesen, R., & Risberg, M.A. (2009). Physical activity for the affected limb and arm lymphedema after breast cancer surgery. A prospective, randomized controlled trial with two years follow-up. *Acta Oncologica, 48,* 1102–1110. doi:10.3109/02841860903061683

65. Clemens, K.E., Jaspers, B., Klaschik, E., & Nieland, P. (2010). Evaluation of the clinical effectiveness of physiotherapeutic management of lymphoedema in palliative care patients. *Japanese Journal of Clinical Oncology, 40,* 1068–1072. doi:10.1093/jjco/hyq093

66. Martin, M.L., Hernandez, M.A., Avendano, C., Rodriguez, F., & Martinez, H. (2011). Manual lymphatic drainage therapy in patients with breast cancer related lymphoedema. *BMC Cancer, 11,* 94. doi:10.1186/1471-2407-11-94

67. McNeely, M.L., Magee, D.J., Lees, A.W., Bagnall, K.M., Haykowsky, M., & Hanson, J. (2004). The addition of manual lymph drainage to compression therapy for breast cancer related lymphedema: A randomized controlled trial. *Breast Cancer Research and Treatment, 86,* 95–106. doi:10.1023/B:BREA.0000032978.67677.9f

68. Devoogdt, N., Christiaens, M.R., Geraerts, I., Truijen, S., Smeets, A., Leunen, K., ... Van Kampen, M. (2011). Effect of manual lymph drainage in addition to guidelines and exercise therapy on arm lymphoedema related to breast cancer: Randomised controlled trial. *BMJ, 343,* d5326. doi:10.1136/bmj.d5326

69. Moseley, A.L., Carati, C.J., & Piller, N.B. (2007). A systematic review of common conservative therapies for arm lymphoedema secondary to breast cancer treatment. *Annals of Oncology, 18,* 639–646. doi:10.1093/annonc/mdl182

70. Zimmermann, A., Wozniewski, M., Szlarska, A., Lipowicz, A., & Szuba, A. (2012). Efficacy of manual lymphatic drainage in preventing secondary lymphedema after breast cancer surgery. *Lymphology, 45,* 103–112.

71. Fife, C.E., Davey, S., Maus, E.A., Guilliod, R., & Mayrovitz, H.N. (2012). A randomized controlled trial comparing two types of pneumatic compression for breast cancer-related lymphedema treatment in the home. *Supportive Care in Cancer, 20,* 3279–3286. doi:10.1007/s00520-012-1455-2

72. Forner-Cordero, I., Muñoz-Langa, J., Forner-Cordero, A., & DeMiguel-Jimeno, J.M. (2010). Predictive factors of response to decongestive therapy in pa-

tients with breast-cancer-related lymphedema. *Annals of Surgical Oncology, 17*, 744–751. doi:10.1245/s10434-009-0778-9

73. Moattari, M., Jaafari, B., Talei, A., Piroozi, S., Tahmasebi, S., & Zakeri, Z. (2012). The effect of combined decongestive therapy and pneumatic compression pump on lymphedema indicators in patients with breast cancer–related lymphedema. *Iranian Red Crescent Medical Journal, 14*, 210–217. Retrieved from http://www.ncbi.nlm.nih.gov/pmc/articles/PMC3385799

74. Pilch, U., Wozniewski, M., & Szuba, A. (2009). Influence of compression cycle time and number of sleeve chambers on upper extremity lymphedema volume reduction during intermittent pneumatic compression. *Lymphology, 42*, 26–35.

75. Ridner, S.H., Fu, M.R., Wanchai, A., Stewart, B.R., Armer, J.M., & Cormier, J.N. (2012). Self-management of lymphedema: A systematic review of the literature from 2004 to 2011. *Nursing Research, 61*, 291–299. doi:10.1097/NNR.0b013e31824f82b2

76. Ridner, S.H., Murphy, B., Deng, J., Kidd, N., Galford, E., & Dietrich, M.S. (2010). Advanced pneumatic therapy in self-care of chronic lymphedema of the trunk. *Lymphatic Research and Biology, 8*, 209–215. doi:10.1089/lrb.2010.0010

77. Rinehart-Ayres, M., Fish, K., Lapp, K., Brown, C.N., & Rucker, B. (2010). Use of compression pumps for treatment of upper extremity lymphedema following treatment for breast cancer: A systematic review. *Rehabilitation Oncology, 28*, 10–18.

78. Szolnoky, G., Lakatos, B., Keskeny, T., Varga, E., Varga, M., Dobozy, A., & Kemeny, L. (2009). Intermittent pneumatic compression acts synergistically with manual lymphatic drainage in complex decongestive physiotherapy for breast cancer treatment-related lymphedema. *Lymphology, 42*, 188–194.

79. Szuba, A., Achalu, R., & Rockson, S.G. (2002). Decongestive lymphatic therapy for patients with breast carcinoma-associated lymphedema. *Cancer, 95*, 2260–2267. doi:10.1002/cncr.10976

80. Cassileth, B.R., Van Zee, K.J., Chan, Y., Coleton, M.I., Hudis, C.A., Cohen, S., ... Vickers, A.J. (2011). A safety and efficacy pilot study of acupuncture for the treatment of chronic lymphoedema. *Acupuncture in Medicine, 29*, 170–172. doi:10.1136/aim.2011.004069

81. Barclay, J., Vestey, J., Lambert, A., & Balmer, C. (2006). Reducing the symptoms of lymphoedema: Is there a role for aromatherapy? *European Journal of Oncology Nursing, 10*, 140–149. doi:10.1016/j.ejon.2005.10.008

82. Maher, J., Refshauge, K., Ward, L., Paterson, R., & Kilbreath, S. (2012). Change in extracellular fluid and arm volumes as a consequence of a single session of lymphatic massage followed by rest with or without compression. *Supportive Care in Cancer, 20*, 3079–3086. doi:10.1007/s00520-012-1433-8

83. Tidhar, D., & Katz-Leurer, M. (2010). Aqua lymphatic therapy in women who suffer from breast cancer treatment–related lymphedema: A randomized controlled study. *Supportive Care in Cancer, 18*, 383–392. doi:10.1007/s00520-009-0669-4

84. Ahmed, R.L., Thomas, W., Yee, D., & Schmitz, K.H. (2006). Randomized controlled trial of weight training and lymphedema in breast cancer survivors. *Journal of Clinical Oncology, 24*, 2765–2772. doi:10.1200/JCO.2005.03.6749

85. Brown, J.C., Troxel, A.B., & Schmitz, K.H. (2012). Safety of weightlifting among women with or at risk for breast cancer-related lymphedema: Musculoskeletal injuries and health care use in a weightlifting rehabilitation trial. *Oncologist, 17*, 1120–1128. doi:10.1634/theoncologist.2012-0035

86. Cormie, P., Galvão, D.A., Spry, N., & Newton, R.U. (2013). Neither heavy nor light load resistance exercise acutely exacerbates lymphedema in breast cancer survivor. *Integrative Cancer Therapies, 12*, 423–432. doi:10.1177/1534735413477194

87. Cormie, P., Pumpa, K., Galvão, D.A., Turner, E., Spry, N., Saunders, C., ... Newton, R.U. (2013). Is it safe and efficacious for women with lymph-

edema secondary to breast cancer to lift heavy weights during exercise: A randomised controlled trial. *Journal of Cancer Survivorship: Research and Practice, 7,* 413–424. doi:10.1007/s11764-013-0284-8

88. Hayes, S.C., Speck, R.M., Reimet, E., Stark, A., & Schmitz, K.H. (2011). Does the effect of weight lifting on lymphedema following breast cancer differ by diagnostic method: Results from a randomized controlled trial. *Breast Cancer Research and Treatment, 130,* 227–234. doi:10.1007/s10549-011-1547-6

89. Schmitz, K.H., Ahmed, R.L., Troxel, A., Cheville, A., Smith, R., Lewis-Grant, L., … Greene, Q.P. (2009). Weight lifting in women with breast-cancer-related lymphedema. *New England Journal of Medicine, 361,* 664–673. doi:10.1056/NEJMoa0810118

90. Schmitz, K.H., Ahmed, R.L., Troxel, A.B., Cheville, A., Lewis-Grant, L., Smith, R., … Chittams, J. (2010). Weight lifting for women at risk for breast cancer–related lymphedema: A randomized trial. *JAMA, 304,* 2699–2705. doi:10.1001/jama.2010.1837

91. Bordin, N.A., Guerreiro Godoy, M.D., & Pereira de Godoy, J.M. (2009). Mechanical lymphatic drainage in the treatment of arm lymphedema. *Indian Journal of Cancer, 46,* 337–339. doi:10.4103/0019-509X.55556

92. Guerreiro Godoy, M.D., Guimaraes, T.D., Oliani, A.H., & Pereira de Godoy, J.M. (2011). Association of Godoy and Godoy contention with mechanism with apparatus-assisted exercises in patients with arm lymphedema after breast cancer. *International Journal of General Medicine, 4,* 373–376. doi:10.2147/IJGM.S17139

93. Guerreiro Godoy, M.D., Oliani, A.H., & Pereira de Godoy, J.M. (2010). Active exercises utilizing a facilitating device in the treatment of lymphedema resulting from breast cancer therapy. *German Medical Science: GMS e-Journal, 8,* Doc31. doi:10.3205/000120

94. Guerreiro Godoy, M.D., Pereira, M.R., Oliani, H.O., & Pereira de Godoy, J.M. (2012). Synergic effect of compression therapy and controlled active exercises using a facilitating device in the treatment of arm lymphedema. *International Journal of Medical Sciences, 9,* 280–284. doi:10.7150/ijms.3272

95. Boneti, C., Badgwell, B., Robertson, Y., Korourian, S., Adkins, L., & Klimberg, V. (2012). Axillary reverse mapping (ARM): Initial results of phase II trial in preventing lymphedema after lymphadenectomy. *Minerva Ginecologica, 64,* 421–430. Retrieved from http://www.minervamedica.it/en/journals/minerva-ginecologica/article.php?cod=R09Y2012N05A0421&acquista=1

96. Schaverien, M.V., Munro, K.J., Baker, P.A., & Munnoch, D.A. (2012). Liposuction for chronic lymphoedema of the upper limb: 5 years of experience. *Journal of Plastic, Reconstructive and Aesthetic Surgery, 65,* 935–942, doi:10.1016/j.bjps.2012.01.021

97. Boccardo, F.M., Casabona, F., Friedman, D., Puglisi, M., De Cian, F., Ansaldi, F., & Campisi, C. (2011). Surgical prevention of arm lymphedema after breast cancer treatment. *Annals of Surgical Oncology, 18,* 2500–2505. doi:10.1245/s10434-011-1624-4

98. Cormier, J.N., Rourke, L., Crosby, M., Chang, D., & Armer, J. (2012). The surgical treatment of lymphedema: A systematic review of the contemporary literature (2004–2010). *Annals of Surgical Oncology, 19,* 642–651. doi:10.1245/s10434-011-2017-4

99. Damstra, R.J., Voesten, H.G., van Schelven, W.D., & van der Lei, B. (2009). Lymphatic venous anastomosis (LVA) for treatment of secondary arm lymphedema. A prospective study of 11 LVA procedures in 10 patients with breast cancer related lymphedema and a critical review of the literature. *Breast Cancer Research and Treatment, 113,* 199–206. doi:10.1007/s10549-008-9932-5

100. Hou, C., Wu, X., & Jin, X. (2008). Autologous bone marrow stromal cells transplantation for the treatment of secondary arm lymphedema: A prospective controlled study in patients with breast cancer related lymphedema. *Japanese Journal of Clinical Oncology, 38,* 670–674. doi:10.1093/jjco/hyn090

101. Maldonado, G.E., Perez, C.A., Covarrubias, E.E., Cabriales, S.A., Leyva, L.A., Perez, J.C., & Almaguer, D.G. (2011). Autologous stem cells for the treatment of post-mastectomy lymphedema: A pilot study. *Cytotherapy, 13,* 1249–1255. doi:10.3109/14653249.2011.594791

102. Penha, T.R., Ijsbrandy, C., Hendrix, N.A., Heuts, E.M., Voogd, A.C., von Meyenfeldt, M.F., & van der Hulst, R.R. (2013). Microsurgical techniques for the treatment of breast cancer-related lymphoedema: A systematic review. *Journal of Reconstructive Microsurgery, 29,* 99–106. doi:10.1055/s-0032-1329919

103. Abbas, S., & Seitz, M. (2009). Systematic review and meta-analysis of the used surgical techniques to reduce leg lymphedema following radical inguinal nodes dissection. *Surgical Oncology, 20,* 88–96. doi:10.1016/j.suronc.2009.11.003

104. Carlson, J.W., Kauderer, J., Walker, J.L., Gold, M.A., O'Malley, D., Tuller, E., ... Clarke-Pearson, D.L. (2008). A randomized phase III trial of VH fibrin sealant to reduce lymphedema after inguinal lymph node dissection: A Gynecologic Oncology Group study. *Gynecologic Oncology, 110,* 76–82. doi:10.1016/j.ygyno.2008.03.005

105. Gothard, L., Haviland, J., Bryson, P., Laden, G., Glover, M., Harrison, S., ... Yarnold, J. (2010). Randomised phase II trial of hyperbaric oxygen therapy in patients with chronic arm lymphoedema after radiotherapy for cancer. *Radiotherapy and Oncology, 97,* 101–107. doi:10.1016/j.radonc.2010.04.026

106. Gothard, L., Stanton, A., MacLaren, J., Lawrence, D., Hall, E., Mortimer, P., ... Yarnold, J. (2004). Non-randomized phase II trial of hyperbaric oxygen therapy in patients with chronic arm lymphedema and tissue fibrosis after radiotherapy for early breast cancer. *Radiotherapy and Oncology, 70,* 217–224. doi:10.1016/S0167-8140(03)00235-4

107. Belmonte, R., Tejero, M., Ferrer, M., Muniesa, J.M., Duarte, E., Cunillera, O., & Escalada, F. (2012). Efficacy of low-frequency low-intensity electrotherapy in the treatment of breast cancer-related lymphoedema: A cross-over randomized trial. *Clinical Rehabilitation, 26,* 607–618. doi:10.1177/0269215511427414

108. Jahr, S., Schoppe, B., & Reisshauer, A. (2008). Effect of treatment with low-intensity and extremely low-frequency electrostatic fields (Deep Oscillation) on breast tissue and pain in patients with secondary breast lymphoedema. *Journal of Rehabilitation Medicine, 40,* 645–650. doi:10.2340/16501977-0225

109. Ahmed Omar, M.T., Abd-El-Guyed Ebid, A., & El Morsy, A.M. (2011). Treatment of post-mastectomy lymphedema with laser therapy: Double blind placebo control randomized study. *Journal of Surgical Research, 165,* 82–90. doi:10.1016/j.jss.2010.03.050

110. Carati, C.J., Anderson, S.N., Gannon, B.J., & Piller, N.B. (2003). Treatment of post-mastectomy lymphedema with low-level laser therapy. *Cancer, 98,* 1114–1122. doi:10.1002/cncr.11641

111. Dirican, A., Andacoglu, O., Johnson, R., McGuire, K., Mager, L., & Soran, A. (2011). The short-term effects of low-level laser therapy in the management of breast-cancer-related lymphedema. *Supportive Care in Cancer, 19,* 685–690. doi:10.1007/s00520-010-0888-8

112. Kaviani, A., Fateh, M., Yousefi Nooraie, R., Alinagi-zadeh, M.R., & Ataie-Fashtami, L. (2006). Low-level laser therapy in management of postmastectomy lymphedema. *Lasers in Medical Science, 21,* 90–94. doi:10.1007/s10103-006-0380-3

113. Kozanoglu, E., Basaran, S., Paydas, S., & Sarpel, T. (2009). Efficacy of pneumatic compression and low-level laser therapy in the treatment of postmastectomy lymphoedema: A randomized controlled trial. *Clinical Rehabilitation, 23,* 117–124. doi:10.1177/0269215508096173

114. Lau, R.W.L., & Cheing, G.L.Y. (2009). Managing postmastectomy lymphedema with low-level laser therapy. *Photomedicine and Laser Surgery, 27,* 763–769. doi:10.1089/pho.2008.2330

115. Omar, M.T., Shaheen, A.A.M., & Zafar, H. (2012). A systematic review of the effect of low-level laser therapy in the management of breast cancer–related lymphedema. *Supportive Care in Cancer, 20,* 2977–2984. doi:10.1007/s00520-012-1546-0

116. Casley-Smith, J.R., & Casley-Smith, J.R. (1996). Lymphedema initiated by aircraft flights. *Aviation, Space, and Environmental Medicine, 67,* 52–56.

117. Graham, P.H. (2002). Compression prophylaxis may increase the potential for flight-associated lymphoedema after breast cancer treatment. *Breast, 11,* 66–71. doi:10.1054/brst.2001.0370

14

Mucositis

Lee Ann Johnson, PhD(c), RN,
Karen S. Henry, ARNP, FNP-BC, MSN, AOCNP®,
Hanan Saca-Hazboun, PhD(c), RN,
Celestine Samuel-Blalock, MSNL-HCS, PHN, RN-BC

Problem and Incidence

Oral mucositis is damage to the epithelium of the oral cavity. Patients receiving chemotherapy, epidermal growth factor receptor inhibitors, tyrosine kinase inhibitors, or radiation to the head and neck are susceptible to the development of oral mucositis. Mucositis causes pain, restricts oral intake, and contributes to malnutrition, interruption of treatment, and increased hospitalizations. Incremental costs of mucositis are usually associated with hospital stays, and these costs more than double when mucositis is severe.[1]

Mucositis occurs in about 40% of patients after standard doses of chemotherapy and in up to 100% of patients receiving high-dose chemotherapy or radiation for head and neck cancer.[2]

Risk Factors and Assessment

Risk factors for mucositis include
- Concurrent radiation and chemotherapy
- Hematopoietic cell transplantation
- High-dose or continuous-infusion chemotherapy and agents containing antimetabolites, such as 5-fluorouracil
- Radiation for head and neck cancer.

Factors contributing to risk include
- Prior poor oral hygiene
- Poor nutritional status.

Assessment approaches for mucositis include physical examination of the mouth and assessment of associated pain and ability to eat.

Commonly used measurement tools include
- World Health Organization scale for mucositis
- National Cancer Institute Cancer Therapy Evaluation Program *Common Terminology Criteria for Adverse Events* (open access)[3]
- Visual analog scale for oral pain.

What interventions are effective in managing mucositis in people with cancer?

Evidence retrieved through August 31, 2013

Recommended for Practice

Cryotherapy using ice water, ice cubes, ice chips, or ice lollipops during chemotherapy infusion reduced symptoms, incidence, severity, and pain associated with mucositis for patients receiving chemotherapy agents with a short half-life.[4-17]

Low-level laser therapy has shown mixed results in individual studies in children and adults; however, the majority of studies demonstrated benefit.[4,18-37] One systematic review in pediatric patients reported conflicting evidence.[38] Two systematic reviews showed effectiveness.[5,39] A meta-analysis showed significant high effect sizes for reducing the prevalence, severity, pain, and duration of mucositis.[40] Current European Society for Medical Oncology (ESMO) guidelines recommend low-level laser treatment before hematopoietic cell transplantation.[41] Research has been restricted to patients with head and neck cancer and those undergoing transplantation.

Oral care protocols to provide consistent frequent oral hygiene, prophylactic mouth rinses, and routine assessment for early detection decreased the incidence, duration, and severity of mucositis.[6,38,42-46] Structure and components of oral care are important.[47]

Palifermin was an effective preventive treatment for patients receiving high-dose chemotherapy.[41,48-62]

Sodium bicarbonate mouth rinses were shown to be effective in systematic reviews.[45,63]

Likely to Be Effective

Benzydamine rinses lowered the severity and pain of mucositis.[6,64-67] A systematic review reported inconsistent results in comparison to chlorhexidine.[45] ESMO guidelines recommend benzydamine oral rinse for patients with head and neck cancer.[44]

Chlorhexidine (prophylactic use only) reduced incidence and pain associated with oral mucositis in three of five individual studies.[43,47,68-70] Two systematic reviews reported moderate support for prophylactic use.[38,71] **Chlorhexidine is not recommended as treatment for existing mucositis.**

Lactobacillus **lozenges** reduced the incidence of oral mucositis compared to placebo in patients with head and neck cancer receiving chemoradiation therapy.[72]

Effectiveness Not Established

Numerous topical and systemic pharmacologic and nonpharmacologic interventions have been studied for efficacy in prevention and management of oral mucositis or management of associated pain. Evidence for these interventions is limited because of inconsistent research results, small studies, and study design limitations.

- Pharmacologic interventions
  - **Allopurinol mouthwash**[73]—Systematic reviews showed no benefit.[6,60,74]

- **Amifostine**[75-81]—A systematic review showed conflicting results, but associated guidelines suggest use of amifostine.[2]
- **Bethanechol**[82]
- **Calcium phosphate mouth rinse (Caphosol®)**[83-85]
- **Colchicine mouthwash**[86]
- **Colony-stimulating factor mouth rinses**[87-89]—Two systematic reviews showed no benefit.[38,39] A meta-analysis showed possible benefit but weak evidence.[5]
- **Colony-stimulating factors** given systemically for prophylaxis[90-95]
- **Doxepin mouthwash**[64]
- **Epithelial growth factor oral spray**[96-98]
- **Folinic acid** given systemically after high-dose methotrexate[99]
- **Glutamine** given orally[100-104]
- **Hyaluronic acid/sodium hyaluronate** and amino acid oral spray[105]—Topical use of a hyaluronic acid compound was associated with reduced pain and pathogen colonization in patients with mucositis in a small study.[106]
- **Intestinal trefoil factor** administered topically[107]
- **Irsogladine maleate** taken orally[108]
- **Phenylbutyrate mouthwash**[109]
- **Pilocarpine**[110,111]
- **Povidone iodine** topical application[112-114]
- **Repifermin**[115]
- **Tetracaine**[116]
- **Triclosan** mouth rinses[117]
- **Zinc/zinc supplements**[118-122]
• **Nonpharmacologic and complementary interventions**
- **Aloe vera**[123]
- **ATL-104**, a plant extract used as an oral rinse[124]
- ***Calendula officinalis* mouthwash**[125]
- **Fluoride chewing gum**[126]
- **Flurbiprofen tooth patch**[127]
- **Honey**[128]—Studies were in children with only low-grade symptoms. Studies in adults show mixed results and had numerous design limitations.[5,129-132]
- **Indigowoad root** gargle[133]
- **Infrared phototherapy**[134]
- **Manuka and kanuka**, plant-derived oils[135]
- **Payayor**, an herbal medicine[136]

- **Professional oral care** by hygienists[114,137]
- **Pycnogenol**®, pine bark extract[138]
- *Rhodiola algida*, an herbal solution taken by mouth[139]
- **Salivary stimulation** with a mechanical chewing device[140]
- **Samital**® mouth rinse[141]
- **Visible light therapy**[142]
- **Vitamin E** applied topically[138]

Effectiveness Unlikely

Iseganan, a peptide, did not improve mucositis compared to placebo.[143,144]

Misoprostol demonstrated no benefit.[145,146]

Traumeel® **S** had no benefit in adults or children.[147,148]

Wobe-Mugos, a concoction of proteolytic enzymes, was associated with an increase in mucositis incidence and duration in one small study.[149]

Not Recommended for Practice

Chlorhexidine (not prophylactic) did not improve existing mucositis and is not recommended in guidelines or systematic reviews for adults or children.[5,41,45,53,63,150]

Sucralfate did not improve oral mucositis.[38,151-154]

Expert Opinion

Avoid irritating foods and beverages, such as spicy, acidic, or very hot or cold substances and dry, hard foods.[155]

When possible, patients should have a professional dental examination and care prior to initiating treatment.

Application to Practice

Patients receiving systemic antitumor therapy may develop oral mucositis. Nurses can educate patients in preventive measures of consistent and frequent oral hygiene and care using appropriate mouth rinse solutions. A solution of sodium bicarbonate is effective, inexpensive, and simple for patients to prepare for their own use.

The efficacy of oral care protocols depends upon consistency and the use of appropriate oral solutions, which can be determined by the level of evidence shown here. It is important to differentiate between topical and oral agents that can be used prior to development of mucositis versus those that are not recommended for the treatment of existing mucositis, such as chlorhexidine.

For patients with poor oral condition, nurses can advocate for professional dental examination and care before treatment when possible.

For patients receiving short-acting chemotherapy, notably 5-fluorouracil, cryotherapy during infusion can be employed.

Management involves assessment and effective management of pain from mucositis and nutritional intake. Interventions to maintain nutritional status and manage pain need to be implemented.

Nurses can educate patients about dietary approaches from expert opinion that may be helpful to reduce pain with eating.

Mucositis Resource Contributors

*Topic leader: June G. Eilers, PhD, APRN, CNS, BC
Yuki Asakura, RN, MS, PhD(c), Carol S. Blecher, RN, MS, AOCN®, CBCN®, Deborah Burgoon, RN, MS, AOCN®, Brenda Robertson Burns, BS, MN, RN, OCN®, Rochelle Chiffelle, RN, BSN, MS, NP, Donna Copeland, MSN, RN, CPON®, Gina DeGennaro, DNP, RN, AOCN®, CNL, Joanne Growney, RN, MA, ANP-BC, OCN®, Dora Hallock, RN, MSN, OCN®, CRNI, CHPN, Debra J. Harris, RN, MSN, OCN®, Karen S. Henry, ARNP, FNP-BC, MSN, AOCNP®, Cathy Maxwell, RN, OCN®, Hanan Saca-Hazboun, PhD(c), RN, Celestine Samuel-Blalock, MSNL-HCS, PHN, RN-BC, and Janice Terlizzi, RN, APN, ACNS-BC, AOCN®*

References

1. Carlotto, A., Hogsett, V.L., Maiorini, E.M., Razulis, J.G., & Sonis, S.T. (2013). The economic burden of toxicities associated with cancer treatment: Review of the literature and analysis of nausea and vomiting, diarrhoea, oral mucositis and fatigue. *PharmacoEconomics, 31,* 753–766. doi:10.1007/s40273-013-0081-2

2. Gibson, R.J., Keefe, D.M.K., Lalla, R.V., Bateman, E., Blijlevens, N., Fijlstra, M., ... Bowen, J.M. (2013). Systematic review of agents for the management of gastrointestinal mucositis in cancer patients. *Supportive Care in Cancer, 21,* 313–326. doi:10.1007/s00520-012-1644-z

3. National Cancer Institute Cancer Therapy Evaluation Program. (2010, June 14). *Common terminology criteria for adverse events* [v.4.03]. Retrieved from http://evs.nci.nih.gov/ftp1/CTCAE/CTCAE_4.03_2010-06-14_QuickReference_5x7.pdf

4. Migliorati, C.A., Oberle-Edwards, L., & Schubert, M. (2006). The role of alternative and natural agents, cryotherapy, and/or laser for management of alimentary mucositis. *Supportive Care in Cancer, 14,* 533–540. doi:10.1007/s00520-006-0049-2

5. Worthington, H.V., Clarkson, J.E., Bryan, G., Furness, S., Glenny, A.M., Littlewood, A., ... Khalid, T. (2011). Interventions for preventing oral mucositis for patients with cancer receiving treatment. *Cochrane Database of Systematic Reviews, 2011*(4). doi:10.1002/14651858.CD000978.pub5

6. Kwong, K.K. (2004). Prevention and treatment of oropharyngeal mucositis following cancer therapy: Are there new approaches? *Cancer Nursing, 27,* 183–205. doi:10.1097/00002820-200405000-00003

7. Aisa, Y., Mori, T., Kudo, M., Yashima, T., Kondo, S., Yokoyama, A., ... Okamoto, S. (2005). Oral cryotherapy for the prevention of high-dose melphalan-induced stomatitis in allogeneic hematopoietic stem cell transplant recipients. *Supportive Care in Cancer, 13,* 266–269. doi:10.1007/s00520-004-0726-y

8. Karagozoğlu, Ş., & Ulusoy, M.F. (2005). Chemotherapy: The effect of oral cryotherapy on the development of mucositis. *Journal of Clinical Nursing, 14,* 754–765. doi:10.1111/j.1365-2702.2005.01128.x

9. Katranci, N., Ovayolu, N., Ovayolu, O., & Sevinc, A. (2012). Evaluation of the effect of cryotherapy in preventing oral mucositis associated with chemotherapy—A randomized controlled trial. *European Journal of Oncology Nursing, 16,* 339–344. doi:10.1016/j.ejon.2011.07.008

10. Lilleby, K., Garcia, P., Gooley, T., McDonnnell, P., Taber, R., Holmberg, L., ... Bensinger, W. (2006). A prospective, randomized study of cryotherapy during administration of high-dose melphalan to decrease the severity and duration of oral mucositis in patients with multiple myeloma undergoing autologous peripheral blood stem cell transplantation. *Bone Marrow Transplantation, 37,* 1031–1035. doi:10.1038/sj.bmt.1705384

11. Mori, T., Hasegawa, K., Okabe, A., Tsujimura, N., Kawata, Y., Yashima, T., ... Okamoto, S. (2008). Efficacy of mouth rinse in preventing oral mucositis in patients receiving high-dose cytarabine for allogeneic hematopoietic stem cell transplantation. *International Journal of Hematology, 88,* 583–587. doi:10.1007/s12185-008-0181-5

12. Mori, T., Yamazaki, R., Aisa, Y., Nakazato, T., Kudo, M., Yashima, T., ... Okamoto, S. (2006). Brief oral cryotherapy for the prevention of high-dose melphalan-induced stomatitis in allogeneic hematopoietic stem cell transplant recipients. *Supportive Care in Cancer, 4,* 392–395. doi:10.1007/s00520-005-0016-3

13. Nikoletti, S., Hyde, S., Shaw, T., Myers, H., & Kristjanson, L.J. (2005). Comparison of plain ice and flavored ice for preventing oral mucositis associated with the use of 5-fluorouracil. *Journal of Clinical Nursing, 14,* 750–753. doi:10.1111/j.1365-2702.2005.01156.x

14. Papadeas, E., Naxakis, S., Riga, M., & Kalofonos, C. (2007). Prevention of 5-fluorouracil-related stomatitis by oral cryotherapy: A randomized controlled study. *European Journal of Oncology Nursing, 11*, 60–65. doi:10.1016/j.ejon.2006.05.002

15. Salvador, P., Azusano, C., Wang, L., & Howell, D. (2012). A pilot randomized controlled trial of an oral care intervention to reduce mucositis severity in stem cell transplant patients. *Journal of Pain and Symptom Management, 44*, 64–73. doi:10.1016/j.jpainsymman.2011.08.012

16. Svanberg, A., Öhrn, K., & Birgegård, G. (2010). Oral cryotherapy reduces mucositis and improves nutrition—A randomised controlled trial. *Journal of Clinical Nursing, 19*, 2146–2151. doi:10.1111/j.1365-2702.2010.03255.x

17. Vokurka, S., Bystřická, E., Sčudlová, J., Mazur, E., Visokaiova, M., Vasilieva, E., ... Streinerova, K. (2011). The risk factors for oral mucositis and the effect of cryotherapy in patients after the BEAM and HD-l-PAM 200 mg/m² autologous hematopoietic stem cell transplantation. *European Journal of Oncology Nursing, 15*, 508–512. doi:10.1016/j.ejon.2011.01.006

18. Antunes, H.S., de Sá Ferreira, E.M., de Matos, V.D., Pinheiro, C.T., & Ferreira, C.G. (2008). The impact of low power laser in the treatment of conditioning-induced oral mucositis: A report of 11 clinical cases and their review. *Medicina Oral, Patología Oral y Cirugía Bucal, 13*, 189–192. Retrieved from http://www.medicinaoral.com/pubmed/medoralv13_i3_p189.pdf

19. Arbabi-Kalati, F., Arbabi-Kalati, F., & Moridi, T. (2013). Evaluation of the effect of low-level laser on prevention of chemotherapy-induced mucositis. *Acta Medica Iranica, 51*, 157–162. Retrieved from http://acta.tums.ac.ir/index.php/acta/article/view/2457

20. Arora, H., Pai, K.M., Maiya, A., Vidyasagar, M.S., & Rajeev, A. (2008). Efficacy of He-Ne laser in the prevention and treatment of radiotherapy-induced oral mucositis in oral cancer patients. *Oral Surgery, Oral Medicine, Oral Pathology, Oral Radiology, and Endodontology, 105*, 180–186. doi:10.1016/j.tripleo.2007.07.043

21. Carvalho, P.A.G., Jaguar, G.C., Pellizzon, A.C., Prado, J.D., Lopes, R.N., & Alves, F.A. (2011). Evaluation of low-level laser therapy in the prevention and treatment of radiation-induced mucositis: A double-blind randomized study in head and neck cancer patients. *Oral Oncology, 47*, 1176–1181. doi:10.1016/j.oraloncology.2011.08.021

22. Cauwels, R.G.E.C., & Martens, L.C. (2011). Low-level laser therapy in oral mucositis: A pilot study. *European Archives of Paediatric Dentistry, 12*, 118–123. doi:10.1007/BF03262791

23. Cruz, L.B., Ribeiro, A.S., Rech, A., Rosa, L.G.N., Castro, C.G., Jr., & Brunetto, A.L. (2007). Influence of low-energy laser in the prevention of oral mucositis in children with cancer receiving chemotherapy. *Pediatric Blood and Cancer, 48*, 435–440. doi:10.1002/pbc.20943

24. Cunha, C.B., Eduardo, F.P., Zezell, D.M., Bezinelli, L.M., Shitara, P.P., & Correa, I. (2012). Effect of irradiation with red and infrared laser in the treatment of oral mucositis: A pilot study with patients undergoing chemotherapy with 5-FU. *Lasers in Medical Science, 27*, 1233–1240. doi:10.1007/s10103-012-1089-0

25. Gautam, A.P., Fernandes, D.J., Vidyasagar, M.S., Maiya, A.G., & Vadhiraja, B.M. (2012). Low-level laser therapy for concurrent chemoradiotherapy induced oral mucositis in head and neck cancer patients—A triple blinded randomized controlled trial. *Radiotherapy and Oncology, 104*, 349–354. doi:10.1016/j.radonc.2012.06.011

26. Gautam, A.P., Fernandes, D.J., Vidyasagar, M.S., & Maiya, G.A. (2012). Low-level helium neon laser therapy for chemoradiotherapy induced oral mucositis in oral cancer patients—A randomized controlled trial. *Oral Oncology, 48*, 893–897. doi:10.1016/j.oraloncology.2012.03.008

27. Genot-Klastersky, M.T., Klastersky, J., Awada, F., Awada, A., Crombez, P., Martinez, M.D., ... Paesmans, M. (2008). The use of low-energy laser (LEL) for the prevention of chemotherapy- and/or radiotherapy-induced oral mucositis in cancer patients: Results from two prospective studies. *Supportive Care in Cancer, 16*, 1381–1387. doi:10.1007/s00520-008-0439-8

28. Gouvêa de Lima, A., Villar, R.C., de Castro, G., Jr., Antequera, R., Gil, E., Rosalmeida, M.C., ... Snitcovsky, I.M.L. (2012). Oral mucositis prevention by low-level laser therapy in head-and-neck cancer patients undergoing concurrent chemoradiotherapy: A phase III randomized study. *International Journal of Radiation Oncology, Biology, Physics, 82*, 270–275. doi:10.1016/j.ijrobp.2010.10.012

29. Jaguar, G.C., Prado, J.D., Nishimoto, I.N., Pinheiro, M.C., De Castro, D.O., Jr., da Cruz Perez, D.E., & Alves, F.A. (2007). Low-energy laser therapy for prevention of oral mucositis in hematopoietic stem cell transplantation. *Oral Diseases, 13*, 538–543. doi:10.1111/j.1601-0825.2006.01330.x

30. Khouri, V.Y., Stracieri, A.B.P.L., Rodrigues, M.C., de Moraes, D.A., Pieroni, F., Simões, B.P., & Voltarelli, J.C. (2009). Use of therapeutic laser for prevention and treatment of oral mucositis. *Brazilian Dental Journal, 20*, 215–220. doi:10.1590/S0103-64402009000300008

31. Kuhn, A., Porto, F.A., Miraglia, P., & Brunetto, A.L. (2009). Low-level infrared laser therapy in chemotherapy-induced oral mucositis: A randomized placebo-controlled trial in children. *Journal of Pediatric Hematology/Oncology, 31*, 33–37. doi:10.1097/MPH.0b013e318192cb8e

32. Maiya, G., Sagar, M., & Fernandes, D. (2006). Effect of low-level helium-neon (He-Ne) laser therapy in the prevention and treatment of radiation induced mucositis in head and neck cancer patients. *Indian Journal of Medical Research, 124*, 399–402.

33. Migliorati, C., Hewson, I., Lalla, R.V., Antunes, H.S., Estilo, C.L., Hodgson, B., ... Elad, S. (2013). Systematic review of laser and other light therapy for the management of oral mucositis in cancer patients. *Supportive Care in Cancer, 21*, 333–341. doi:10.1007/s00520-012-1605-6

34. Nes, A.G., & Posso, M.B.S. (2005). Patients with moderate chemotherapy-induced mucositis: Pain therapy using low intensity lasers. *International Nursing Review, 52*, 68–72. doi:10.1111/j.1466-7657.2004.00401.x

35. Schubert, M.M., Eduardo, F.P., Guthrie, K.A., Franquin, J.-C., Bensadoun, R.J., Migliorati, C.A., ... Hamdi, M. (2007). A phase III randomized double-blind placebo-controlled clinical trial to determine the efficacy of low-level laser therapy for the prevention of oral mucositis in patients undergoing hematopoietic cell transplantation. *Supportive Care in Cancer, 15*, 1145–1154. doi:10.1007/s00520-007-0238-7

36. Simões, A., Eduardo, F.P., Luiz, A.C., Campos, L., Sá, P.H., Cristófaro, M., ... Eduardo, C.P. (2009). Laser phototherapy as topical prophylaxis against head and neck cancer radiotherapy-induced oral mucositis: Comparison between low and high/low power lasers. *Lasers in Surgery and Medicine, 41*, 264–270. doi:10.1002/lsm.20758

37. Zanin, T., Zanin, F., Carvalhosa, A.A., de Souza Castro, P.H., Pacheco, M.T., Zanin, I.C., & Brugnera, A. (2010). Use of 660-nm diode laser in the prevention and treatment of human oral mucositis induced by radiotherapy and chemotherapy. *Photomedicine and Laser Surgery, 28*, 233–237. doi:10.1089/pho.2008.2242

38. Qutob, A.F., Gue, S., Revesz, T., Logan, R.M., & Keefe, D. (2013). Prevention of oral mucositis in children receiving cancer therapy: A systematic review and evidence-based analysis. *Oral Oncology, 49*, 102–107. doi:10.1016/j.oraloncology.2012.08.008

39. Clarkson, J.E., Worthington, H.V., Furness, S., McCabe, M., Khalid, T., & Meyer, S. (2010). Interventions for treating oral mucositis for patients with cancer receiving treatment. *Cochrane Database of Systematic Reviews, 2010*(8). doi:10.1002/14651858.CD001973.pub4

40. Bjordal, J.M., Bensadoun, R.-J., Tunèr, J., Frigo, L., Gjerde, K., & Lopes-Martins, R.A.B. (2011). A systematic review with meta-analysis of the effect of low-level laser therapy (LLLT) in cancer therapy-induced oral mucositis. *Supportive Care in Cancer, 19*, 1069–1077. doi:10.1007/s00520-011-1202-0

41. Peterson, D.E., Bensadoun, R.-J., & Roila, F. (2010). Management of oral and gastrointestinal mucositis: ESMO clinical practice guidelines. *Annals of Oncology, 21*(Suppl. 5), v261–v265. doi:10.1093/annonc/mdq197

42. Bhatt, V., Vendrell, N., Nau, K., Crumb, D., & Roy, V. (2010). Implementation of a standardized protocol for prevention and management of oral mucositis in patients undergoing hematopoietic cell transplantation. *Journal of Oncology Pharmacy Practice, 16,* 195–204. doi:10.1177/1078155209348721

43. Cheng, K.K.F., Molassiotis, A., Chang, A.M., Wai, W.C., & Cheung, S.S. (2001). Evaluation of an oral care protocol intervention in the prevention of chemotherapy-induced oral mucositis in pediatric cancer patients. *European Journal of Cancer, 37,* 2056–2063. doi:10.1016/S0959-8049(01)00098-3

44. Peterson, D.E., Bensadoun, R.-J., & Roila, F. (2011). Management of oral and gastrointestinal mucositis: ESMO clinical practice guidelines. *Annals of Oncology, 22*(Suppl. 6), vi78–vi84. doi:10.1093/annonc/mdr391

45. Shih, A., Miaskowski, C., Dodd, M.J., Stotts, N.A., & MacPhail, L. (2002). A research review of the current treatments for radiation-induced oral mucositis in patients with head and neck cancer. *Oncology Nursing Forum, 29,* 1063–1078. doi:10.1188/02.ONF.1063-1080

46. Yamagata, K., Arai, C., Sasaki, H., Takeuchi, Y., Onizawa, K., Yanagawa, T., ... Bukawa, H. (2012). The effect of oral management on the severity of oral mucositis during hematopoietic SCT. *Bone Marrow Transplantation, 47,* 725–730. doi:10.1038/bmt.2011.171

47. Dodd, M.J., Dibble, S.L., Miaskowski, C., MacPhail, L., Greenspan, D., Paul, S.M., ... Larson, P. (2000). Randomized clinical trial of the effectiveness of 3 commonly used mouthwashes to treat chemotherapy-induced mucositis. *Oral Surgery, Oral Medicine, Oral Pathology, Oral Radiology, and Endodontology, 90,* 39–47. doi:10.1067/moe.2000.105713

48. Blijlevens, N., de Château, M., Krivan, G., Rabitsch, W., Szomor, A., Pytlik, R., ... Niederwieser, D. (2013). In a high-dose melphalan setting, palifermin compared with placebo had no effect on oral mucositis or related patient's burden. *Bone Marrow Transplantation, 48,* 966–971. doi:10.1038/bmt.2012.257

49. Henke, M., Alfonsi, M., Foa, P., Giralt, J., Bardet, E., Cerezo, L., ... Berger, D. (2011). Palifermin decreases severe oral mucositis of patients undergoing postoperative radiochemotherapy for head and neck cancer: A randomized, placebo-controlled trial. *Journal of Clinical Oncology, 29,* 2815–2820. doi:10.1200/JCO.2010.32.4103

50. Langner, S., Staber, P.B., Schub, N., Gramatzki, M., Grothe, W., Behre, G., ... Neumeister, P. (2008). Palifermin reduces incidence and severity of oral mucositis in allogeneic stem-cell transplant recipients. *Bone Marrow Transplantation, 42,* 275–279. doi:10.1038/bmt.2008.157

51. Le, Q.T., Kim, H.E., Schneider, C.J., Muraközy, G., Skladowski, K., Reinisch, S., ... Henke, M. (2011). Palifermin reduces severe mucositis in definitive chemoradiotherapy of locally advanced head and neck cancer: A randomized, placebo-controlled study. *Journal of Clinical Oncology, 29,* 2808–2814. doi:10.1200/JCO.2010.32.4095

52. Nasilowska-Adamska, B., Rzepecki, P., Manko, J., Czyz, A., Markieweicz, M., Federowicz, I., ... Marianska, B. (2007). The influence of palifermin (Kepivance) on oral mucositis and acute graft versus host disease in patients with hematological diseases undergoing hematopoietic stem cell transplant. *Bone Marrow Transplantation, 40,* 983–988. doi:10.1038/sj.bmt.1705846

53. Niscola, P., Scaramucci, L., Giovannini, M., Ales, M., Bondanini, F., Cupelli, L., ... de Fabritiis, P. (2009). Palifermin in the management of mucositis in hematological malignancies: Current evidences and future perspectives. *Cardiovascular and Hematological Agents in Medicinal Chemistry, 7,* 305–312. doi:10.2174/187152509789541873

54. Raber-Durlacher, J.E., von Bültzingslöwen, I., Logan, R.M., Bowen, J., Al-Azri, A.R., Everaus, H., ... Lalla, R.V. (2013). Systematic review of cytokines and growth factors for the management of oral mucositis in cancer patients. *Supportive Care in Cancer, 21,* 343–355. doi:10.1007/s00520-012-1594-5

55. Rosen, L.S., Abdi, E., Davis, I.D., Gutheil, J., Schnell, F.M., Zalcberg, J., ... Clarke, S. (2006). Palifermin reduces the incidence of oral mucositis in

patients with metastatic coloroctal cancer treated with fluorouracil-based chemotherapy. *Journal of Clinical Oncology, 24,* 5194–5200. doi:10.1200/JCO.2005.04.1152

56. Schmidt, E., Thoennissen, N.H., Rudat, A., Bieker, R., Schliemann, C., Mesters, R.M., ... Berdel, W.E. (2008). Use of palifermin for the prevention of high-dose methotrexate-induced oral mucositis. *Annals of Oncology, 19,* 1644–1649. doi:10.1093/annonc/mdn179

57. Shea, T.C., Kewalramani, T., Mun, Y., Jayne, G., & Dreiling, L.K. (2007). Evaluation of single-dose palifermin to reduce oral mucositis in fractionated total-body irradiation and high-dose chemotherapy with autologous peripheral blood progenitor cell transplantation. *Journal of Supportive Oncology, 5*(4, Suppl. 2), 60–61. Retrieved from http://www.oncologypractice.com/jso/journal/articles/0504s260.pdf

58. Sonis, S.T. (2009). Efficacy of palifermin (keratinocyte growth factor-1) in the amelioration of oral mucositis. *Core Evidence, 4,* 199–205. doi:10.2147/CE.S5995

59. Spielberger, R., Stiff, P., Bensinger, W., Gentile, T., Weisdorf, D., Kewalramani, T., ... Emmanouilides, C. (2004). Palifermin for oral mucositis after intensive therapy for hematologic cancers. *New England Journal of Medicine, 351,* 2590–2598. doi:10.1056/NEJMoa040125

60. Stokman, M.A., Spijkervet, F.K.L., Boezen, H.M., Schouten, J.P., Roodenburg, J.L.N., & deVries, E.G.E. (2006). Preventive intervention possibilities in radiotherapy and chemotherapy-induced oral mucositis: Results of meta-analysis. *Journal of Dental Research, 85,* 690–700. doi:10.1177/154405910608500802

61. Vadhan-Raj, S., Trent, J., Patel, S., Zhou, X., Johnson, M.M., Araujo, D., ... Benjamin, R.S. (2010). Single-dose palifermin prevents severe oral mucositis during multicycle chemotherapy in patients with cancer: A randomized trial. *Annals of Internal Medicine, 153,* 358–367. doi:10.7326/0003-4819-153-6-201009210-00003

62. von Bültzingslöwen, I., Brennan, M.T., Spijkervet, F.K., Logan, R., Stringer, A., Raber-Durlacher, J.E., & Keefe, D. (2006). Growth factors and cytokines in the prevention and treatment of oral and gastrointestinal mucositis. *Supportive Care in Cancer, 14,* 519–527. doi:10.1007/s00520-006-0052-7

63. Potting, C.M.J., Uitterhoeve, R., Scholte Op Reimer, W., & Van Achterberg, T. (2006). The effectiveness of commonly used mouthwashes for the prevention of chemotherapy-induced oral mucositis: A systematic review. *European Journal of Cancer Care, 15,* 431–439. doi:10.1111/j.1365-2354.2006.00684.x

64. Epstein, J.B., Epstein, J.D., Epstein, M.S., Oien, H., & Truelove, E.L. (2008). Doxepin rinse for management of mucositis pain in patients with cancer: One week follow-up of topical therapy. *Special Care in Dentistry, 28,* 73–77. doi:10.1111/j.1754-4505.2008.00015.x

65. Epstein, J.B., Silverman, S., Paggiarino, D.A., Crockett, S., Schubert, M.M., Senzer, N.N., ... Leveque, F.G. (2001). Benzydamine HCl for prophylaxis of radiation-induced oral mucositis: Results from a multicenter, randomized, double-blind, placebo-controlled clinical trial. *Cancer, 92,* 875–885. doi:10.1002/1097-0142(20010815)92:4<875::AID-CNCR1396>3.0.CO;2-1

66. Kazemian, A., Kamian, S., Aghili, M., Hashemi, F.A., & Haddad, P. (2009). Benzydamine for prophylaxis of radiation-induced oral mucositis in head and neck cancers: A double-blind placebo-controlled randomized clinical trial. *European Journal of Cancer Care, 18,* 174–178. doi:10.1111/j.1365-2354.2008.00943.x

67. Roopashri, G., Jayanthi, K., & Guruprasad, R. (2011). Efficacy of benzydamine hydrochloride, chlorhexidine, and povidone iodine in the treatment of oral mucositis among patients undergoing radiotherapy in head and neck malignancies: A drug trial. *Contemporary Clinical Dentistry, 2,* 8–12. doi:10.4103/0976-237X.79292

68. Cheng, K.K.F., Chang, A.M., & Yuen, M.P. (2004). Prevention of oral mucositis in pediatric patients treated with chemotherapy: A randomized

crossover trial comparing two protocols of oral care. *European Journal of Cancer, 40,* 1208–1216. doi:10.1016/j.ejca.2003.10.023

69. Pitten, F.-A., Kiefer, T., Buth, C., Doelken, G., & Kramer, A. (2003). Do cancer patients with chemotherapy-induced leukopenia benefit from an antiseptic chlorhexidine-based oral rinse? A double-blind, block-randomized, controlled study. *Journal of Hospital Infection, 53,* 283–291. doi:10.1053/jhin.2002.1391

70. Sorensen, J.B., Skovsgaard, T., Bork, E., Damstrup, L., & Ingeberg, S. (2008). Double-blind, placebo-controlled, randomized study of chlorhexidine prophylaxis for 5-fluorouracil–based chemotherapy-induced oral mucositis with nonblinded randomized comparison to oral cooling (cryotherapy) in gastrointestinal malignancies. *Cancer, 112,* 1600–1606. doi:10.1002/cncr.23328

71. Donnelly, J.P., Bellm, L.A., Epstien, J.B., Sonis, S.T., & Symonds, R.P. (2003). Antimicrobial therapy to prevent or treat oral mucositis. *Lancet Infectious Diseases, 3,* 405–412. doi:10.1016/S1473-3099(03)00668-6

72. Sharma, A., Rath, G.K., Chaudhary, S.P., Thakar, A., Mohanti, B.K., & Bahadur, S. (2012). *Lactobacillus brevis* CD2 lozenges reduce radiation- and chemotherapy-induced mucositis in patients with head and neck cancer: A randomized double-blind placebo-controlled study. *European Journal of Cancer, 48,* 875–881. doi:10.1016/j.ejca.2011.06.010

73. Panahi, Y., Ala, S., Saeedi, M., Okhovatian, A., Bazzaz, N., & Naghizadeh, M. (2010). Allopurinol mouth rinse for prophylaxis of fluorouracil-induced mucositis. *European Journal of Cancer Care, 19,* 308–312. doi:10.1111/j.1365-2354.2008.01042.x

74. Worthington, H.V., Clarkson, J.E., & Eden, O.B. (2004). Interventions for treating oral mucositis for patients with cancer receiving treatment. *Cochrane Database of Systematic Reviews, 2004*(2). doi:10.1002/14651858.CD001973.pub2

75. Antonadou, D., Pepelassi, M., Synodinou, M., Puglisi, M., & Throuvalas, N. (2002). Prophylactic use of amifostine to prevent radiochemotherapy-induced mucositis and xerostomia in head-and-neck cancer. *International Journal of Radiation Oncology, Biology, Physics, 52,* 739–747. doi:10.1016/S0360-3016(01)02683-9

76. Buentzel, J., Micke, O., Adamietz, I.A., Monnier, A., Glatzel, M., & deVries, A. (2006). Intravenous amifostine during chemoradiotherapy for head-and-neck cancer: A randomized placebo-controlled phase III study. *International Journal of Radiation Oncology, Biology, Physics, 64,* 684–691. doi:10.1016/j.ijrobp.2005.08.005

77. Hwang, W.Y., Koh, L.P., Ng, H.J., Tan, P.H., Chuah, C.T., Fook, S.C., ... Goh, Y.T. (2004). A randomized trial of amifostine as a cytoprotectant for patients receiving myeloablative therapy for allogeneic hematopoietic stem cell transplantation. *Bone Marrow Transplantation, 34,* 51–56. doi:10.1038/sj.bmt.1704521

78. Jantunen, E., Kuittinen, T., & Nousiainen, T. (2002). A pilot study on feasibility and efficacy of amifostine preceding high-dose melphalan with autologous stem cell support in myeloma patients. *Leukemia and Lymphoma, 43,* 1961–1965. doi:10.1080/1042819021000015907

79. Lorusso, D., Ferrandina, G., Greggi, S., Gadducci, A., Pignata, S., Tateo, S., ... Scambia, G. (2003). Phase III multicenter randomized trial of amifostine as cytoprotectant in first-line chemotherapy in ovarian cancer patients. *Annals of Oncology, 14,* 1086–1093. doi:10.1093/annonc/mdg301

80. Spencer, A., Horvath, N., Gibson, J., Prince, H.M., Herrmann, R., Bashford, J., ... Taylor, K. (2005). Prospective randomized trial of amifostine cytoprotection in myeloma patients undergoing high-dose melphalan conditioned autologous stem cell transplantation. *Bone Marrow Transplantation, 35,* 971–977. doi:10.1038/sj.bmt.1704946

81. Thieblemont, V.C., Dumontet, C., Saad, H., Roch, N., Bouafia, F., Arnaud, P., ... Coiffier, B. (2002). Amifostine reduces mucosal damage after high-dose melphalan conditioning and autologous peripheral blood progenitor

cell transplantation for patients with multiple myeloma. *Bone Marrow Transplantation, 30,* 769–775. doi:10.1038/sj.bmt.1703757

82. Jham, B.C., Chen, H., Carvalho, A.L., & Freire, A.R. (2009). A randomized phase III prospective trial of bethanechol to prevent mucositis, candidiasis, and taste loss in patients with head and neck cancer undergoing radiotherapy: A secondary analysis. *Journal of Oral Science, 51,* 565–572. doi:10.2334/josnusd.51.565

83. Markiewicz, M., Dzierzak-Mietla, M., Frankiewicz, A., Zielinska, P., Koclega, A., Kruszelnicka, M., & Kyrcz-Krzemien, S. (2012). Treating oral mucositis with a supersaturated calcium phosphate rinse: Comparison with control in patients undergoing allogeneic hematopoietic stem cell transplantation. *Supportive Care in Cancer, 20,* 2223–2229. doi:10.1007/s00520-012-1489-5

84. Papas, A.S., Clark, R.E., Martuscelli, G., O'Loughlin, K.T., Johansen, E., & Miller, K.B. (2003). A prospective, randomized trial for the prevention of mucositis in patients undergoing hematopoietic stem cell transplantation. *Bone Marrow Transplantation, 31,* 705–712. doi:10.1038/sj.bmt.1703870

85. Stokman, M.A., Burlage, F.R., & Spijkervet, F.K. (2012). The effect of a calcium phosphate mouth rinse on (chemo) radiation induced oral mucositis in head and neck cancer patients: A prospective study. *International Journal of Dental Hygiene, 10,* 175–180. doi:10.1111/j.1601-5037.2012.00574.x

86. Garavito, A.A., Cardona, A.F., Reveiz, L., Ospina, E., Yepes, A., & Ospina, V. (2008). Colchicine mouth washings to improve oral mucositis in patients with hematological malignancies: A clinical trial. *Palliative and Supportive Care, 6,* 371–376. doi:10.1017/S147895150800059X

87. Hejna, M., Köstler, W.J., Raderer, M., Steger, G.G., Brodowicz, T., Scheithauer, W., … Zielinski, C.C. (2001). Decrease of duration and symptoms in chemotherapy-induced oral mucositis by topical GM-CSF: Results of a prospective randomized trial. *European Journal of Cancer, 37,* 1994–2002. doi:10.1016/S0959-8049(01)00132-0

88. Mantovani, G., Massa, E., Astara, G., Murgia, V., Gramignano, G., Lusso, M.R., … Macciò, A. (2003). Phase II clinical trial of local use of GM-CSF for prevention and treatment of chemotherapy and concomitant chemoradiotherapy-induced severe oral mucositis in advanced head and neck cancer patients: An evaluation of effectiveness, safety and costs. *Oncology Reports, 10,* 197–206. doi:10.3892/or.10.1.197

89. Nicolatou-Galitis, O., Dardoufas, K., Markoulatos, P., Sotiropoulou-Lontou, A., Kyprianou, K., Kolitsi, G., … Velegraki, A. (2001). Oral pseudomembranous candidiasis, herpes simplex virus-1 infection, and oral mucositis in head and neck cancer patients receiving radiotherapy and granulocyte-macrophage colony-stimulating factor (GM-CSF) mouthwash. *Journal of Oral Pathology and Medicine, 30,* 471–480. doi:10.1034/j.1600-0714.2001.030008471.x

90. Crawford, J., Tomita, D.K., Mazanet, R., Glaspy, J., & Ozer, H. (1999). Reduction of oral mucositis by filgrastim (r-metHuG-CSF) in patients receiving chemotherapy. *Cytokines, Cellular and Molecular Therapy, 5,* 187–193.

91. McAleese, J.J., Bishop, K.M., A'Hern, R., & Henk, J.M. (2006). Randomized phase II study of GM-CSF to reduce mucositis caused by accelerated radiotherapy of laryngeal cancer. *British Journal of Radiology, 79,* 608–613. doi:10.1259/bjr/55190439

92. Rossi, A., Rosati, G., Colarusso, D., & Manzione, L. (2003). Subcutaneous granulocyte–macrophage colony-stimulating factor in mucositis induced by an adjuvant 5-fluorouracil plus leucovorin regimen. *Oncology, 64,* 353–360. doi:10.1159/000070293

93. Ryu, J.K., Swann, S., LeVeque, F., Scarantino, C.W., Johnson, D., Chen, A., … Ang, K.K. (2007). The impact of concurrent granulocyte–colony stimulating factor on radiation-induced mucositis in head and neck cancer patients: A double-blind placebo-controlled prospective phase III study by Radiation Therapy Oncology Group 9901. *International Journal of Radiation Oncology, Biology, Physics, 67,* 643–650. doi:10.1016/j.ijrobp.2006.09.043

94. Sprinzl, G.M., Glavan, O., de Vries, A., Ulmer, H., Gunkel, A.R., Lukas, P., & Thumfart, W.F. (2001). Local application of granulocyte-macrophage colony stimulating factor (GM-CSF) for the treatment of oral mucositis. *European Journal of Cancer, 37,* 2003–2009. doi:10.1016/S0959-8049(01)00170-8

95. Valcárcel, D., Sanz, M.A., Jr., Sureda, A., Sala, M., Muñoz, L., Subirá, M., … Sierra, J. (2002). Mouth-washings with recombinant human granulocyte–macrophage colony stimulating factor (rhGM-CSF) do not improve grade III–IV oropharyngeal mucositis (OM) in patients with hematological malignancies undergoing stem cell transplantation. Results of a randomized, double-blind, placebo-controlled study. *Bone Marrow Transplantation, 29,* 783–787. doi:10.1038/sj.bmt.1703543

96. Hong, J.P., Lee, S.-W., Song, S.Y., Ahn, S.D., Shin, S.S., Choi, E.K., & Kim, J.H. (2009). Recombinant human epidermal growth factor treatment of radiation-induced severe oral mucositis in patients with head and neck malignancies. *European Journal of Cancer Care, 18,* 636–641. doi:10.1111/j.1365-2354.2008.00971.x

97. Kim, K.I., Kim, J.W., Lee, H.J., Kim, B.S., Bang, S.M., Kim, I., … Kim, B.K. (2013). Recombinant human epidermal growth factor on oral mucositis induced by intensive chemotherapy with stem cell transplantation. *American Journal of Hematology, 88,* 107–112. doi:10.1002/ajh.23359

98. Wu, H.G., Song, S.Y., Kim, Y.S., Oh, Y.T., Lee, C.G., Keum, K.C., … Lee, S.-W. (2009). Therapeutic effect of recombinant human epidermal growth factor (RhEGF) on mucositis in patients undergoing radiotherapy, with or without chemotherapy, for head and neck cancer: A double-blind placebo-controlled prospective phase 2 multi-institutional clinical trial. *Cancer, 115,* 3699–3708. doi:10.1002/cncr.24414

99. Sugita, J., Matsushita, T., Kashiwazaki, H., Kosugi, M., Takahashi, S., Wakasa, K., … Imamura, M. (2012). Efficacy of folinic acid in preventing oral mucositis in allogeneic hematopoietic stem cell transplant patients receiving MTX as prophylaxis for GVHD. *Bone Marrow Transplantation, 47,* 258–264. doi:10.1038/bmt.2011.53

100. Blijlevens, N.M.A., Donnelly, J.P., Naber, A.H.J., Schattenberg, A.V.M.B., & dePauw, B.E. (2005). A randomised, double-blinded, placebo-controlled, pilot study of parenteral glutamine for allogeneic stem cell transplant patients. *Supportive Care in Cancer, 13,* 790–796. doi:10.1007/s00520 -005-0790-y

101. Cerchietti, L.C.A., Navigante, A.H., Lutteral, M.A., Castro, M.A., Kirchuck, R., Bonomi, M., … Uchima, P. (2006). Double-blinded, placebo-controlled trial on intravenous L-alanyl-L-glutamine in the incidence of oral mucositis following chemoradiotherapy in patients with head-and-neck cancer. *International Journal of Radiation Oncology, Biology, Physics, 65,* 1330–1337. doi:10.1016/j.ijrobp.2006.03.042

102. Peterson, D.E., Jones, J.B., & Petit, R.G., II. (2006). Randomized, placebo-controlled trial of Saforis for prevention and treatment of oral mucositis in breast cancer patients receiving anthracycline-based chemotherapy. *Cancer, 109,* 322–331. doi:10.1002/cncr.22384

103. Vidal-Casariego, A., Calleja-Fernández, A., Ballesteros-Pomar, M.D., & Cano-Rodríguez, I. (2013). Efficacy of glutamine in the prevention of oral mucositis and acute radiation-induced esophagitis: A retrospective study. *Nutrition and Cancer, 65,* 424–429. doi:10.1080/01635581.2013.765017

104. Ward, E., Smith, M., Henderson, M., Reid, U., Lewis, I., Kinsey, S., … Picton, S.V. (2009). The effect of high-dose enteral glutamine on the incidence and severity of mucositis in paediatric oncology patients. *European Journal of Clinical Nutrition, 63,* 134–140. doi:10.1038/sj.ejcn.1602894

105. Colella, G., Cannavale, R., Vicidomini, A., Rinaldi, G., Compilato, D., & Campisi, G. (2010). Efficacy of a spray compound containing a pool of collagen precursor synthetic aminoacids (l-proline, l-leucine, l-lysine and glycine) combined with sodium hyaluronate to manage chemo/radiotherapy-induced oral mucositis: Preliminary data of an open trial. *International Journal of Immunopathology and Pharmacology, 23,* 143–151.

106. Vokurka, S., Skardova, J., Hruskova, R., Kabatova-Maxova, K., Svoboda, T., Bystricka, E., ... Koza, V. (2011). The effect of polyvinylpyrrolidone-sodium hyaluronate gel (Gelclair) on oral microbial colonization and pain control compared with other rinsing solutions in patients with oral mucositis after allogeneic stem cells transplantation. *Medical Science Monitor, 17,* CR572–CR576. doi:10.12659/MSM.881983

107. Peterson, D.E., Barker, N.P., Akhmadullina, L.I., Rodionova, I., Sherman, N.Z., Davidenko, I.S., ... Woon, C.-W. (2009). Phase II, randomized, double-blind, placebo-controlled study of recombinant human intestinal trefoil factor oral spray for prevention of oral mucositis in patients with colorectal cancer who are receiving fluorouracil-based chemotherapy. *Journal of Clinical Oncology, 27,* 4333–4338. doi:10.1200/JCO.2008.21.2381

108. Nomura, M., Kamata, M., Kojima, H., Hayashi, K., & Sawada, S. (2013). Irsogladine maleate reduces the incidence of fluorouracil-based chemotherapy-induced oral mucositis. *Annals of Oncology, 24,* 1062–1066. doi:10.1093/annonc/mds584

109. Yen, S.-H., Wang, L.-W., Lin, Y.-H., Jen, Y.-M., & Chung, Y.-L. (2012). Phenylbutyrate mouthwash mitigates oral mucositis during radiotherapy or chemoradiotherapy in patients with head-and-neck cancer. *International Journal of Radiation Oncology, Biology, Physics, 82,* 1463–1470. doi:10.1016/j.ijrobp.2011.04.029

110. Awidi, A., Homsi, U., Kakail, R.I., Mubarak, A., Hassan, A., Kelta, M., ... El-Alossy, A.S. (2001). Double-blind, placebo-controlled cross-over study of oral pilocarpine for the prevention of chemotherapy-induced oral mucositis in adult patients with cancer. *European Journal of Cancer, 37,* 2010–2014. doi:10.1016/S0959-8049(01)00189-7

111. Lockhart, P.B., Brennan, M.T., Kent, M.L., Packman, C.H., Norton, H.J., Fox, P.C., & Frenette, G. (2005). Randomized controlled trial of pilocarpine hydrochloride for the moderation of oral mucositis during autologous blood stem cell transplantation. *Bone Marrow Transplantation, 35,* 713–720. doi:10.1038/sj.bmt.1704820

112. Kumar, P.D.M., Sequeira, P.S., Shenoy, K., & Shetty, J. (2008). The effect of three mouthwashes on radiation-induced oral mucositis in patients with head and neck malignancies: A randomized control trial. *Journal of Cancer Research and Therapeutics, 4,* 3–8. doi:10.4103/0973-1482.39597

113. Vokurka, S., Bystřická, E., Koza, V., Sčudlová, J., Pavlicová, V., Valentová, D., ... Mišaniová, L. (2005). The comparative effects of povidone-iodine and normal saline mouthwashes on oral mucositis in patients after high-dose chemotherapy and APBSCT—Results of a randomized multicentre study. *Supportive Care in Cancer, 13,* 554–558. doi:10.1007/s00520-005-0792-9

114. Yoneda, S., Imai, S., Hanada, N., Yamazaki, T., Senpuku, H., Ota, Y., & Uematsu, H. (2007). Effects of oral care on development of oral mucositis and microorganisms in patients with esophageal cancer. *Japanese Journal of Infectious Diseases, 60,* 23–28. Retrieved from http://www0.nih.go.jp/JJID/60/23.pdf

115. Freytes, C.O., Ratanatharathorn, V., Taylor, C., Abboud, C., Chesser, N., Restrepoo, A., ... Odenheimer, D. (2004). Phase I/II randomized trial evaluating the safety and clinical effects of repifermin administered to reduce mucositis in patients undergoing autologous hematopoietic stem cell transplantation. *Clinical Cancer Research, 10,* 8318–8324. doi:10.1158/1078-0432.CCR-04-1118

116. Alterio, D., Jereczek-Fossa, B.A., Zuccotti, G.F., Leon, M.E., Sale, E.O., Pasetti, M., ... Orecchia, R. (2006). Tetracaine oral gel in patients treated with radiotherapy for head-and-neck cancer: Final results of a phase II study. *International Journal of Radiation Oncology, Biology, Physics, 64,* 392–395. doi:10.1016/j.ijrobp.2005.07.301

117. Satheeshkumar, P.S., Chamba, M.S., Balan, A., Sreelatha, K.T., Bhatathiri, V.N., & Bose, T. (2010). Effectiveness of triclosan in the management of radiation-induced oral mucositis: A randomized clinical trial. *Journal of Cancer Research and Therapeutics, 6,* 466–472. doi:10.4103/0973-1482.77109

118. Arbabi-kalati, F., Arbabi-kalati, F., Deghatipour, M., & Moghadam, A.A. (2012). Evaluation of the efficacy of zinc sulfate in the prevention of chemotherapy-induced mucositis: A double-blind randomized clinical trial. *Archives of Iranian Medicine, 15,* 413–417. Retrieved from http://www.ams .ac.ir/AIM/NEWPUB/12/15/7/008.pdf

119. Ertekin, M.V., Koç, M., Karslio lu, I., & Sezen, O. (2003). Zinc sulfate in the prevention of radiation-induced oropharyngeal mucositis: A prospective, placebo-controlled, randomized study. *International Journal of Radiation Oncology, Biology, Physics, 58,* 167–174. doi:10.1016/S0360 -3016(03)01562-1

120. Lin, L.-C., Que, J., Lin, L.-K., & Lin, F.-C. (2006). Zinc supplementation to improve mucositis and dermatitis in patients after radiotherapy for head-and-neck cancers: A double-blind, randomized study. *International Journal of Radiation Oncology, Biology, Physics, 65,* 745–750. doi:10.1016/ j.ijrobp.2006.01.015

121. Lin, Y., Lin, L., Lin, S., & Chang, C. (2010). Discrepancy of the effects of zinc supplementation on the prevention of radiotherapy-induced mucositis between patients with nasopharyngeal carcinoma and those with oral cancers: Subgroup analysis of a double-blind, randomized study. *Nutrition and Cancer, 62,* 682–691. doi:10.1080/01635581003605532

122. Mansouri, A., Hadjibabaie, M., Iravani, M., Shamshiri, A.R., Hayatshahi, A., Javadi, M.R., ... Ghavamzadeh, A. (2011). The effect of zinc sulfate in the prevention of high-dose chemotherapy-induced mucositis: A double-blind, randomized, placebo-controlled study. *Hematological Oncology, 30,* 22–26. doi:10.1002/hon.999

123. Su, C.K., Mehta, V., Ravikumar, L., Shah, R., Pinto, H., Halpern, J., ... Le, Q.-T. (2004). Phase II double-blind randomized study comparing oral aloe vera versus placebo to prevent radiation-related mucositis in patients with head-and-neck neoplasms. *International Journal of Radiation Oncology, Biology, Physics, 60,* 171–177. doi:10.1016/j.ijrobp.2004.02.012

124. Hunter, A., Mahendra, P., Wilson, K., Fields, P., Cook, G., Peniket, A., ... Marcus, R. (2009). Treatment of oral mucositis after peripheral blood SCT with ATL-104 mouthwash: Results from a randomized, double-blind, placebo-controlled trial. *Bone Marrow Transplantation, 43,* 563–569. doi:10.1038/bmt.2008.363

125. Babaee, N., Moslemi, D., Khalilpour, M., Vejdani, F., Moghadamnia, Y., Bijani, A., ... Moghadamnia, A.A. (2013). Antioxidant capacity of *Calendula officinalis* flowers extract and prevention of radiation induced oropharyngeal mucositis in patients with head and neck cancers: A randomized controlled clinical study. *Daru Journal of Pharmaceutical Sciences, 21,* 18. doi:10.1186/2008-2231-21-18

126. Gandemer, V., Le Deley, M., Dollfus, C., Auvrignon, A., Bonnaure-Mallet, M., Duval, M., ... Schmitt, C. (2007). Multicenter randomized trial of chewing gum for preventing oral mucositis in children receiving chemotherapy. *Journal of Pediatric Hematology/Oncology, 29,* 86–94. doi:10.1097/ MPH.0b013e318030a3e4

127. Stokman, M.A., Spijkervet, F.K., Burlage, F.R., & Roodenburg, J.L. (2005). Clinical effects of flurbiprofen tooth patch on radiation-induced oral mucositis. A pilot study. *Supportive Care in Cancer, 13,* 42–48. doi:10.1007/ s00520-004-0674-6

128. Abdulrhman, M., Elbarbary, N.S., Amin, D.A., & Ebrahim, R.S. (2012). Honey and a mixture of honey, beeswax, and olive oil-propolis extract in treatment of chemotherapy-induced oral mucositis: A randomized controlled pilot study. *Pediatric Hematology-Oncology, 29,* 285–292. doi:10.3109/ 08880018.2012.669026

129. Bardy, J., Molassiotis, A., Ryder, W.D., Mais, K., Sykes, A., Yap, B., ... Slevin, N. (2011). A double-blind, placebo-controlled, randomised trial of active manuka honey and standard oral care for radiation-induced oral mucositis. *British Journal of Oral and Maxillofacial Surgery, 50,* 221–226. doi:10.1016/j.bjoms.2011.03.005

130. Jayachandran, S., & Balaji, N. (2012). Evaluating the effectiveness of topical application of natural honey and benzydamine hydrochloride in the management of radiation mucositis. *Indian Journal of Palliative Care, 18,* 190–195. doi:10.4103/0973-1075.105689

131. Maiti, P.K., Ray, A., Mitra, T.N., Jana, U., Bhattacharya, J., & Ganguly, S. (2012). The effect of honey on mucositis induced by chemoradiation in head and neck cancer. *Journal of the Indian Medical Association, 110,* 453–456.

132. Song, J.J., Twumasi-Ankrah, P., & Salcido, R. (2012). Systematic review and meta-analysis on the use of honey to protect from the effects of radiation-induced oral mucositis. *Advances in Skin and Wound Care, 25,* 23–28. doi:10.1097/01.ASW.0000410687.14363.a3

133. You, W.C., Hsieh, C.C., & Huang, J.T. (2009). Effect of extracts from indigowood root (*Isatis indigotica Fort.*) on immune responses in radiation-induced mucositis. *Journal of Alternative and Complementary Medicine, 15,* 771–778. doi:10.1089/acm.2008.0322

134. Hodgson, B.D., Margolis, D.M., Salzman, D.E., Eastwood, D., Tarima, S., Williams, L.D., ... Whelan, H.T. (2011). Amelioration of oral mucositis pain by NASA near-infrared light-emitting diodes in bone marrow transplant patients. *Supportive Care in Cancer, 20,* 1405–1415. doi:10.1007/s00520-011-1223-8

135. Maddocks-Jennings, W., Wilkinson, J.M., Cavanagh, H.M., & Shillington, D. (2009). Evaluating the effects of the essential oils *Leptospermum scoparium* (manuka) and *Kunzea ericoides* (kanuka) on radiotherapy induced mucositis: A randomized, placebo controlled feasibility study. *European Journal of Oncology Nursing, 13,* 87–93. doi:10.1016/j.ejon.2009.01.002

136. Putwatana, P., Sanmanowong, P., Oonprasertpong, L., Junda, T., Pitiporn, S., & Narkwong, L. (2009). Relief of radiation-induced oral mucositis in head and neck cancer. *Cancer Nursing, 32,* 82–87. doi:10.1097/01.NCC.0000343362.68129.ed

137. Kashiwazaki, H., Matsushita, T., Sugita, J., Shigematsu, A., Kasashi, K., Yamazaki, Y., ... Inoue, N. (2011). Professional oral health care reduces oral mucositis and febrile neutropenia in patients treated with allogeneic bone marrow transplantation. *Supportive Care in Cancer, 20,* 367–373. doi:10.1007/s00520-011-1116-x

138. Khurana, H., Pandey, R., Saksena, A.K., & Kumar, A. (2013). An evaluation of vitamin E and Pycnogenol in children suffering from oral mucositis during cancer chemotherapy. *Oral Diseases, 19,* 456–464. doi:10.1111/odi.12024

139. Loo, W.T.Y., Jin, L.J., Chow, L.W., Cheung, M.N.B., & Wang, M. (2010). *Rhodiola algida* improves chemotherapy-induced oral mucositis in breast cancer patients. *Expert Opinion on Investigational Drugs, 19*(Suppl. 1), S91–S100. doi:10.1517/13543781003727057

140. Amaral, T.M.P., Campos, C.C., Moreira dos Santos, T.P., Leles, C.R., Teixeira, A.L., Teixeira, M.M., ... Silva, T.A. (2012). Effect of salivary stimulation therapies on salivary flow and chemotherapy-induced mucositis: A preliminary study. *Oral Surgery, Oral Medicine, Oral Pathology and Oral Radiology, 113,* 628–637. doi:10.1016/j.oooo.2011.10.012

141. Pawar, D., Neve, R.S., Kalgane, S., Riva, A., Bombardelli, E., Ronchi, M., ... Morazzoni, P. (2013). SAMITAL® improves chemo/radiotherapy–induced oral mucositis in patients with head and neck cancer: Results of a randomized, placebo-controlled, single-blind phase II study. *Supportive Care in Cancer, 21,* 827–834. doi:10.1007/s00520-012-1586-5

142. Elad, S., Luboshitz-Shon, N., Cohen, T., Wainchwaig, E., Shapira, M.Y., Resnick, I.B., ... Or, R. (2011). A randomized controlled trial of visible-light therapy for the prevention of oral mucositis. *Oral Oncology, 47,* 125–130. doi:10.1016/j.oraloncology.2010.11.013

143. Giles, F.J., Rodriguez, R., Weisdorf, D., Wingard, J.R., Martin, P.J., Fleming, T.R., ... Hurd, D.D. (2004). A phase III, randomized, double-blind, placebo-controlled study of iseganan for the reduction of stomatitis in patients receiving stomatotoxic chemotherapy. *Leukemia Research, 28,* 559–565. doi:10.1016/j.leukres.2003.10.021

144. Trotti, A., Garden, A., Warde, P., Symonds, P., Langer, C., Redman, R., ... Ang, K.K. (2004). A multinational, randomized phase III trial of iseganan HCl oral solution for reducing the severity of oral mucositis in patients receiving radiotherapy for head-and-neck malignancy. *International Journal of Radiation Oncology, Biology, Physics, 58*, 674–681. doi:10.1016/S0360-3016(03)01627-4

145. Lalla, R.V., Gordon, G.B., Schubert, M., Silverman, S., Jr., Hutten, M., Sonis, S.T., ... Peterson, D.E. (2012). A randomized, double-blind, placebo-controlled trial of misoprostol for oral mucositis secondary to high-dose chemotherapy. *Supportive Care in Cancer, 20*, 1797–1804. doi:10.1007/s00520-011-1277-7

146. Veness, M.J., Foroudi, F., Gebski, V., Timms, I., Sathiyaseelan, Y., Cakir, B., & Tiver, K.W. (2006). Use of topical misoprostol to reduce radiation-induced mucositis: Results of a randomized, double-blind, placebo-controlled trial. *Australasian Radiology, 50*, 468–474. doi:10.1111/j.1440-1673.2006.01628.x

147. Sencer, S.F., Zhou, T., Freedman, L.S., Ives, J.A., Chen, Z., Wall, D., ... Oberbaum, M. (2012). Traumeel S in preventing and treating mucositis in young patients undergoing SCT: A report of the Children's Oncology Group. *Bone Marrow Transplantation, 47*, 1409–1414. doi:10.1038/bmt.2012.30

148. Steinmann, D., Eilers, V., Beynenson, D., Buhck, H., & Fink, M. (2012). Effect of Traumeel S on pain and discomfort in radiation-induced oral mucositis: A preliminary observational study. *Alternative Therapies in Health and Medicine, 18*, 12–18.

149. Dörr, W., & Herrmann, T. (2007). Efficacy of Wobe-Mugos® E for reduction of oral mucositis after radiotherapy: Results of a prospective, randomized, placebo-controlled, triple-blind phase III multicenter study. *Strahlentherapie und Onkologie, 183*, 121–127. doi:10.1007/s00066-007-1634-0

150. Nashwan, A.J. (2011). Use of chlorhexidine mouthwash in children receiving chemotherapy: A review of literature. *Journal of Pediatric Oncology Nursing, 28*, 295–299. doi:10.1177/1043454211408103

151. Castagna, L., Benhamou, E., Pedraza, E., Luboinski, M., Forni, M., Brandes, I., ... Dietrich, P.-Y. (2001). Prevention of mucositis in bone marrow transplantation: A double blind randomised controlled trial of sucralfate. *Annals of Oncology, 12*, 953–955. doi:10.1023/A:1011119721267

152. Dodd, M.J., Miaskowski, C., Greenspan, D., MacPhail, L., Shih, A., Shiba, G., ... Paul, S.M. (2003). Radiation-induced mucositis: A randomized clinical trial of micronized sucralfate versus salt and soda mouthwashes. *Cancer Investigation, 21*, 21–33. doi:10.1081/CNV-120016400

153. Etiz, D., Erkal, H.Ş., Serin, M., Küçük, B., Heparl, A., Elhan, A.H., ... Cakmak, A. (2000). Clinical and histopathological evaluation of sucralfate in prevention of oral mucositis induced by radiation therapy in patients with head and neck malignancies. *Oral Oncology, 36*, 116–120. doi:10.1016/S1368-8375(99)00075-5

154. Nottage, M., McLachlan, S.A., Brittain, M.A., Oza, A., Hedley, D., Feld, R., ... Moore, M.J. (2003). Sucralfate mouthwash for prevention and treatment of 5-fluorouracil-induced mucositis: A randomized, placebo-controlled trial. *Supportive Care in Cancer, 11*, 41–47. doi:10.1007/s00520-002-0378-8

155. Grünwald, V., Kalanovic, D., & Merseburger, A.S. (2010). Management of sunitinib-related adverse events: An evidence- and expert-based consensus approach. *World Journal of Urology, 28*, 343–351. doi:10.1007/s00345-010-0565-z

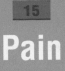

15

Pain

Jeannine M. Brant, PhD, APRN, AOCN®,
Karen L. Visich, MSN, ANP-BC, AOCNP®,
Bethany Sterling, MSN, CRNP, ANP-BC, OCN®, CHPN,
and Margaret Irwin, PhD, RN, MN

Problem and Incidence

Pain is one of the most common and feared experiences for patients with cancer. Approximately 33% of patients receiving treatment and 60%–90% of patients with metastatic disease experience moderate to severe pain.[1] Pain may be acute (usually related to procedures and treatment), chronic (lasting three months or more), breakthrough (sudden increase in the setting of generally controlled pain), or refractory (uncontrolled pain despite aggressive treatment). Breakthrough pain prevalence ranges from 19%–95%.[2,3] Cancer-related pain tends to be undertreated, which has a negative effect on patients' mood, quality of life, and functional status.[4] The most common barrier to optimal treatment of cancer pain is inadequate assessment and failure to act upon the assessment.[1]

Risk Factors and Assessment

Major risk factors include
- Advanced disease[5]
- Cancers of the head and neck,[5] cervix, or prostate and rectal or sigmoid tumors[6]
- Invasive procedures
- Treatment and supportive therapies that cause pain (e.g., bone pain associated with colony-stimulating factors, mucositis).

Patient self-report is the standard for pain assessment.[7] Comprehensive assessment includes medical history, psychosocial aspects, physical exam, laboratory results, and imaging studies to evaluate the etiology and pathophysiology of pain.[7-9]

Assessment instruments include
- Numeric rating scale
- Visual analog scale
- Multidimensional tools, such as the Edmonton Classification System for Cancer Pain[8] and the MD Anderson Symptom Inventory.[10]

What interventions are effective in managing pain in people with cancer?

Evidence retrieved through May 31, 2013

Acute Pain

Recommended for Practice

Local anesthetic infusion at the surgical site reduced pain and opioid consumption.[11-16]

Postoperative epidural anesthetics were superior to patient-controlled analgesia (PCA) in surgical patients.[17]

Likely to Be Effective

Continuous-release tramadol demonstrated efficacy in patients undergoing breast cancer surgery.[18]

Hypnosis/hypnotherapy showed mixed results in small studies.[19-21] Systematic reviews[22,23] and a meta-analysis[24] showed positive effects in adults and children.

Music/music therapy reduced procedural pain[23,25-27] and was beneficial for patients during chemotherapy.[28]

Naproxen decreased acute bone pain associated with peg-filgrastim.[29]

Perioperative gabapentin as a co-analgesic decreased opioid requirements and pain intensity,[30,31] anesthesia with craniotomy,[32] and bladder discomfort in patients undergoing transurethral resection of a bladder tumor.[33]

Effectiveness Not Established

Several pharmacologic and nonpharmacologic interventions have shown inconsistent results, or research findings were inconclusive because of small samples and other study limitations.

- **Pharmacologic interventions**
  - **Ketamine** prior to surgery[34]
  - **Morphine mouthwash** for mucositis pain[35,36]
  - **Paravertebral block**[37,38]
  - **Perioperative drugs** in various combinations of acetaminophen, dexamethasone, dextromethorphan, celecoxib, pregabalin, morphine, ketoprofen, naproxen, and gabapentin[30-41]
  - **Pregabalin**[42]
  - **Preoperative dexamethasone**[43]
  - **Remifentanil PCA**[44]
  - **Topical local anesthetics** via patch[45] or topical cream[46]
- **Nonpharmacologic interventions**
  - **Acupuncture/acupressure**[47-53]
  - **Massage**[54,55]
  - **Progressive muscle relaxation and imagery**[56]—A systematic review concluded evidence was insufficient to show efficacy.[48]
  - **Reflexology**[57]
  - **Therapeutic touch**[58]—Systematic reviews concluded that there was inadequate evidence to recommend use.[48,59-61]

Refractory and Intractable Pain

Recommended for Practice

Intraspinal analgesia (epidural or intrathecal) is supported by evidence[62-66] and recommended for consideration in guidelines.[7]

Effectiveness Not Established

Additional interventions have been examined in small studies or showed inconsistent results in larger trials.
- **Dimethyl sulfoxide**[67]
- **Ketamine**[68-70]
- **KRN5500**, an experimental spicamycin derivative[71]
- **IV lidocaine**[72]
- **Opioid rotation** from one opioid to another[73-76]

Breakthrough Pain

Recommended for Practice

Oral, transmucosal, and intranasal opioids are effective.[77-80] Transmucosal or intranasal fentanyl may provide more rapid relief.[81-95]

Proportional immediate-release opioids at 10%–20% of the basal 24-hour dose are recommended for breakthrough pain.[7,96,97]

Effectiveness Not Established

Interventions with insufficient evidence for breakthrough pain include the following.
- **Flurbiprofen**, a nonsteroidal anti-inflammatory drug (NSAID)[98]
- **Intranasal sufentanil**[99] (currently not U.S. Food and Drug Administration approved)
- **Tramadol and acetaminophen** combination[100]

Chronic Pain

Recommended for Practice

Acetaminophen is recommended for mild pain.[7,77]

Bone-modifying agents (bisphosphonates, denosumab) reduced pain in patients with bone metastases, although their primary indication is to reduce skeletal-related events.[101-106]

Celiac plexus block reduced pain associated with pancreatic cancer.[107-112]

Local anesthetics infusion (IV lidocaine) controlled neuropathic pain.[113]

NSAIDs are recommended for mild pain or as a co-analgesic for pain with inflammation.[7,114]

Opioids are recommended.[77,96,115-117] Most opioids are comparable in efficacy and adverse events.[80]
- **Transdermal buprenorphine** may be used alone or as an adjunct in the management of neuropathic pain.[118-121]
- **Methadone** is an alternative to traditional opioids. The long half-life of the drug can lead to toxic accumulation, so prescribing should be done by experienced clinicians.[77,116,122]
- **Oxycodone/naloxone** produces less constipation.[123,124]
- **Tramadol** is an alternative to traditional opioids[77,125] but may have more side effects.[126] A synergistic effect may also exist with transdermal fentanyl.[127]
- **Transdermal opioids** are effective with potentially less constipation.[118,127-132]

Psychoeducation was beneficial in multiple research studies and systematic reviews.[133-148] Mixed findings have been reported by others.[149-156] Meta-analyses showed small to moderate effect sizes.[143,157] Education for patients with cancer-related pain is recommended by the National Comprehensive Cancer Network.[7]

Sustained, continuous-release, and long-acting opioids were effective.[158-166] Once-daily dosing formulations of morphine[167] and hydromorphone[166,168] may be advantageous for some patients.

Likely to Be Effective

Abiraterone acetate reduced pain and pain interference in patients with castrate-resistant prostate cancer.[169]

Cannabis/cannabinoids as an adjunct to opioids reduced pain.[170,171]

Duloxetine decreased chemotherapy-induced painful neuropathy.[172,173]

Early opioid use, earlier than proposed by the World Health Organization Analgesic Ladder, was more effective than standard approaches for chronic pain.[174-176]

Gabapentin in combination with other medications showed mixed results for neuropathic pain.[177-183] Guidelines recommend consideration of gabapentin for neuropathic pain.[7,184]

Effectiveness Not Established

Several pharmacologic, medical, and nonpharmacologic interventions have been examined for chronic pain. Results have been inconsistent or were inconclusive due to limited study designs and small samples.

- **Pharmacologic interventions**
  - **Around-the-clock acetaminophen**[185-189] often is used and is recommended in some guidelines.[116,184,190] Research has shown lack of benefit.
  - **Antidepressants**[172]
  - **Caffeine**[191]
  - **Prednisolone**[192]
  - **Pregabalin**[193]
- **Medical interventions**
  - **Autologous fat graft** in patients with severe scar retraction and postmastectomy pain syndrome[194]

- **Celiac ganglion irradiation** for unresectable pancreatic cancer[195]
- **Focused ultrasound** with magnetic resonance imaging guidance to areas of painful bone metastases[196]
- **Gene therapy** via intradermal injection of a herpes simplex virus vector[197]
- Nonpharmacologic interventions
  - **Acupuncture**[117,198]—Multiple systematic reviews did not show effectiveness.[49,51-53,199]
  - **Biofield interventions (therapeutic touch, Reiki, healing touch)**[48,200,201]
  - **Exercise**, such as walking[202]—Appropriate physical therapy in patients with head and neck cancer improved neck and shoulder pain and function.[203,204]
  - **Expressive writing**[205]
  - **Herbal medicines**[48,206-208]
  - **Hypnosis/hypnotherapy**[209]—A systematic review concluded that hypnosis could not be recommended for chronic pain.[48]
  - **Institutional initiatives** to improve pain management[210,211]
  - **Massage**[54,55,201,212,213]
  - **Palliative care consultation**[214,215]
  - **Progressive muscle relaxation and imagery**[48,56,216]—Evidence regarding guided imagery alone was inconclusive.[217]
  - **Transcutaneous electrical nerve stimulation**[218-221]
  - **Yoga**[222]

Not Recommended for Practice

Calcitonin use to control pain from bone metastases is not supported by evidence.[223]

Application to Practice

Nurses need to identify patients at risk for pain, assess pain, and ensure that evidence-based interventions are implemented to optimally manage pain. Identification of frequency and timing of breakthrough pain episodes is critical for effective chronic pain management.

Nurses can use and advocate use of pharmacologic and nonpharmacologic interventions that have strong evidence of effectiveness for relief of the type of pain experienced by patients.

Nurses can provide psychoeducational interventions to patients and caregivers to ensure effective use and monitoring of medications and should address any misconceptions and barriers to self-management, such as fears about opioid use. Nurses need to ensure that patients and caregivers have the knowledge and skills needed for ongoing pain management.

Nurses can be instrumental in assessment of patient and caregiver needs and capabilities and appropriate patient selection when implementing invasive interventions such as intraspinal therapy for long-term use.

Pain Resource Contributors

Topic leader: Christine A. Miaskowski, RN, PhD, FAAN
Jeannine M. Brant, PhD, APRN, AOCN®, Pamela Caldwell, RN-BC, MS, OCN®, Linda Eaton, MN, RN, AOCN®, Natalie Gallagher, RN, MPH, Zehra Habib, RN, BSN, Josie Howard-Ruben, MS, RN, APN-CNS, AOCN®, Sharon S. Kilbride, RN, BSN, OCN®, Lynne M. Kuhl, RN, Dawn M. Kunz, RN, MSN, AOCN®, CHPN, Karen McLeod, MSN, RN, OCN®, CNL, Barbara B. Rogers, CRNP, MN, AOCN®, ANP-BC, Wendy J. Smith, RN, MSN, ACNP, AOCN®, Malgorzata Sokolowski, MSN, APN, OCN®, AOCNS®, Evie Sprague, MSN, RN, OCN®, CCRP, Bethany Sterling, MSN, CRNP, ANP-BC, OCN®, CHPN, Julie A. Summers, RN, BSN, OCN®, Mary Lou Sylwestrak, RN, MS, OCN®, CWOCN, Linda M. Truty, RN, Fabienne G. Ulysse, DNP, RN, MSN, ANP, AOCNP®, Kimberly L. Valochovic, APN, MSN, AOCNS®, and Karen L. Visich, MSN, ANP-BC, AOCNP®

References

1. Vogel, W.H., & Rosiak, J.M. (2009). Pain, fatigue, and cognitive dysfunction. In B.H. Gobel, S. Triest-Robertson, & W.H. Vogel (Eds.), *Advanced oncology nursing certification review and resource manual* (pp. 357–403). Pittsburgh, PA: Oncology Nursing Society.
2. Mercadante, S., Radbruch, I., Caraceni, A., Cherny, N., Kassa, S., Nauck, F., ... De Conno, F. (2002). Episodic (breakthrough) pain: Consensus

conference of an expert working group of the European Association for Palliative Care. *Cancer, 94,* 832–839. doi:10.1002/cncr.10249

3. Zeppetella, G., & Ribeiro, M.D.C. (2003). The pharmacotherapy of cancer-related episodic pain. *Expert Opinion on Pharmacotherapy, 4,* 493–502. doi:10.1517/14656566.4.4.493

4. Miaskowski, C. (2010). Cancer pain. In C.G. Brown (Ed.), *A guide to oncology symptom management* (pp. 389–403). Pittsburgh, PA: Oncology Nursing Society.

5. Van den Beuken-van Everdingen, M.H.J., de Rijke, J.M., Kessels, A.G., Schouten, H.C., van Kleef, M., & Patijn, J. (2007). Prevalence of pain in patients with cancer: A systematic review of the past 40 years. *Annals of Oncology, 18,* 1437–1449. doi:10.1093/annonc/mdm056

6. Brescia, F.J., Portenoy, R.K., Ryan, M., Krasnoff, L., & Gray, G. (1992). Pain, opioid use, and survival in hospitalized patients with advanced cancer. *Journal of Clinical Oncology, 10,* 149–155. Retrieved from http://jco.ascopubs.org/content/10/1/149.long

7. National Comprehensive Cancer Network. (2013). *NCCN Clinical Practice Guidelines in Oncology: Adult cancer pain* [v. 2.2013]. Retrieved from http://www.nccn.org/professionals/physician_gls/pdf/pain.pdf

8. Campbell, V. (2011). The challenges of cancer pain assessment and management. *Ulster Medical Journal, 80,* 104–106. Retrieved from http://www.ncbi.nlm.nih.gov/pmc/articles/PMC3229856/pdf/umj8002-104.pdf

9. National Cancer Institute. (2013). Pain (PDQ®): Pain assessment [Health professional version]. Retrieved from http://www.cancer.gov/cancertopics/pdq/supportivecare/pain/HealthProfessional/page2

10. University of Texas MD Anderson Cancer Center. (n.d.). The MD Anderson symptom inventory. Retrieved from http://www.mdanderson.org/education-and-research/departments-programs-and-labs/departments-and-divisions/symptom-research/symptom-assessment-tools/mdanderson-symptom-inventory.html

11. Albi-Feldzer, A., Mouret-Fourme, E.E., Hamouda, S., Motamed, C., Dubois, P.-Y., Jouanneau, L., & Jayr, C. (2013). A double-blind randomized trial of wound and intercostal space infiltration with ropivacaine during breast cancer surgery: Effects on chronic postoperative pain. *Anesthesiology, 118,* 318–326. doi:10.1097/ALN.0b013e31827d88d8

12. Bertoglio, S., Fabiani, F., Negri, P.D., Corcione, A., Merlo, D.F., Cafiero, F., … Zappi, L. (2012). The postoperative analgesic efficacy of preperitoneal continuous wound infusion compared to epidural continuous infusion with local anesthetics after colorectal cancer surgery: A randomized controlled multicenter study. *Anesthesia and Analgesia, 115,* 1442–1450. doi:10.1213/ANE.0b013e31826b4694

13. Demmy, T.L., Nwogu, C., Solan, P., Yendamuri, S., Wilding, G., & DeLeon, O. (2009). Chest tube–delivered bupivacaine improves pain and decreases opioid use after thoracoscopy. *Annals of Thoracic Surgery, 87,* 1040–1041. doi:10.1016/j.athoracsur.2008.12.099

14. Heller, L., Kowalski, A.M., Wei, C., & Butler, C.E. (2008). Prospective, randomized, double-blind trial of local anesthetic infusion and intravenous narcotic patient-controlled anesthesia pump for pain management after free TRAM flap breast reconstruction. *Plastic and Reconstructive Surgery, 122,* 1010–1018. doi:10.1097/PRS.0b013e3181858c09

15. Legeby, M., Jurell, G., Beausang-Linder, M., & Olofsson, C. (2009). Placebo-controlled trial of local anaesthesia for treatment of pain after breast reconstruction. *Scandinavian Journal of Plastic and Reconstructive Surgery and Hand Surgery, 43,* 315–319. doi:10.1080/02844310903259108

16. Zielinski, J., Jaworski, R., Smietanska, I., Irga, N., Wujtewicz, M., & Jaskiewicz, J. (2011). A randomized, double-blind, placebo-controlled trial of preemptive analgesia with bupivacaine in patients undergoing mastectomy for carcinoma of the breast. *Medical Science Monitor, 17,* CR589–CR597. doi:10.12659/MSM.881986

17. Ferguson, S.E., Malhotra, T., Seshan, V.E., Levine, D.A., Sonoda, Y., Chi, D.S., ... Abu-Rustum, N.R. (2009). A prospective randomized trial comparing patient-controlled epidural analgesia to patient-controlled intravenous analgesia on postoperative pain control and recovery after major open gynecologic cancer surgery. *Gynecologic Oncology, 114,* 111–116. doi:10.1016/j.ygyno.2009.03.014

18. Kampe, S., Wolter, K., Warm, M., Dagtekin, O., Shaheen, S., & Landwehr, S. (2009). Clinical equivalence of controlled-release oxycodone 20 mg and controlled-release tramadol 200 mg after surgery for breast cancer. *Pharmacology, 84,* 276–281. doi:10.1159/000242998

19. Lew, M.W., Kravits, K., Garberoglio, C., & Williams, A.C. (2011). Use of preoperative hypnosis to reduce postoperative pain and anesthesia-related side effects. *International Journal of Clinical and Experimental Hypnosis, 59,* 406–423. doi:10.1080/00207144.2011.594737

20. Liossi, C., White, P., & Hatira, P. (2009). A randomized clinical trial of a brief hypnosis intervention to control venipuncture-related pain of paediatric cancer patients. *Pain, 142,* 255–263. doi:10.1016/j.pain.2009.01.017

21. Snow, A., Dorfman, D., Warbet, R., Cammarata, M., Eisenman, S., Zilberfein, F., ... Navada, S. (2012). A randomized trial of hypnosis for relief of pain and anxiety in adult cancer patients undergoing bone marrow procedures. *Journal of Psychosocial Oncology, 30,* 281–293. doi:10.1080/07347332.2012.664261

22. Richardson, J., Smith, J.E., McCall, G., & Pilkington, K. (2006). Hypnosis for procedure-related pain and distress in pediatric cancer patients: A systematic review of effectiveness and methodology related to hypnosis interventions. *Journal of Pain and Symptom Management, 31,* 70–84. doi:10.1016/j.jpainsymman.2005.06.010

23. Rheingans, J.I. (2007). A systematic review of nonpharmacologic adjunctive therapies for symptom management in children with cancer. *Journal of Pediatric Oncology Nursing, 24,* 81–94. doi:10.1177/1043454206298837

24. Montgomery, G.H., Weltz, C.R., Seltz, M., & Bovbjerg, D.H. (2002). Brief presurgery hypnosis reduces distress and pain in excisional breast biopsy patients. *International Journal of Clinical and Experimental Hypnosis, 50,* 17–32. doi:10.1080/00207140208410088

25. Bradt, J., Dileo, C., Grocke, D., & Magill, L. (2011). Music interventions for improving psychological and physical outcomes in cancer patients. *Cochrane Database of Systematic Reviews, 2011*(8). doi:10.1002/14651858.CD006911.pub2

26. Cepeda, M.S., Carr, D.B., Lau, J., & Alvarez, H. (2010). Music for pain relief. *Cochrane Database of Systematic Reviews, 2010*(8). doi:10.1002/14651858.CD004843.pub2

27. Tsivian, M., Qi, P., Kimura, M., Chen, V.H., Chen, S.H., Gan, T.J., & Polascik, T.J. (2012). The effect of noise-cancelling headphones or music on pain perception and anxiety in men undergoing transrectal prostate biopsy. *Urology, 79,* 32–36. doi:10.1016/j.urology.2011.09.037

28. Li, X.M., Yan, H., Zhou, K.N., Dang, S.N., Wang, D.L., & Zhang, Y.P. (2011). Effects of music therapy on pain among female breast cancer patients after radical mastectomy: Results from a randomized controlled trial. *Breast Cancer Research and Treatment, 128,* 411–419. doi:10.1007/s10549-011-1533-z

29. Kirshner, J.J., Heckler, C.E., Janelsins, M.C., Dakhil, S.R., Hopkins, J.O., Coles, C., & Morrow, G.R. (2012). Prevention of pegfilgrastim-induced bone pain: A phase III double-blind placebo-controlled randomized clinical trial of the University of Rochester Cancer Center Clinical Community Oncology Program Research Base. *Journal of Clinical Oncology, 30,* 1974–1979. doi:10.1200/JCO.2011.37.8364

30. Bharti, N., Bala, I., Narayan, V., & Singh, G. (2013). Effect of gabapentin pretreatment on propofol consumption, hemodynamic variables, and postoperative pain relief in breast cancer surgery. *Acta Anaesthesiologica Taiwanica, 51,* 10–13. doi:10.1016/j.aat.2013.03.009

31. Grover, V.K., Mathew, P.J., Yaddanapudi, S., & Sehgal, S. (2009). A single dose of preoperative gabapentin for pain reduction and requirement of morphine after total mastectomy and axillary dissection: Randomized placebo-controlled double-blind trial. *Journal of Postgraduate Medicine, 55*, 257–260. doi:10.4103/0022-3859.58928

32. Türe, H., Sayin, M., Karlikaya, G., Bingol, C.A., Aykac, B., & Türe, U. (2009). The analgesic effect of gabapentin as a prophylactic anticonvulsant drug on postcraniotomy pain: A prospective randomized study. *Anesthesia and Analgesia, 109*, 1625–1631. doi:10.1213/ane.0b013e3181b0f18b

33. Bala, I., Bharti, N., Chaubey, V.K., & Mandal, A.K. (2012). Efficacy of gabapentin for prevention of postoperative catheter-related bladder discomfort in patients undergoing transurethral resection of bladder tumor. *Urology, 79*, 853–857. doi:10.1016/j.urology.2011.11.050

34. Mikesell, C.E., Atkinson, D.E., & Rachman, B.R. (2011). Prolonged QT syndrome and sedation: A case report and a review of the literature. *Pediatric Emergency Care, 27*, 129–131. doi:10.1097/PEC.0b013e318209bef4

35. Nielsen, B.N., Aagaard, G., Henneberg, S.W., Schmiegelow, K., Hansen, S.H., & Rømsing, J. (2012). Topical morphine for oral mucositis in children: Dose finding and absorption. *Journal of Pain and Symptom Management, 44*, 117–123. doi:10.1016/j.jpainsymman.2011.06.029

36. Vayne-Bossert, P., Escher, M., de Vautibault, C.G., Dulguerov, P., Allal, A., Desmeules, J., ... Pautex, S. (2010). Effect of topical morphine (mouthwash) on oral pain due to chemotherapy- and/or radiotherapy-induced mucositis: A randomized double-blinded study. *Journal of Palliative Medicine, 13*, 125–128. doi:10.1089/jpm.2009.0195

37. Aufforth, R., Jain, J., Morreale, J., Baumgarten, R., Falk, J., & Wesen, C. (2012). Paravertebral blocks in breast cancer surgery: Is there a difference in postoperative pain, nausea, and vomiting? *Annals of Surgical Oncology, 19*, 548–552. doi:10.1245/s10434-011-1899-5

38. Li, N.L., Yu, B.L., Tseng, S.C., Hsu, C.C., Lai, W.J., Hsieh, P.F., ... Chen, C.M. (2011). The effect on improvement of recovery and pain scores of paravertebral block immediately before breast surgery. *Acta Anaesthesiologica Taiwanica, 49*, 91–95. doi:10.1016/j.aat.2011.08.006

39. Gärtner, R., Kroman, N., Callesen, T., & Kehlet, H. (2010). Multimodal prevention of pain, nausea and vomiting after breast cancer surgery. *Minerva Anestesiologica, 76*, 805–813. Retrieved from http://www.minervamedica.it/en/journals/minerva-anestesiologica/article.php?cod=R02Y2010N10A0805

40. Gomez, H., Camacho, J., Yelicich, B., Moraes, L., Biestro, A., & Puppo, C. (2010). Development of a multimodal monitoring platform for medical research. *Conference Proceedings: Engineering in Medicine and Biology Society, 2010*, 2358–2361. doi:10.1109/IEMBS.2010.5627936

41. Samulak, D., Michalska, M., Gaca, M., Wilczak, M., Mojs, E., & Chuchracki, M. (2011). Efficiency of postoperative pain management after gynecological oncological surgeries with the use of morphine + acetaminophen + ketoprofen versus morphine + metamizol + ketoprofen. *European Journal of Gynaecological Oncology, 32*, 168–170.

42. Kim, S.Y., Song, J.W., Park, B., Park, S., An, Y.J., & Shim, Y.H. (2011). Pregabalin reduces post-operative pain after mastectomy: A double-blind, randomized, placebo-controlled study. *Acta Anaesthesiologica Scandinavica, 55*, 290–296. doi:10.1111/j.1399-6576.2010.02374.x

43. Gomez-Hernandez, J., Orozco-Alatorre, A.L., Dominguez-Contreras, M., Oceguera-Villanueva, A., Gomez-Romo, S., Alvarez Villasenor, A.S., ... Gonzalez-Ojeda, A. (2010). Preoperative dexamethasone reduces postoperative pain, nausea and vomiting following mastectomy for breast cancer. *BMC Cancer, 10*, 692. doi:10.1186/1471-2407-10-692

44. Lipszyc, M., Winters, E., Engelman, E., Baurain, M., & Barvais, L. (2011). Remifentanil patient-controlled analgesia effect-site target-controlled infusion compared with morphine patient-controlled analgesia for treatment of acute pain after uterine artery embolization. *British Journal of Anaesthesia, 106*, 724–731. doi:10.1093/bja/aer041

45. Cheville, A.L., Sloan, J.A., Northfelt, D.W., Jillella, A.P., Wong, G.Y., Bearden, J.D., ... Loprinzi, C.L. (2009). Use of a lidocaine patch in the management of postsurgical neuropathic pain in patients with cancer: A phase III double-blind crossover study (N01CB). *Supportive Care in Cancer, 17,* 451–460. doi:10.1007/s00520-008-0542-x

46. O'Connor, J.M., Helmer, S.D., Osland, J.S., Cusick, T.E., & Tenofsky, P.L. (2011). Do topical anesthetics reduce periareolar injectional pain before sentinel lymph node biopsy? *American Journal of Surgery, 202,* 707–712. doi:10.1016/j.amjsurg.2011.06.040

47. Bao, T., Ye, X., Skinner, J., Cao, B., Fisher, J., Nesbit, S., & Grossman, S.A. (2011). The analgesic effect of magnetic acupressure in cancer patients undergoing bone marrow aspiration and biopsy: A randomized, blinded, controlled trial. *Journal of Pain and Symptom Management, 41,* 995–1002. doi:10.1016/j.jpainsymman.2010.08.012

48. Bardia, A., Barton, D.L., Prokop, L.J., Bauer, B.A., & Moynihan, T.J. (2006). Efficacy of complementary and alternative medicine therapies in relieving cancer pain: A systematic review. *Journal of Clinical Oncology, 24,* 5457–5464. doi:10.1200/JCO.2006.08.3725

49. Choi, T.-Y., Lee, M.S., Kim, T.-H., Zaslawski, C., & Ernst, E. (2012). Acupuncture for the treatment of cancer pain: A systematic review of randomised clinical trials. *Supportive Care in Cancer, 20,* 1147–1158. doi:10.1007/s00520-012-1432-9

50. Deng, G., Rusch, V., Vickers, A., Malhotra, V., Ginex, P., Downey, R., ... Cassileth, B. (2008). Randomized controlled trial of a special acupuncture technique for pain after thoracotomy. *Journal of Thoracic and Cardiovascular Surgery, 136,* 1464–1469. doi:10.1016/j.jtcvs.2008.07.053

51. Garcia, M.K., McQuade, J., Haddad, R., Patel, S., Lee, R., Yang, P., ... Cohen, L. (2013). Systematic review of acupuncture in cancer care: A synthesis of the evidence. *Journal of Clinical Oncology, 31,* 952–960. doi:10.1200/JCO.2012.43.5818

52. Lee, H., Schmidt, K., & Ernst, E. (2005). Acupuncture for the relief of cancer-related pain—A systematic review. *European Journal of Pain, 9,* 437–444. doi:10.1016/j.ejpain.2004.10.004

53. Paley, C.A., Johnson, M.I., Tashani, O.A., & Bagnall, A.-M. (2011). Acupuncture for cancer pain in adults. *Cochrane Database of Systematic Reviews, 2011*(1). doi:10.1002/14651858.CD007753.pub2

54. Currin, J., & Meister, E.A. (2008). A hospital-based intervention using massage to reduce distress among oncology patients. *Cancer Nursing, 31,* 214–221. doi:10.1097/01.NCC.0000305725.65345.f3

55. Wilkinson, S., Barnes, K., & Storey, L. (2008). Massage for symptom relief in patients with cancer: Systematic review. *Journal of Advanced Nursing, 63,* 430–439. doi:10.1111/j.1365-2648.2008.04712.x

56. Kwekkeboom, K.L., Wanta, B., & Bumpus, M. (2008). Individual difference variables and the effects of progressive muscle relaxation and analgesic imagery interventions on cancer pain. *Journal of Pain and Symptom Management, 36,* 604–615. doi:10.1016/j.jpainsymman.2007.12.011

57. Tsay, S.L., Chen, H.L., Chen, S.C., Lin, H.R., & Lin, K.C. (2008). Effects of reflexotherapy on acute postoperative pain and anxiety among patients with digestive cancer. *Cancer Nursing, 31,* 109–115. doi:10.1097/01.NCC.0000305694.74754.7b

58. Aghabati, N., Mohammadi, E., & Esmaiel, Z.P. (2010). The effect of therapeutic touch on pain and fatigue of cancer patients undergoing chemotherapy. *Evidence-Based Complementary and Alternative Medicine, 7,* 375–381. doi:10.1093/ecam/nen006

59. Fraih Sahawneh, L.J. (2011). Effectiveness of therapeutic touch on pain management among patients with cancer—Literature review. *Middle East Journal of Nursing, 5,* 21–24. doi:10.5742/MEJN.2011.54047

60. Jackson, E., Kelley, M., McNeil, P., Meyer, E., Schlegel, L., & Eaton, M. (2008). Does therapeutic touch help reduce pain and anxiety in patients with cancer? *Clinical Journal of Oncology Nursing, 12,* 113–120. doi:10.1188/08.CJON.113-120

61. Jain, S., & Mills, P. (2010). Biofield therapies: Helpful or full of hype? A best evidence synthesis. *International Journal of Behavioral Medicine, 17,* 1–16. doi:10.1007/s12529-009-9062-4

62. Deer, T.R., Smith, H.S., Burton, A.W., Pope, J.E., Doleys, D.M., Levy, R.M., ... Cousins, M. (2011). Comprehensive consensus based guidelines on intrathecal drug delivery systems in the treatment of pain caused by cancer pain. *Pain Physician, 14,* E283–E312. Retrieved from http://www .painphysicianjournal.com/2011/may/2011;14;E283-E312.pdf

63. Hayek, S.M., Deer, T.R., Pope, J.E., Panchal, S.J., & Patel, V.B. (2011). Intrathecal therapy for cancer and non-cancer pain. *Pain Physician, 14,* 219–248. http://www.painphysicianjournal.com/2011/may/2011;14;219-248.pdf

64. Jeon, Y.S., Lee, J.A., Choi, J.W., Kang, E.G., Jung, H.S., Kim, H.K., ... Joo, J.D. (2012). Efficacy of epidural analgesia in patients with cancer pain: A retrospective observational study. *Yonsei Medical Journal, 53,* 649–653. doi:10.3349/ymj.2012.53.3.649

65. Mercadante, S., Intravaia, G., Villari, P., Ferrera, P., Riina, S., David, F., & Mangione, S. (2007). Intrathecal treatment in cancer patients unresponsive to multiple trials of systemic opioids. *Clinical Journal of Pain, 23,* 793–798. doi:10.1097/AJP.0b013e3181565d17

66. Myers, J., Chan, V., Jarvis, V., & Walker-Dilks, C. (2010). Intraspinal techniques for pain management in cancer patients: A systematic review. *Supportive Care in Cancer, 18,* 137–149. doi:10.1007/s00520-009-0784-2

67. Hoang, B.X., Le, B.T., Tran, H.D., Hoang, C., Tran, H.Q., Tran, D.M., ... Shaw, D.G. (2011). Dimethyl sulfoxide–sodium bicarbonate infusion for palliative care and pain relief in patients with metastatic prostate cancer. *Journal of Pain and Palliative Care Pharmacotherapy, 25,* 350–355. doi:10 .3109/15360288.2011.606294

68. Bell, R.F., Eccleston, C., & Kalso, E.A. (2012). Ketamine as an adjuvant to opioids for cancer pain. *Cochrane Database of Systematic Reviews, 2012*(11). doi:10.1002/14651858.CD003351.pub2

69. Hardy, J., Quinn, S., Fazekas, B., Plummer, J., Eckermann, S., Agar, M., ... Currow, D.C. (2012). Randomized, double-blind, placebo-controlled study to assess the efficacy and toxicity of subcutaneous ketamine in the management of cancer pain. *Journal of Clinical Oncology, 30,* 3611–3617. doi:10.1200/JCO.2012.42.1081

70. Jackson, K., Ashby, M., Howell, D., Petersen, J., Brumley, D., Good, P., ... Woodruff, R. (2010). The effectiveness and adverse effects profile of "burst" ketamine in refractory cancer pain: The VCOG PM 1-00 study. *Journal of Palliative Care, 26,* 176–183.

71. Weinstein, S.M., Abernethy, A.P., Spruill, S.E., Pike, I.M., Kelly, A.T., & Jett, L.G. (2012). A Spicamycin derivative (KRN5500) provides neuropathic pain relief in patients with advanced cancer: A placebo-controlled, proof-of-concept trial. *Journal of Pain and Symptom Management, 43,* 679–693. doi:10.1016/j.jpainsymman.2011.05.003

72. Sharma, S., Rajagopal, M.R., Palat, G., Singh, C., Haji, A.G., & Jain, D. (2009). A phase II pilot study to evaluate use of intravenous lidocaine for opioid-refractory pain in cancer patients. *Journal of Pain and Symptom Management, 37,* 85–93. doi:10.1016/j.jpainsymman.2007.12.023

73. Aurilio, C., Pace, M.C., Pota, V., Sansone, P., Barbarisi, M., Grella, E., & Passavanti, M.B. (2009). Opioids switching with transdermal systems in chronic cancer pain. *Journal of Experimental and Clinical Cancer Research, 28,* 61. doi:10.1186/1756-9966-28-61

74. Mercadante, S., & Bruera, E. (2006). Opioid switching: A systematic and critical review. *Cancer Treatment Reviews, 32,* 304–315. doi:10.1016/j.ctrv .2006.03.001

75. Mercadante, S., Ferrera, P., Villari, P., & Casuccio, A. (2005). Rapid switching between transdermal fentanyl and methadone in cancer patients. *Journal of Clinical Oncology, 23,* 5229–5234. doi:10.1200/JCO.2005.13.128

76. Narabayashi, M., Saijo, Y., Takenoshita, S., Chida, M., Shimoyama, N., Miura, T., ... Tsushima, T. (2008). Opioid rotation from oral morphine to

oral oxycodone in cancer patients with intolerable adverse effects: An open-label trial. *Japanese Journal of Clinical Oncology, 38*, 296–304. doi:10.1093/jjco/hyn010

77. Aiello-Laws, L., Reynolds, J., Deizer, N., Peterson, M., Ameringer, S., & Bakitas, M. (2009). Putting evidence into practice: What are the pharmacologic interventions for nociceptive and neuropathic cancer pain in adults? *Clinical Journal of Oncology Nursing, 13*, 649–655. doi:10.1188/09 .CJON.649-655

78. Ripamonti, C.I., Bandieri, E., & Roila, F. (2011). Management of cancer pain: ESMO clinical practice guidelines. *Annals of Oncology, 22*(Suppl. 6), vi69–vi77. doi:10.1093/annonc/mdr390

79. Virizuela, J.A., Escobar, Y., Cassinello, J., & Borrega, P. (2012). Treatment of cancer pain: Spanish Society of Medical Oncology (SEOM) recommendations for clinical practice. *Clinical and Translational Oncology, 14*, 499–504. doi:10.1007/s12094-012-0831-1

80. Wiffen, P.J., & McQuay, H.J. (2007). Oral morphine for cancer pain. *Cochrane Database of Systematic Reviews, 2007*(4). doi:10.1002/14651858 .CD003868.pub2

81. Davies, A., Sitte, T., Elsner, F., Reale, C., Espinosa, J., Brooks, D., & Fallon, M. (2011). Consistency of efficacy, patient acceptability, and nasal tolerability of fentanyl pectin nasal spray compared with immediate-release morphine sulfate in breakthrough cancer pain. *Journal of Pain and Symptom Management, 41*, 358–366. doi:10.1016/j.jpainsymman.2010.11 .004

82. Fallon, M., Reale, C., Davies, A., Lux, A.E., Kumar, K., Stachowiak, A., & Galvez, R. (2011). Efficacy and safety of fentanyl pectin nasal spray compared with immediate-release morphine sulfate tablets in the treatment of breakthrough cancer pain: A multicenter, randomized, controlled, double-blind, double-dummy multiple-crossover study. *Journal of Supportive Oncology, 9*, 224–231. doi:10.1016/j.suponc.2011.07.004

83. Kress, H.G., Orońska, A., Kaczmarek, Z., Kaasa, S., Colberg, T., & Nolte, T. (2009). Efficacy and tolerability of intranasal fentanyl spray 50 to 200 mcg for breakthrough pain in patients with cancer: A phase III, multinational, randomized, double-blind, placebo-controlled, crossover trial with a 10-month, open-label extension treatment period. *Clinical Therapeutics, 31*, 1177–1191. doi:10.1016/j.clinthera.2009.05.022

84. Lennernas, B., Frank-Lissbrant, I., Lennernas, H., Kalkner, K.M., Derrick, R., & Howell, J. (2010). Sublingual administration of fentanyl to cancer patients is an effective treatment for breakthrough pain: Results from a randomized phase II study. *Palliative Medicine, 24*, 286–293. doi:10.1177/0269216309356138

85. Mercadante, S., Radbruch, L., Davies, A., Poulain, P., Sitte, T., Perkins, P., … Camba, M.A. (2009). A comparison of intranasal fentanyl spray with oral transmucosal fentanyl citrate for the treatment of breakthrough cancer pain: An open-label, randomised, crossover trial. *Current Medical Research and Opinion, 25*, 2805–2815. doi:10.1185/03007990903336135

86. Nalamachu, S., Hassman, D., Wallace, M.S., Dumble, S., Derrick, R., & Howell, J. (2011). Long-term effectiveness and tolerability of sublingual fentanyl orally disintegrating tablet for the treatment of breakthrough cancer pain. *Current Medical Research and Opinion, 27*, 519–530. doi:10.1185/ 03007995.2010.545380

87. Portenoy, R.K., Raffaeli, W., Torres, L.M., Sitte, T., Deka, A.C., Herrera, I.G., & Wallace, M.S. (2010). Long-term safety, tolerability, and consistency of effect of fentanyl pectin nasal spray for breakthrough cancer pain in opioid-tolerant patients. *Journal of Opioid Management, 6*, 319–328. doi:10.5055/jom.2010.0029

88. Radbruch, L., Torres, L.M., Ellershaw, J.E., Gatti, A., Luis Lerzo, G., Revnic, J., & Taylor, D. (2011). Long-term tolerability, efficacy and acceptability of fentanyl pectin nasal spray for breakthrough cancer pain. *Supportive Care in Cancer, 20*, 565–573. doi:10.1007/s00520-011-1124-x

89. Rauck, R., North, J., Gever, L.N., Tagarro, I., & Finn, A.L. (2010). Fentanyl buccal soluble film (FBSF) for breakthrough pain in patients with cancer: A randomized, double-blind, placebo-controlled study. *Annals of Oncology, 21,* 1308–1314. doi:10.1093/annonc/mdp541

90. Slatkin, N.E., Xie, F., Messina, J., & Segal, T.J. (2007). Fentanyl buccal tablet for relief of breakthrough pain in opioid-tolerant patients with cancer-related chronic pain. *Journal of Supportive Oncology, 5,* 327–334. Retrieved from http://www.oncologypractice.com/jso/journal/articles/0507327.pdf

91. Taylor, D., Galan, V., Weinstein, S.M., Reyes, E., Pupo-Araya, A.R., & Rauck, R. (2010). Fentanyl pectin nasal spray in breakthrough cancer pain. *Journal of Supportive Oncology, 8,* 184–190. Retrieved from http://www.oncologypractice.com/jso/journal/articles/0804184.pdf

92. Überall, M.A., & Müller-Schwefe, G.H. (2011). Sublingual fentanyl orally disintegrating tablet in daily practice: Efficacy, safety and tolerability in patients with breakthrough cancer pain. *Current Medical Research and Opinion, 27,* 1385–1394. doi:10.1185/03007995.2011.583231

93. Vissers, D., Stam, W., Nolte, T., Lenre, M., & Jansen, J. (2010). Efficacy of intranasal fentanyl spray versus other opioids for breakthrough pain in cancer. *Current Medical Research and Opinion, 26,* 1037–1045. doi:10.1185/03007991003694340

94. Weinstein, S.M., Messina, J., & Xie, F. (2009). Fentanyl buccal tablet for the treatment of breakthrough pain in opioid-tolerant patients with chronic cancer pain: A long-term, open-label safety study. *Cancer, 115,* 2571–2579. doi:10.1002/cncr.24279

95. Zeppetella, G., & Ribeiro, M.D.C. (2006). Opioids for the management of breakthrough (episodic) pain in cancer patients. *Cochrane Database of Systematic Reviews, 2006*(1). doi:10.1002/14651858.CD004311.pub2

96. Green, E., Zwaal, C., Beals, C., Fitzgerald, B., Harle, I., Jones, J., ... Wiernikowski, J. (2010). Cancer-related pain management: A report of evidence-based recommendations to guide practice. *Clinical Journal of Pain, 26,* 449–462. doi:10.1097/AJP.0b013e3181dacd62

97. Mercadante, S., Villari, P., Ferrera, P., Mangione, S., & Casuccio, A. (2010). The use of opioids for breakthrough pain in acute palliative care unit by using doses proportional to opioid basal regimen. *Clinical Journal of Pain, 26,* 306–309. doi:10.1097/AJP.0b013e3181c4458a

98. Hao, J., Wang, K., Shao, Y., Cheng, X., & Yan, Z. (2013). Intravenous flurbiprofen axetil to relieve cancer-related multiple breakthrough pain: A clinical study. *Journal of Palliative Medicine, 16,* 190–192. doi:10.1089/jpm.2012.0353

99. Good, P., Jackson, K., Brumley, D., & Ashby, M. (2009). Intranasal sufentanil for cancer-associated breakthrough pain. *Palliative Medicine, 23,* 54–58. doi:10.1177/0269216308100249

100. Ho, M.-L., Chung, C.-Y., Wang, C.-C., Lin, H.-Y., Hsu, N.C., & Chang, C.-S. (2010). Efficacy and safety of tramadol/acetaminophen in the treatment of breakthrough pain in cancer patients. *Saudi Medical Journal, 31,* 1315–1319. Retrieved from http://www.smj.org.sa/PDFFiles/Dec10/03Efficacy20100456.pdf

101. Cleeland, C.S., Body, J.J., Stopeck, A., von Moos, R., Fallowfield, L., Mathias, S.D., ... Chung, K. (2013). Pain outcomes in patients with advanced breast cancer and bone metastases: Results from a randomized, double-blind study of denosumab and zoledronic acid. *Cancer, 119,* 832–838. doi:10.1002/cncr.27789

102. Heras, P., Hatzopoulos, A., Heras, V., Kritikos, N., Karagiannis, S., & Kritikos, K. (2011). A comparative study of intravenous ibandronate and pamindronate in patients with bone metastases from breast or lung cancer: Effect on metastatic bone pain. *American Journal of Therapeutics, 18,* 340–342. doi:10.1097/MJT.0b013e3181e70c38

103. Saad, F., & Eastham, J. (2010). Zoledronic acid improves clinical outcomes when administered before onset of bone pain in patients with prostate cancer. *Urology, 76,* 1175–1181. doi:10.1016/j.urology.2010.05.026

104. Van Poznak, C.H., Temin, S., Yee, G.C., Janjan, N.A., Barlow, W.E., Biermann, J.S., ... Von Roenn, J.H. (2011). American Society of Clinical Oncology executive summary of the clinical practice guideline update on the role of bone-modifying agents in metastatic breast cancer. *Journal of Clinical Oncology, 29,* 1221–1227. doi:10.1200/JCO.2010.32.5209

105. Wong, R.K.S., & Wiffen, P.J. (2009). Bisphosphonates for the relief of pain secondary to bone metastases. *Cochrane Database of Systematic Reviews, 2009*(4). doi:10.1002/14651858.CD002068

106. Yuen, K.K., Shelley, M., Sze, W.M., Wilt, T., & Mason, M.D. (2006). Bisphosphonates for advanced prostate cancer. *Cochrane Database of Systematic Reviews, 2006*(4). doi:10.1002/14651858.CD006250

107. Arcidiacono, P.G., Calori, G., Carrara, S., McNicol, E.D., & Testoni, P.A. (2011). Celiac plexus block for pancreatic cancer pain in adults. *Cochrane Database of Systematic Reviews, 2011*(3). doi:10.1002/14651858 .CD007519.pub2

108. Johnson, C.D., Berry, D.P., Harris, S., Pickering, R.M., Davis, C., George, S., ... Sutton, R. (2009). An open randomized comparison of clinical effectiveness of protocol-driven opioid analgesia, celiac plexus block or thoracoscopic splanchnicectomy for pain management in patients with pancreatic and other abdominal malignancies. *Pancreatology, 9,* 755–763. doi:10.1159/000199441

109. Kaufman, M., Singh, G., Das, S., Concha-Parra, R., Erber, J., Micames, C., & Gress, F. (2010). Efficacy of endoscopic ultrasound-guided celiac plexus block and celiac plexus neurolysis for managing abdominal pain associated with chronic pancreatitis and pancreatic cancer. *Journal of Clinical Gastroenterology, 44,* 127–134. doi:10.1097/MCG.0b013e3181bb854d

110. Puli, S.R., Reddy, J.B.K., Bechtold, M.L., Antillon, M.R., & Brugge, W.R. (2009). EUS-guided celiac plexus neurolysis for pain due to chronic pancreatitis or pancreatic cancer pain: A meta-analysis and systematic review. *Digestive Diseases and Sciences, 54,* 2330–2337. doi:10.1007/s10620-008-0651-x

111. Wyse, J.M., Carone, M., Paquin, S.C., Usatii, M., & Sahai, A.V. (2011). Randomized, double-blind, controlled trial of early endoscopic ultrasound-guided celiac plexus neurolysis to prevent pain progression in patients with newly diagnosed, painful, inoperable pancreatic cancer. *Journal of Clinical Oncology, 29,* 3541–3546. doi:10.1200/JCO.2010.32.2750

112. Yan, B.M., & Myers, R.P. (2007). Neurolytic celiac plexus block for pain control in unresectable pancreatic cancer. *American Journal of Gastroenterology, 102,* 430–438. doi:10.1111/j.1572-0241.2006.00967.x

113. Challapalli, V., Tremont-Lukats, I.W., McNicol, E.D., Lau, J., & Carr, D.D. (2005). Systemic administration of local anesthetic agents to relieve neuropathic pain. *Cochrane Database of Systematic Reviews, 2005*(4). doi:10.1002/14651858.CD003345.pub2

114. McNicol, E., Strassels, S.A., Goudas, L., Lau, J., & Carr, D.B. (2005). NSAIDs or paracetamol, alone or combined with opioids for cancer pain. *Cochrane Database of Systematic Reviews, 2005*(2). doi:10.1002/14651858. CD005180

115. Colson, J., Koyyalagunta, D., Falco, F.J., & Manchikanti, L. (2011). A systematic review of observational studies on the effectiveness of opioid therapy for cancer pain. *Pain Physician, 14,* E85–E102. Retrieved from http://www.painphysicianjournal.com/2011/march/2011;14;E85-E102.pdf

116. Miaskowski, C., Bair, M., Chou, R., D'Arcy, Y., Hartwick, C., Huffman, L., ... Manworren, R. (2008). *Principles of analgesic use in the treatment of acute pain and cancer pain* (6th ed.). Glenview, IL: American Pain Society.

117. Qaseem, A., Snow, V., Shekelle, P., Casey, D.E., Jr., Cross, J.T., Jr., & Owens, D.K., Jr. (2008). Evidence-based interventions to improve the palliative care of pain, dyspnea, and depression at the end of life: A clinical practice guideline from the American College of Physicians. *Annals of Internal Medicine, 148,* 141–146. doi:10.7326/0003-4819-148-2-200801150 -00009

118. Tassinari, D., Sartori, S., Tamburini, E., Scarpi, E., Raffaeli, W., Tombesi, P., & Maltoni, M. (2008). Adverse effects of transdermal opiates treating moderate-severe cancer pain in comparison to long-acting morphine: A meta-analysis and systematic review of the literature. *Journal of Palliative Medicine, 11,* 492–501. doi:10.1089/jpm.2007.0200

119. Pergolizzi, J.V., Jr., Mercadante, S., Echaburu, A.V., Van den Eynden, B., Fragoso, R.M., Mordarski, S., ... Slama, O. (2009). The role of transdermal buprenorphine in the treatment of cancer pain: An expert panel consensus. *Current Medical Research and Opinion, 25,* 1517–1528. doi:10.1185/03007990902920731

120. Przeklasa-Muszyńska, A., & Dobrogowski, J. (2011). Transdermal buprenorphine in the treatment of cancer and non-cancer pain—The results of multicenter studies in Poland. *Pharmacological Reports, 63,* 935–948. Retrieved from http://www.if-pan.krakow.pl/pjp/pdf/2011/4_935.pdf

121. Ruggiero, A., Coccia, P., Arena, R., Maurizi, P., Battista, A., Ridola, V., ... Riccardi, R. (2013). Efficacy and safety of transdermal buprenorphine in the management of children with cancer-related pain. *Pediatric Blood and Cancer, 60,* 433–437. doi:10.1002/pbc.24332

122. Nicholson, A.B. (2007). Methadone for cancer pain. *Cochrane Database of Systematic Reviews, 2007*(4). doi:10.1002/14651858.CD003971.pub3

123. Meissner, W., Leyendecker, P., Mueller-Lissner, S., Nadstawek, J., Hopp, M., Ruckes, C., ... Reimer, K. (2009). A randomised controlled trial with prolonged-release oral oxycodone and naloxone to prevent and reverse opioid-induced constipation. *European Journal of Pain, 13,* 56–64. doi:10.1016/j.ejpain.2008.06.012

124. Schutter, U., Grunert, S., Meyer, C., Schmidt, T., & Nolte, T. (2010). Innovative pain therapy with a fixed combination of prolonged-release oxycodone/naloxone: A large observational study under conditions of daily practice. *Current Medical Research and Opinion, 26,* 1377–1387. doi:10.1185/03007991003787318

125. Leppert, W., & Majkowicz, M. (2010). The impact of tramadol and dihydrocodeine treatment on quality of life of patients with cancer pain. *International Journal of Clinical Practice, 64,* 1681–1687. doi:10.1111/j.1742-1241.2010.02422.x

126. Rodriguez, R.F., Castillo, J.M., Castillo, M.P., Montoya, O., Daza, P., Rodriguez, M.F., ... Angel, A.M. (2008). Hydrocodone/acetaminophen and tramadol chlorhydrate combination tablets for the management of chronic cancer pain: A double-blind comparative trial. *Clinical Journal of Pain, 24,* 1–4. doi:10.1097/AJP.0b013e318156ca4d

127. Marinangeli, F., Ciccozzi, A., Aloisio, L., Colangeli, A., Paladini, A., Bajocco, C., ... Varrassi, G. (2007). Improved cancer pain treatment using combined fentanyl-TTS and tramadol. *Pain Practice, 7,* 307–312. doi:10.1111/j.1533-2500.2007.00155.x

128. Cai, Q., Huang, H., Sun, X., Xia, Z., Li, Y., Lin, X., & Guo, Y. (2008). Efficacy and safety of transdermal fentanyl for treatment of oral mucositis pain caused by chemotherapy. *Expert Opinion on Pharmacotherapy, 9,* 3137–3144. doi:10.1517/14656560802504508

129. Chang, J.T.-C., Lin, C.-Y., Lin, J.C., Lee, M.S., Chen, Y.-J., & Wang, H.-M. (2010). Transdermal fentanyl for pain caused by radiotherapy in head and neck cancer patients treated in an outpatient setting: A multicenter trial in Taiwan. *Japanese Journal of Clinical Oncology, 40,* 307–312. doi:10.1093/jjco/hyp166

130. Kress, H.G. (2008). Clinical update on the pharmacology, efficacy and safety of transdermal buprenorphine. *European Journal of Pain, 13,* 219–230. doi:10.1016/j.ejpain.2008.04.011

131. Miyazaki, T., Hanaoka, K., Namiki, A., Ogawa, S., Kitajima, T., Hosokawa, T., ... Mashimo, S. (2008). Efficacy, safety and pharmacokinetic study of a novel fentanyl-containing matrix transdermal patch system in Japanese patients with cancer pain. *Clinical Drug Investigation, 28,* 313–325. doi:10.2165/00044011-200828050-00005

132. Pergolizzi, J., Boger, R.H., Budd, K., Dahan, A., Erdine, S., Hans, G., … Sacerdote, P. (2008). Opioids and the management of chronic severe pain in the elderly: Consensus statement of an International Expert Panel with focus on the six clinically most often used World Health Organization step III opioids (buprenorphine, fentanyl, hydromorphone, methadone, morphine, oxycodone). *Pain Practice, 8,* 287–313. doi:10.1111/j.1533 -2500.2008.00204.x

133. Bennett, M.I., Bagnall, A.M., & Closs, S.J. (2009). How effective are patient-based educational interventions in the management of cancer pain? Systematic review and meta-analysis. *Pain, 143,* 192–199. doi:10.1016/j.pain .2009.01.016

134. Devine, E.C. (2003). Meta-analysis of the effect of psychoeducational interventions on pain in adults with cancer. *Oncology Nursing Forum, 30,* 75–89. doi:10.1188/03.ONF.75-89

135. Flemming, K. (2010). The use of morphine to treat cancer-related pain: A synthesis of quantitative and qualitative research. *Journal of Pain and Symptom Management, 39,* 139–154. doi:10.1016/j.jpainsymman.2009.05.014

136. Kravitz, R.L., Tancredi, D.J., Grennan, T., Kalauokalani, D., Street, R.L., Jr., Slee, C.K., … Franks, P. (2011). Cancer Health Empowerment for Living without Pain (Ca-HELP): Effects of a tailored education and coaching intervention on pain and impairment. *Pain, 152,* 1572–1582. doi:10.1016/j.pain .2011.02.047

137. Kravitz, R.L., Tancredi, D.J., Jerant, A., Saito, N., Street, R.L., Grennan, T., & Franks, P. (2012). Influence of patient coaching on analgesic treatment adjustment: Secondary analysis of a randomized controlled trial. *Journal of Pain and Symptom Management, 43,* 874–884. doi:10.1016/ j.jpainsymman.2011.05.020

138. Kroenke, K., Theobald, D., Wu, J., Norton, K., Morrison, G., Carpenter, J., & Tu, W. (2010). Effect of telecare management on pain and depression in patients with cancer: A randomized trial. *JAMA, 304,* 163–171. doi:10.1001/ jama.2010.944

139. Kwekkeboom, K.L., Abbott-Anderson, K., Cherwin, C., Roiland, R., Serlin, R.C., & Ward, S.E. (2012). Pilot randomized controlled trial of a patient-controlled cognitive-behavioral intervention for the pain, fatigue, and sleep disturbance symptom cluster in cancer. *Journal of Pain and Symptom Management, 44,* 810–822. doi:10.1016/j.jpainsymman.2011.12 .281

140. Ling, C.-C., Lui, L.Y.Y., & So, W.K.W. (2012). Do educational interventions improve cancer patients' quality of life and reduce pain intensity? Quantitative systematic review. *Journal of Advanced Nursing, 68,* 511–520. doi:10.1111/j.1365-2648.2011.05841.x

141. Lovell, M.R., Forder, P.M., Stockler, M.R., Butow, P., Briganti, E.M., Chye, R., … Boyle, F.M. (2010). A randomized controlled trial of a standardized educational intervention for patients with cancer pain. *Journal of Pain and Symptom Management, 40,* 49–59. doi:10.1016/j.jpainsymman.2009.12.013

142. Oldenmenger, W.H., Sillevis Smitt, P.A.E., van Montfort, C.A.G.M., de Raaf, P.J., & van der Rijt, C.C.D. (2011). A combined pain consultation and pain education program decreases average and current pain and decreases interference in daily life by pain in oncology outpatients: A randomized controlled trial. *Pain, 152,* 2632–2639. doi:10.1016/j.pain.2011.08.009

143. Sheinfeld Gorin, S., Krebs, P., Badr, H., Janke, E.A., Jim, H.S., Spring, B., … Jacobsen, P.B. (2012). Meta-analysis of psychosocial interventions to reduce pain in patients with cancer. *Journal of Clinical Oncology, 30,* 539–547. doi:10.1200/JCO.2011.37.0437

144. Syrjala, K.L., Abrams, J.R., Polissar, N.L., Hansberry, J., Robison, J., DuPen, S., … DuPen, A. (2008). Patient training in cancer pain management using integrated print and video materials: A multisite randomized controlled trial. *Pain, 135,* 175–186. doi:10.1016/j.pain.2007.10.026

145. Tulipani, C., Morelli, F., Spedicato, M.R., Maiello, E., Todarello, O., & Porcelli, P. (2010). Alexithymia and cancer pain: The effect of psycho-

logical intervention. *Psychotherapy and Psychosomatics, 79,* 156–163. doi:10.1159/000286960

146. van der Peet, E.H., van den Beuken-van Everdingen, M.H., Patijn, J., Schouten, H.C., van Kleef, M., & Courtens, A.M. (2009). Randomized clinical trial of an intensive nursing-based pain education program for cancer outpatients suffering from pain. *Supportive Care in Cancer, 17,* 1089–1099. doi:10.1007/s00520-008-0564-4

147. Ward, S., Donovan, H., Gunnarsdottir, S., Serlin, R.C., Shapiro, G.R., & Hughes, S. (2008). A randomized trial of a representational intervention to decrease cancer pain (RIDcancerPain). *Health Psychology, 27,* 59–67. doi:10.1037/0278-6133.27.1.59

148. Yildirim, Y.K., Cicek, F., & Uyar, M. (2009). Effects of pain education program on pain intensity, pain treatment satisfaction, and barriers in Turkish cancer patients. *Pain Management Nursing, 10,* 220–228. doi:10.1016/j.pmn.2007.09.004

149. Anderson, K.O., Cohen, M.Z., Mendoza, T.R., Guo, H., Harle, M.T., & Cleeland, C.S. (2006). Brief cognitive-behavioral audiotape interventions for cancer-related pain: Immediate but not long-term effectiveness. *Cancer, 107,* 207–214. doi:10.1002/cncr.21964

150. Given, B., Given, C.W., McCorkle, R., Kozachik, S., Cimprich, B., Rahbar, M.H., & Wojcik, C. (2002). Pain and fatigue management: Results of a nursing randomized clinical trial. *Oncology Nursing Forum, 29,* 949–956. doi:10.1188/02.ONF.949-956

151. Kim, H.S., Shin, S.J., Kim, S.C., An, S., Rha, S.Y., Ahn, J.B., ... Lee, S. (2013). Randomized controlled trial of standardized education and telemonitoring for pain in outpatients with advanced solid tumors. *Supportive Care in Cancer, 21,* 1751–1759. doi:10.1007/s00520-013-1722-x

152. Koller, A., Miaskowski, C., De Geest, S., Opitz, O., & Spichiger, E. (2012). A systematic evaluation of content, structure, and efficacy of interventions to improve patients' self-management of cancer pain. *Journal of Pain and Symptom Management, 44,* 264–284. doi:10.1016/j.jpainsymman.2011.08.015

153. Kwekkeboom, K.L., Abbott-Anderson, K., & Wanta, B. (2010). Feasibility of a patient-controlled cognitive-behavioral intervention for pain, fatigue, and sleep disturbance in cancer [Online exclusive]. *Oncology Nursing Forum, 37,* E151–E159. doi:10.1188/10.ONF.E151-E159

154. Thomas, M.L., Elliott, J.E., Rao, S.M., Fahey, K.F., Paul, S.M., & Miaskowski, C. (2012). A randomized, clinical trial of education or motivational-interviewing–based coaching compared to usual care to improve cancer pain management. *Oncology Nursing Forum, 39,* 39–49. doi:10.1188/12.ONF.39-49

155. Ward, S.E., Serlin, R.C., Donovan, H.S., Ameringer, S.W., Hughes, S., Pe-Romashko, K., & Wang, K.K. (2009). A randomized trial of a representational intervention for cancer pain: Does targeting the dyad make a difference? *Health Psychology, 28,* 588–597. doi:10.1037/a0015216

156. Ward, S.E., Wang, K.K., Serlin, R.C., Peterson, S.L., & Murray, M.E. (2009). A randomized trial of a tailored barriers intervention for Cancer Information Service (CIS) callers in pain. *Pain, 144,* 49–56. doi:10.1016/j.pain.2009.02.021

157. Tatrow, K., & Montgomery, G.H. (2006). Cognitive behavioral therapy techniques for distress and pain in breast cancer patients: A meta-analysis. *Journal of Behavioral Medicine, 29,* 17–27. doi:10.1007/s10865-005-9036-1

158. Currow, D.C., Plummer, J.L., Cooney, N.J., Gorman, D., & Glare, P.A. (2007). A randomized, double-blind, multi-site, crossover, placebo-controlled equivalence study of morning versus evening once-daily sustained-release morphine sulfate in people with pain from advanced cancer. *Journal of Pain and Symptom Management, 34,* 17–23. doi:10.1016/j.jpainsymman.2006.10.011

159. De Conno, F., Ripamonti, C., Fagnoni, E., Brunelli, C., Luzzani, M., Maltoni, M., ... Bertetto, O. (2008). The MERITO Study: A multicentre trial of the analgesic effect and tolerability of normal-release oral morphine during

'titration phase' in patients with cancer pain. *Palliative Medicine, 22,* 214–221. doi:10.1177/0269216308088692

160. Homsi, J., Walsh, D., Lasheen, W., Nelson, K.A., Rybicki, L.A., Bast, J., & LeGrand, S.B. (2010). A comparative study of 2 sustained-release morphine preparations for pain in advanced cancer. *American Journal of Hospice and Palliative Care, 27,* 99–105. doi:10.1177/1049909109345146

161. Liguori, S., Gottardi, M., Micheletto, G., & Bruno, L. (2010). Pharmacological approach to chronic visceral pain. Focus on oxycodone controlled release: An open multicentric study. *European Review for Medical and Pharmacological Sciences, 14,* 185–190. Retrieved from http://www.europeanreview.org/wp/wp-content/uploads/722.pdf

162. Mayyas, F., Fayers, P., Kaasa, S., & Dale, O. (2010). A systematic review of oxymorphone in the management of chronic pain. *Journal of Pain and Symptom Management, 39,* 296–308. doi:10.1016/j.jpainsymman.2009.07.010

163. Mercadante, S., Tirelli, W., David, F., Arcara, C., Fulfaro, F., Casuccio, A., & Gebbia, V. (2010). Morphine versus oxycodone in pancreatic cancer pain: A randomized controlled study. *Clinical Journal of Pain, 26,* 794–797. doi:10.1097/AJP.0b013e3181ecd895

164. Silvestri, B., Bandieri, E., Del Prete, S., Ianniello, G.P., Micheletto, G., Dambrosio, M., ... Spanu, P. (2008). Oxycodone controlled-release as first-choice therapy for moderate-to-severe cancer pain in Italian patients: Results of an open-label, multicentre, observational study. *Clinical Drug Investigation, 28,* 399–407. doi:10.2165/00044011-200828070-00001

165. Slatkin, N.E., Rhiner, M.I., Gould, E.M., Ma, T., & Ahdieh, H. (2010). Long-term tolerability and effectiveness of oxymorphone extended release in patients with cancer. *Journal of Opioid Management, 6,* 181–191. doi:10.5055/jom.2010.0016

166. Wallace, M., Moulin, D.E., Rauck, R.L., Khanna, S., Tudor, I.C., Skowronski, R., & Thipphawong, J. (2009). Long-term safety, tolerability, and efficacy of OROS hydromorphone in patients with chronic pain. *Journal of Opioid Management, 5,* 97–105.

167. Ridgway, D., Sopata, M., Burneckis, A., Jespersen, L., & Andersen, C. (2010). Clinical efficacy and safety of once-daily dosing of a novel, prolonged-release oral morphine tablet compared with twice-daily dosing of a standard controlled-release morphine tablet in patients with cancer pain: A randomized, double-blind, exploratory crossover study. *Journal of Pain and Symptom Management, 39,* 712–720. doi:10.1016/j.jpainsymman.2009.08.013

168. Lee, K.H., Kim, M.K., Hyun, M.S., Kim, J.Y., Park, K.U., Song, H.S., ... Cho, Y.Y. (2012). Clinical effectiveness and safety of OROS® hydromorphone in break-through cancer pain treatment: A multicenter, prospective, open-label study in Korean patients. *Journal of Opioid Management, 8,* 243–252. doi:10.5055/jom.2012.0122

169. Logothetis, C.J., Basch, E., Molina, A., Fizazi, K., North, S.A., Chi, K.N., ... de Bono, J.S. (2012). Effect of abiraterone acetate and prednisone compared with placebo and prednisone on pain control and skeletal-related events in patients with metastatic castration-resistant prostate cancer: Exploratory analysis of data from the COU-AA-301 randomised trial. *Lancet Oncology, 13,* 1210–1217. doi:10.1016/S1470-2045(12)70473-4

170. Johnson, J.R., Burnell-Nugent, M., Lossignol, D., Ganae-Motan, E.D., Potts, R., & Fallon, M.T. (2010). Multicenter, double-blind, randomized, placebo-controlled, parallel-group study of the efficacy, safety, and tolerability of THC:CBD extract and THC extract in patients with intractable cancer-related pain. *Journal of Pain and Symptom Management, 39,* 167–179. doi:10.1016/j.jpainsymman.2009.06.008

171. Portenoy, R.K., Ganae-Motan, E.D., Allende, S., Yanagihara, R., Shaiova, L., Weinstein, S., ... Fallon, M.T. (2012). Nabiximols for opioid-treated cancer patients with poorly-controlled chronic pain: A randomized, placebo-controlled, graded-dose trial. *Journal of Pain, 13,* 438–449. doi:10.1016/j.jpain.2012.01.003

172. Matsuoka, H., Makimura, C., Koyama, A., Otsuka, M., Okamoto, W., Fujisaka, Y., ... Nakagawa, K. (2012). Pilot study of duloxetine for cancer patients with neuropathic pain non-responsive to pregabalin. *Anticancer Research, 32,* 1805–1809. Retrieved from http://ar.iiarjournals.org/content/32/5/1805.long

173. Smith, E.M., Pang, H., Cirrincione, C., Fleishman, S., Paskett, E.D., Ahles, T., ... Shapiro, C.L. (2013). Effect of duloxetine on pain, function, and quality of life among patients with chemotherapy-induced painful peripheral neuropathy: A randomized clinical trial. *JAMA, 309,* 1359–1367. doi:10.1001/jama.2013.2813

174. Maltoni, M., Scarpi, E., Modonesi, C., Passardi, A., Calpona, S., Turriziani, A., ... Ferrario, S. (2005). A validation study of the WHO analgesic ladder: A two-step vs three-step strategy. *Supportive Care in Cancer, 13,* 888–894. doi:10.1007/s00520-005-0807-6

175. Takase, H., Sakata, T., Yamano, T., Sueta, T., Nomoto, S., & Nakagawa, T. (2011). Advantage of early induction of opioid to control pain induced by irradiation in head and neck cancer patients. *Auris Nasus Larynx, 38,* 495–500. doi:10.1016/j.anl.2010.12.012

176. Tessaro, L., Bandieri, E., Costa, G., Fornasier, G., Iorno, V., Pizza, C., ... Micheletto, G. (2010). Use of oxycodone controlled-release immediately after NSAIDs: A new approach to obtain good pain control. *European Review for Medical and Pharmacological Sciences, 14,* 113–121.

177. Arai, Y.-C., Matsubara, T., Shimo, K., Suetomi, K., Nishihara, M., Ushida, T., ... Arakawa, M. (2010). Low-dose gabapentin as useful adjuvant to opioids for neuropathic cancer pain when combined with low-dose imipramine. *Journal of Anesthesia, 24,* 407–410. doi:10.1007/s00540-010-0913-6

178. Dworkin, R.H., O'Connor, A.B., Backonja, M., Farrar, J.T., Finnerup, N.B., Jensen, T.S., ... Wallace, M.S. (2007). Pharmacologic management of neuropathic pain: Evidence-based recommendations. *Pain, 132,* 237–251. doi:10.1016/j.pain.2007.08.033

179. Keskinbora, K., Pekel, A.F., & Aydinli, I. (2007). Gabapentin and an opioid combination versus opioid alone for the management of neuropathic cancer pain: A randomized open trial. *Journal of Pain and Symptom Management, 34,* 183–189. doi:10.1016/j.jpainsymman.2006.11.013

180. Mishra, S., Bhatnagar, S., Goyal, G.N., Rana, S.P., & Upadhya, S.P. (2012). A comparative efficacy of amitriptyline, gabapentin, and pregabalin in neuropathic cancer pain: A prospective randomized double-blind placebo-controlled study. *American Journal of Hospice and Palliative Care, 29,* 177–182. doi:10.1177/1049909111412539

181. Patarica-Huber, E., Boskov, N., & Pjevic, M. (2011). Multimodal approach to therapy-related neuropathic pain in breast cancer. *Journal of B.U.ON., 16,* 40–45.

182. Ross, J.R., Goller, K., Hardy, J., Riley, J., Broadley, K., A'Hern, R., & Williams, J. (2005). Gabapentin is effective in the treatment of cancer-related neuropathic pain: A prospective, open-label study. *Journal of Palliative Medicine, 8,* 1118–1126. doi:10.1089/jpm.2005.8.1118

183. Takahashi, H., & Shimoyama, N. (2010). A prospective open-label trial of gabapentin as an adjuvant analgesic with opioids for Japanese patients with neuropathic cancer pain. *International Journal of Clinical Oncology, 15,* 46–51. doi:10.1007/s10147-009-0009-1

184. Caraceni, A., Hanks, G., Kaasa, S., Bennett, M.I., Brunelli, C., Cherny, N., ... Zeppetella, G. (2012). Use of opioid analgesics in the treatment of cancer pain: Evidence-based recommendations from the EAPC. *Lancet Oncology, 13,* e58–e68. doi:10.1016/S1470-2045(12)70040-2

185. Axelsson, B., Stellborn, P., & Ström, G. (2008). Analgesic effect of paracetamol on cancer related pain in concurrent strong opioid therapy. A prospective clinical study. *Acta Oncologica, 47,* 891–895. doi:10.1080/02841860701687259

186. Cubero, D.I., & del Giglio, A. (2010). Early switching from morphine to methadone is not improved by acetaminophen in the analgesia of onco-

logic patients: A prospective, randomized, double-blind, placebo-controlled study. *Supportive Care in Cancer, 18,* 235–242. doi:10.1007/s00520 -009-0649-8

187. Israel, F.J., Parker, G., Charles, M., & Reymond, L. (2010). Lack of benefit from paracetamol (acetaminophen) for palliative cancer patients requiring high-dose strong opioids: A randomized, double-blind, placebo-controlled, crossover trial. *Journal of Pain and Symptom Management, 39,* 548–554. doi:10.1016/j.jpainsymman.2009.07.008

188. Sima, L., Fang, W.X., Wu, X.M., & Li, F. (2012). Efficacy of oxycodone/paracetamol for patients with bone-cancer pain: A multicenter, randomized, double-blinded, placebo-controlled trial. *Journal of Clinical Pharmacy and Therapeutics, 37,* 27–31. doi:10.1111/j.1365-2710.2010.01239.x

189. Tasmacioglu, B., Aydinli, I., Keskinbora, K., Pekel, A.F., Salihoglu, T., & Sonsuz, A. (2009). Effect of intravenous administration of paracetamol on morphine consumption in cancer pain control. *Supportive Care in Cancer, 17,* 1475–1481. doi:10.1007/s00520-009-0612-8

190. American Geriatrics Society Panel on the Pharmacological Management of Persistent Pain in Older Persons. (2009). Pharmacological management of persistent pain in older persons. *Pain Medicine, 10,* 1062–1083. doi:10.1111/j.1526-4637.2009.00699.x

191. Suh, S.-Y., Choi, Y.S., Oh, S.C., Kim, Y.S., Cho, K., Bae, W.K., … Ahn, H.-Y. (2013). Caffeine as an adjuvant therapy to opioids in cancer pain: A randomized, double-blind, placebo-controlled trial. *Journal of Pain and Symptom Management, 46,* 474–482. doi:10.1016/j.jpainsymman.2012.10.232

192. Kubo, N., Suzuki, H., Kobayashi, T., Araki, K., Sasaki, S., Wada, W., & Kuwano, H. (2012). Usefulness of steroid administration for diagnosis of IgG4-related sclerosing cholangitis. *International Surgery, 97,* 145–149. doi:10.9738/CC78.1

193. Mañas, A., Ciria, J.P., Fernández, M.C., Gonzálvez, M.L., Morillo, V., Perez, M., … López-Gómez, V. (2011). Post hoc analysis of pregabalin vs. non-pregabalin treatment in patients with cancer-related neuropathic pain: Better pain relief, sleep and physical health. *Clinical and Translational Oncology, 13,* 656–663. doi:10.1007/s12094-011-0711-0

194. Caviggioli, F., Maione, L., Forcellini, D., Klinger, F., & Klinger, M. (2011). Autologous fat graft in postmastectomy pain syndrome. *Plastic and Reconstructive Surgery, 128,* 349–352. doi:10.1097/PRS.0b013e31821e70e7

195. Wang, K.X., Jin, Z.D., Du, Y.Q., Zhan, X.B., Zou, D.W., Liu, Y., … Li, Z.S. (2012). EUS-guided celiac ganglion irradiation with iodine-125 seeds for pain control in pancreatic carcinoma: A prospective pilot study. *Gastrointestinal Endoscopy, 76,* 945–952. doi:10.1016/j.gie.2012.05.032

196. Liberman, B., Gianfelice, D., Inbar, Y., Beck, A., Rabin, T., Shabshin, N., … Catane, R. (2009). Pain palliation in patients with bone metastases using MR-guided focused ultrasound surgery: A multicenter study. *Annals of Surgical Oncology, 16,* 140–146. doi:10.1245/s10434-008-0011-2

197. Fink, D.J., Wechuck, J., Mata, M., Glorioso, J.C., Goss, J., Krisky, D., & Wolfe, D. (2011). Gene therapy for pain: Results of a phase I clinical trial. *Annals of Neurology, 70,* 207–212. doi:10.1002/ana.22446

198. Lim, J.T.W., Wong, E.T., & Aung, S.K.H. (2011). Is there a role for acupuncture in the symptom management of patients receiving palliative care for cancer? A pilot study of 20 patients comparing acupuncture with nurse-led supportive care. *Acupuncture in Medicine, 29,* 173–179. doi:10.1136/aim.2011.004044

199. Hollis, A.H. (2010). Acupuncture as a treatment modality for the management of cancer pain: The state of the science [Online exclusive]. *Oncology Nursing Forum, 37,* E344–E348. doi:10.1188/10.ONF.E344-E348

200. Birocco, N., Guillame, C., Storto, S., Ritorto, G., Catino, C., Gir, N., … Ciuffreda, L. (2012). The effects of Reiki therapy on pain and anxiety in patients attending a day oncology and infusion services unit. *American Journal of Hospice and Palliative Care, 29,* 290–294. doi:10.1177/1049909111420859

201. Post White, J., Kinney, M.E., Savik, K., Gau, J.B., Wilcox, C., & Lerner, I. (2003). Therapeutic massage and healing touch improve symptoms in cancer. *Integrative Cancer Therapies, 2,* 332–344. doi:10.1177/1534735403259064

202. Cheville, A.L., Kollasch, J., Vandenberg, J., Shen, T., Grothey, A., Gamble, G., & Basford, J.R. (2013). A home-based exercise program to improve function, fatigue, and sleep quality in patients with stage IV lung and colorectal cancer: A randomized controlled trial. *Journal of Pain and Symptom Management, 45,* 811–821. doi:10.1016/j.jpainsymman.2012.05.006

203. Fernández-Lao, C., Cantarero-Villanueva, I., Fernández-de-Las-Peñas, C., del Moral-Ávila, R., Castro-Sanchez, A.M., & Arroyo-Morales, M. (2012). Effectiveness of a multidimensional physical therapy program on pain, pressure hypersensitivity, and trigger points in breast cancer survivors: A randomized controlled clinical trial. *Clinical Journal of Pain, 28,* 113–121. doi:10.1097/AJP.0b013e318225dc02

204. McNeely, M.L., Parliament, M.B., Seikaly, H., Jha, N., Magee, D.J., Haykowsky, M.J., & Courneya, K.S. (2008). Effect of exercise on upper extremity pain and dysfunction in head and neck cancer survivors: A randomized controlled trial. *Cancer, 113,* 214–222. doi:10.1002/cncr.23536

205. Cepeda, M.S., Chapman, C.R., Miranda, N., Sanchez, R., Rodriguez, C.H., Restrepo, A.E., ... Carr, D.B. (2008). Emotional disclosure through patient narrative may improve pain and well-being: Results of a randomized controlled trial in patients with cancer pain. *Journal of Pain and Symptom Management, 35,* 623–631. doi:10.1016/j.jpainsymman.2007.08.011

206. Bao, Y.-J., Hua, B.-J., Hou, W., Lin, H.-S., Zhang, X.-B., & Yang, G.-X. (2010). Alleviation of cancerous pain by external compress with Xiaozheng Zhitong Paste. *Chinese Journal of Integrative Medicine, 16,* 309–314. doi:10.1007/s11655-010-0501-5

207. Wu, T.-H., Chiu, T.-Y., Tsai, J.-S., Chen, C.-Y., Chen, L.-C., & Yang, L.-L. (2008). Effectiveness of Taiwanese traditional herbal diet for pain management in terminal cancer patients. *Asia Pacific Journal of Clinical Nutrition, 17,* 17–22. Retrieved from http://apjcn.nhri.org.tw/server/APJCN/17/1/17.pdf

208. Xu, L., Lao, L.X., Ge, A., Yu, S., Li, J., & Mansky, P.J. (2007). Chinese herbal medicine for cancer pain. *Integrative Cancer Therapies, 6,* 208–234. doi:10.1177/1534735407305705

209. Butler, L.D., Koopman, C., Neri, E., Giese-Davis, J., Palesh, O., Thorne-Yocam, K.A., ... Spiegel, D. (2009). Effects of supportive-expressive group therapy on pain in women with metastatic breast cancer. *Health Psychology, 28,* 579–587. doi:10.1037/a0016124

210. Cummings, G.G., Olivo, S.A., Biondo, P.D., Stiles, C.R., Yurtseven, O., Fainsinger, R.L., & Hagen, N.A. (2011). Effectiveness of knowledge translation interventions to improve cancer pain management. *Journal of Pain and Symptom Management, 41,* 915–939. doi:10.1016/j.jpainsymman.2010.07.017

211. Goldberg, G.R., & Morrison, R.S. (2007). Pain management in hospitalized cancer patients: A systematic review. *Journal of Clinical Oncology, 25,* 1792–1801. doi:10.1200/JCO.2006.07.9038

212. Jane, S.-W., Chen, S.-L., Wilkie, D.J., Lin, Y.C., Foreman, S.W., Beaton, R.D., ... Liao, M.-N. (2011). Effects of massage on pain, mood status, relaxation, and sleep in Taiwanese patients with metastatic bone pain: A randomized clinical trial. *Pain, 152,* 2432–2442. doi:10.1016/j.pain.2011.06.021

213. Kutner, J.S., Smith, M.C., Corbin, L., Hemphill, L., Benton, K., Mellis, B.K., ... Fairclough, D.L. (2008). Massage therapy versus simple touch to improve pain and mood in patients with advanced cancer: A randomized trial. *Annals of Internal Medicine, 149,* 369–379. doi:10.7326/0003-4819-149-6-200809160-00003

214. Bandieri, E., Sichetti, D., Romero, M., Fanizza, C., Belfiglio, M., Buonaccorso, L., ... Luppi, M. (2012). Impact of early access to a palliative/supportive care intervention on pain management in patients with cancer. *Annals of Oncology, 23,* 2016–2020. doi:10.1093/annonc/mds103

215. Yennurajalingam, S., Kang, J.H., Hui, D., Kang, D.H., Kim, S.H., & Bruera, E. (2012). Clinical response to an outpatient palliative care consultation in patients with advanced cancer and cancer pain. *Journal of Pain and Symptom Management, 44,* 340–350. doi:10.1016/j.jpainsymman.2011.09.014

216. Kwekkeboom, K.L., Cherwin, C.H., Lee, J.W., & Wanta, B. (2010). Mind-body treatments for the pain-fatigue-sleep disturbance symptom cluster in persons with cancer. *Journal of Pain and Symptom Management, 39,* 126–138. doi:10.1016/j.jpainsymman.2009.05.022

217. King, K. (2010). A review of the effects of guided imagery on cancer patients with pain. *Journal of Evidence-Based Complementary and Alternative Medicine, 15,* 98–107. doi:10.1177/1533210110388113

218. Bennett, M.I., Johnson, M.I., Brown, S.R., Radford, H., Brown, J.M., & Searle, R.D. (2010). Feasibility study of transcutaneous electrical nerve stimulation (TENS) for cancer bone pain. *Journal of Pain, 11,* 351–359. doi:10.1016/j.jpain.2009.08.002

219. Hurlow, A., Bennett, M.I., Robb, K.A., Johnson, M.I., Simpson, K.H., & Oxberry, S.G. (2012). Transcutaneous electric nerve stimulation (TENS) for cancer pain in adults. *Cochrane Database of Systematic Reviews, 2012*(3). doi:10.1002/14651858.CD006276.pub3

220. Ricci, M., Pirotti, S., Scarpi, E., Burgio, M., Maltoni, M., Sansoni, E., & Amadori, D. (2012). Managing chronic pain: Results from an open-label study using MC5-A Calmare® device. *Supportive Care in Cancer, 20,* 405–412. doi:10.1007/s00520-011-1128-6

221. Robb, K.A., Bennett, M.I., Johnson, M.I., Simpson, K.J., & Oxberry, S.G. (2008). Transcutaneous electric nerve stimulation (TENS) for cancer pain in adults. *Cochrane Database of Systematic Reviews, 2008*(3). doi:10.1002/14651858.CD006276.pub2

222. Galantino, M.L., Desai, K., Greene, L., Demichele, A., Stricker, C.T., & Mao, J.J. (2012). Impact of yoga on functional outcomes in breast cancer survivors with aromatase inhibitor-associated arthralgias. *Integrative Cancer Therapies, 11,* 313–320. doi:10.1177/1534735411413270

223. Martinez-Zapata, M.J., Roqué i Figules, M., Alonso-Coello, P., Roman, Y., & Català, E. (2006). Calcitonin for metastatic bone pain. *Cochrane Database of Systematic Reviews, 2006*(3). doi:10.1002/14651858.CD003223.pub2

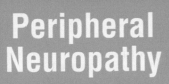

16

Peripheral Neuropathy

Cindy Tofthagen, PhD, ARNP, AOCNP®, FAANP, and Margaret Irwin, PhD, RN, MN

Problem and Incidence

Peripheral neuropathy is a chronic side effect of many chemotherapeutic agents and can also be caused by radiation therapy or malignant and paraneoplastic processes.[1,2] Chemotherapy-induced peripheral neuropathy (CIPN) can result in dose reductions, delays, or early cessation of treatment, compromising efficacy of cancer treatment. CIPN has significant deleterious effects on physical functioning and quality of life.[3,4] Symptoms of CIPN are usually bilateral, involving loss of sensation and/or hypersensitivity that begin in the fingers and toes and progress from distal to proximal in a stocking-glove pattern.[5] CIPN is predominantly sensory, but motor and autonomic neuropathy also can occur. The incidence of neuropathy varies based upon the drugs, dose, and administration schedule, with 64%–86% of people receiving neurotoxic chemotherapy developing neuropathy.[6-8]

Risk Factors and Assessment

The major risk factor for CIPN is treatment with neurotoxic chemotherapy, such as taxanes, platinum-based agents, vinca alkaloids, thalidomide, or bortezomib. Risk escalates as the cumulative dose increases. Patients at risk should be assessed for CIPN development.

Assessment includes evaluation of symptoms and interference with physical function using both subjective and objective data.[9-11]

Assess for
- Neuropathic pain
- Numbness, tingling, or itching
- Impairments in fine motor function
- Impairments in gross motor function
- Impaired balance
- Loss of sensation, reflexes, and vibration.

Assessment tools include
- National Cancer Institute Cancer Therapy Evaluation Program *Common Terminology Criteria for Adverse Events* (open access)[12]
- Total Neuropathy Score–reduced[13] (A pediatric version of this tool is available.[14])
- Functional Assessment of Cancer Therapy/Gynecologic Oncology Group—Neurotoxicity subscale[15]
- Rasch-Built Overall Disability Scale for patients with CIPN[16]
- Visual analog scale for pain or numbness.[17]

What interventions are effective in preventing and managing peripheral neuropathy in people with cancer?

Evidence retrieved through December 31, 2013

Likely to Be Effective

Duloxetine improved pain associated with peripheral neuropathy.[18,19] Both studies had relatively high dropout rates and did not address other analgesic use.

Effectiveness Not Established

Several pharmacologic and complementary and alternative interventions had mixed results, or evidence was inconclusive due to small samples and study limitations.

- **Pharmacologic interventions**
  - **Amifostine**[20]—A systematic review concluded there was insufficient evidence to show effectiveness.[21]
  - **BAK**, a topical gel containing baclofen, ketamine, and amitriptyline[22]
  - **Calcium and magnesium infusion**[23-26]
  - **Gabapentin monotherapy**[27-29]
  - **Gabapentin-opioid combination**[27,30]—Adjuvant medication, such as gabapentin, for neuropathic pain is suggested in guidelines.[31]
  - **Glutamine** oral supplements[32-37]
  - **Glutathione** infusions or injections[38-40]
  - **KRN5500**, an agent that inhibits some enzymes that may modulate neuropathic pain[41]
  - **Pregabalin**[42-44]
  - **Tricyclic antidepressants amitriptyline**[45,46] and **nortriptyline**[46]
  - **Venlafaxine**[47]
- **Complementary and alternative interventions**
  - **Acupuncture**[48]
  - **Bee venom** injections at acupuncture points[49]
  - **Cannabis/cannabinoids**[50]
  - **Cutaneous electrostimulation** applied to areas of CIPN[51]
  - **Goshajinkigan**, a combination of several Japanese medicinal herbs[52]
  - **Omega-3 fatty acid** supplementation[53]
  - **Palmitoylethanolamide**, an endogenous bioactive lipid[54]
  - **Vitamin E** supplements[55-59]

Effectiveness Unlikely

Carbamazepine had no effect.[60]

Lamotrigine did not affect CIPN in one large double-blind placebo-controlled trial.[61]

Not Recommended for Practice

Carnitine/acetyl-L-carnitine was examined in two small observational trials[62,63] showing possible benefit. However, a systematic review concluded evidence was insufficient to show effectiveness for CIPN.[21] One trial in patients receiving sagopilone did not show any benefit,[64] and a large multisite study showed more CIPN symptoms and functional status decline in patients receiving acetyl-L-carnitine compared to patients given placebo.[65]

Human leukemia inhibitory factor did not prevent or diminish CIPN in a study of patients receiving carboplatin/paclitaxel.[66]

Expert Opinion

Managing pain, enhancing physical functioning, and promoting safety are important goals for nursing management of CIPN.[11,67-69]

Despite limited data in CIPN, medications approved to treat neuropathic pain can be used to treat painful CIPN.[70]

A multidisciplinary approach to managing physical limitations caused by CIPN includes rehabilitation medicine, physical therapy, and occupational therapy.

Use of assistive devices may improve patient safety, prevent falls and other injuries, and help compensate for sensory deficits.[71]

Application to Practice

Patients at risk need to be consistently monitored and assessed for symptoms of peripheral neuropathy for early identification and management.

Based upon scope of practice, nurses can prescribe or advocate use of those medications that have the strongest evidence to support effectiveness for prevention and management of symptoms.

Patients with impaired balance can benefit from physical and occupational therapy to improve balance, learn the use of assistive devices, maintain or improve function, and prevent further disability.

Patients with peripheral neuropathy are at greater risk for falls. Nurses need to identify this risk for fall prevention in clinical care settings, and patients and caregivers need to be educated about actions to improve safety in the home.

Peripheral Neuropathy Resource Contributors

Topic leader: Constance Visovsky, RN, PhD, ACNP
Mary L. Collins, RN, MSN, OCN®, Emily K. Olson, RN, MSN,
OCN®, and Cindy Tofthagen, PhD, ARNP, AOCNP®, FAANP

References

1. Englander, E.W. (2013). DNA damage response in peripheral nervous system: Coping with cancer therapy-induced DNA lesions. *DNA Repair, 12,* 685–690. doi:10.1016/j.dnarep.2013.04.020

2. Ocean, A.J., & Vahdat, L.T. (2004). Chemotherapy-induced peripheral neuropathy: Pathogenesis and emerging therapies. *Supportive Care In Cancer, 12,* 619–625. doi:10.1007/s00520-004-0657-7

3. Mols, F., Beijers, T., Lemmens, V., van den Hurk, C.J., Vreugdenhil, G., & van de Poll-Franse, L.V. (2013). Chemotherapy-induced neuropathy and its association with quality of life among 2- to 11-year colorectal cancer survivors: Results from the population-based PROFILES registry. *Journal of Clinical Oncology, 31,* 2699–2707. doi:10.1200/JCO.2013.49.1514

4. Tofthagen, C. (2010). Patient perceptions associated with chemotherapy-induced peripheral neuropathy [Online exclusive]. *Clinical Journal of Oncology Nursing, 14,* E22–E28. doi:10.1188/10.CJON.E22-E28

5. Visovsky, C. (2003). Chemotherapy-induced peripheral neuropathy. *Cancer Investigation, 21,* 439–451. doi:10.1081/CNV-120018236

6. Argyriou, A.A., Polychronopoulos, P., Iconomou, G., Koutras, A., Kalofonos, H.P., & Chroni, E. (2005). Paclitaxel plus carboplatin–induced peripheral neuropathy. *Journal of Neurology, 252,* 1459–1464. doi:10.1007/s00415-005-0887-8

7. Osmani, K., Vignes, S., Aissi, M., Wade, F., Milani, P., Lévy, B.I., & Kubis, N. (2012). Taxane-induced peripheral neuropathy has good long-term prognosis: A 1- to 13-year evaluation. *Journal of Neurology, 259,* 1936–1943. doi:10.1007/s00415-012-6442-5

8. Ramanathan, R.K., Rothenberg, M.L., de Gramont, A., Tournigand, C., Goldberg, R.M., Gupta, S., & André, T. (2010). Incidence and evolution of

oxaliplatin-induced peripheral sensory neuropathy in diabetic patients with colorectal cancer: A pooled analysis of three phase III studies. *Annals of Oncology, 21,* 754–758. doi:10.1093/annonc/mdp509

9. Cavaletti, G., Cornblath, D.R., Merkies, I.S.J., Postma, T.J., Rossi, E., Frigeni, B., ... Valsecchi, M.G. (2013). The chemotherapy-induced peripheral neuropathy outcome measures standardization study: From consensus to the first validity and reliability findings. *Annals of Oncology, 24,* 454–462. doi:10.1093/annonc/mds329

10. Smith, E.M.L., Cohen, J.A., Pett, M.A., & Beck, S.L. (2011). The validity of neuropathy and neuropathic pain measures in patients with cancer receiving taxanes and platinums. *Oncology Nursing Forum, 38,* 133–142. doi:10.1188/11.ONF.133-142

11. Tofthagen, C., Visovsky, C.M., & Hopgood, R. (2013). Chemotherapy-induced peripheral neuropathy: An algorithm to guide nursing management. *Clinical Journal of Oncology Nursing, 17,* 138–144. doi:10.1188/13.CJON.138-144

12. National Cancer Institute Cancer Therapy Evaluation Program. (2010, June 14). *Common terminology criteria for adverse events* [v.4.03]. Retrieved from http://evs.nci.nih.gov/ftp1/CTCAE/CTCAE_4.03_2010-06-14_QuickReference_5x7.pdf

13. Smith, E.M.L., Cohen, J.A., Pett, M.A., & Beck, S.L. (2010). The reliability and validity of a modified total neuropathy score-reduced and neuropathic pain severity items when used to measure chemotherapy-induced peripheral neuropathy in patients receiving taxanes and platinums. *Cancer Nursing, 33,* 173–183. doi:10.1097/NCC.0b013e3181c989a3

14. Gilchrist, L.S., & Tanner, L. (2013). The pediatric-modified total neuropathy score: A reliable and valid measure of chemotherapy-induced peripheral neuropathy in children with non-CNS cancers. *Supportive Care in Cancer, 21,* 847–856. doi:10.1007/s00520-012-1591-8

15. Calhoun, E.A., Welshman, E.E., Chang, C.H., Lurain, J.R., Fishman, D.A., Hunt, T.L., & Cella, D. (2003). Psychometric evaluation of the Functional Assessment of Cancer Therapy/Gynecologic Oncology Group—Neurotoxicity (FACT/GOG-Ntx) questionnaire for patients receiving systemic chemotherapy. *International Journal of Gynecological Cancer, 13,* 741–748. doi:10.1111/j.1525-1438.2003.13603.x

16. Binda, D., Vanhoutte, E.K., Cavaletti, G., Cornblath, D.R., Postma, T.J., Fringeni, B., ... Dorsey, S.G. (2013). Rasch-built Overall Disability Scale for patients with chemotherapy-induced peripheral neuropathy (CIPN-R-ODS). *European Journal of Cancer, 49,* 2910–2918. doi:10.1016/j.ejca.2013.04.004

17. Takemoto, S., Ushijima, K., Honda, K., Wada, H., Terada, A., Imaishi, H., & Kamura, T. (2012). Precise evaluation of chemotherapy-induced peripheral neuropathy using the visual analogue scale: A quantitative and comparative analysis of neuropathy occurring with paclitaxel–carboplatin and docetaxel–carboplatin therapy. *International Journal of Clinical Oncology, 17,* 367–372. doi:10.1007/s10147-011-0303-6

18. Smith, E.M.L., Pang, H., Cirrincione, C., Fleishman, S., Paskett, E.D., Ahles, T., ... Shapiro, C.L. (2013). Effect of duloxetine on pain, function, and quality of life among patients with chemotherapy-induced painful peripheral neuropathy: A randomized clinical trial. *JAMA, 309,* 1359–1367. doi:10.1001/jama.2013.2813

19. Yang, Y.-H., Lin, J.-K., Chen, W.-S., Lin, T.-C., Yang, S.-H., Jiang, J.-K., ... Teng, H.-W. (2012). Duloxetine improves oxaliplatin-induced neuropathy in patients with colorectal cancer: An open-label pilot study. *Supportive Care in Cancer, 20,* 1491–1497. doi:10.1007/s00520-011-1237-2

20. Hilpert, F., Stähle, A., Tomé, O., Burges, A., Rossner, D., Späthe, K., ... du Bois, A. (2005). Neuroprotection with amifostine in the first-line treatment of advanced ovarian cancer with carboplatin/paclitaxel-based chemotherapy—A double-blind, placebo-controlled, randomized phase II study from the Arbeitsgemeinschaft Gynäkologische Onkologoie (AGO)

Ovarian Cancer Study Group. *Supportive Care in Cancer, 13*, 797–805. doi:10.1007/s00520-005-0782-y

21. Albers, J.W., Chaudhry, V., Cavaletti, G., & Donehower, R.C. (2011). Interventions for preventing neuropathy caused by cisplatin and related compounds. *Cochrane Database of Systematic Reviews, 2011*(2). doi:10.1002/14651858.CD005228.pub3

22. Barton, D.L., Wos, E.J., Qin, R., Mattar, B.I., Green, N.B., Lanier, K.S., ... Loprinzi, C.L. (2011). A double-blind, placebo-controlled trial of a topical treatment for chemotherapy-induced peripheral neuropathy: NCCTG trial N06CA. *Supportive Care in Cancer, 19*, 833–841. doi:10.1007/s00520 -010-0911-0

23. Chay, W.-Y., Tan, S.-H., Lo, Y.-L., Ong, S.Y.-K., Ng, H.-C., Gao, F., ... Choo, S.-P. (2010). Use of calcium and magnesium infusions in prevention of oxaliplatin induced sensory neuropathy. *Asia-Pacific Journal of Clinical Oncology, 6*, 270–277. doi:10.1111/j.1743-7563.2010.01344.x

24. Gamelin, L., Boisdron-Celle, M., Delva, R., Geurin-Meyer, V., Ifrah, N., Morel, A., & Gamelin, E. (2004). Prevention of oxaliplatin-related neurotoxicity by calcium and magnesium infusions: A retrospective study of 161 patients receiving oxaliplatin combined with 5-fluorouracil and leucovorin for advanced colorectal cancer. *Clinical Cancer Research, 10*(12, Pt. 1), 4055–4061. doi:10.1158/1078-0432.CCR-03-0666

25. Grothey, A., Nikcevich, D.A., Sloan, J.A., Kugler, J.W., Silberstein, P.T., Dentchev, T., ... Loprinzi, C.L. (2011). Intravenous calcium and magnesium for oxaliplatin-induced sensory neurotoxicity in adjuvant colon cancer: NCCTG N04C7. *Journal of Clinical Oncology, 29*, 412–427. doi:10.1200/ JCO.2010.31.5911

26. Knijn, N., Tol, J., Koopman, M., Werter, M.J., Imholz, A.L.T., Valster, F.A.A., ... Punt, C.J.A. (2011). The effect of prophylactic calcium and magnesium infusions on the incidence of neurotoxicity and clinical outcome of oxaliplatin-based systemic treatment in advanced colorectal cancer patients. *European Journal of Cancer, 47*, 369–374. doi:10.1016/j.ejca.2010.10.006

27. Arai, Y.-C., Matsubara, T., Shimo, K., Suetomi, K., Nishihara, M., Ushida, T., ... Arakawa, M. (2010). Low-dose gabapentin as useful adjuvant to opioids for neuropathic cancer pain when combined with low-dose imipramine. *Journal of Anesthesia, 24*, 407–410. doi:10.1007/s00540-010-0913-6

28. Rao, R.D., Michalak, J.C., Sloan, J.A., Loprinzi, C.L., Soori, G.S., Nikcevich, D.A., ... Wong, G.Y. (2007). Efficacy of gabapentin in the management of chemotherapy-induced peripheral neuropathy: A phase 3 randomized, double-blind, placebo-controlled, crossover trial (N00C3). *Cancer, 110*, 2110–2118. doi:10.1002/cncr.23008

29. Takahashi, H., & Shimoyama, N. (2010). A prospective open-label trial of gabapentin as an adjuvant analgesic with opioids for Japanese patients with neuropathic cancer pain. *International Journal of Clinical Oncology, 15*, 46–51. doi:10.1007/s10147-009-0009-1

30. Keskinbora, K., Pekel, A.F., & Aydinli, I. (2007). Gabapentin and an opioid combination versus opioid alone for the management of neuropathic cancer pain: A randomized open trial. *Journal of Pain and Symptom Management, 34*, 183–189. doi:10.1016/j.jpainsymman.2006.11.013

31. National Comprehensive Cancer Network. (2013). *NCCN Clinical Practice Guidelines in Oncology: Adult cancer pain* [v.2.2013]. Retrieved from http:// www.nccn.org/professionals/physician_gls/pdf/pain.pdf

32. Amara, S. (2008). Oral glutamine for the prevention of chemotherapy-induced peripheral neuropathy. *Annals of Pharmacotherapy, 42*, 1481–1485. doi:10.1345/aph.1L179

33. Loven, D., Levavi, H., Sabach, G., Zart, R., Andras, M., Fishman, A., ... Gadoth, N. (2009). Long-term glutamate supplementation failed to protect against peripheral neurotoxicity of paclitaxel. *European Journal of Cancer Care, 18*, 78–83. doi:10.1111/j.1365-2354.2008.00996.x

34. Mokhtar, G.M., Shaaban, S.Y., Elbarbary, N.S., & Fayed, W.A. (2010). A trial to assess the efficacy of glutamic acid in prevention of vincristine-induced

neurotoxicity in pediatric malignancies: A pilot study. *Journal of Pediatric Hematology/Oncology, 32,* 594–600. doi:10.1097/MPH.0b013e3181e9038d

35. Stubblefield, M.D., Vahdat, L.T., Balmaceda, C.M., Troxel, A.B., Hesdorffer, C.S., & Gooch, C.L. (2005). Glutamine as a neuroprotective agent in high-dose paclitaxel-induced peripheral neuropathy: A clinical and electrophysio-logic study. *Clinical Oncology, 17,* 271–276. doi:10.1016/j.clon.2004.11.014

36. Vahdat, L., Papadopoulos, K., Lange, D., Leuin, S., Kaufman, E., Donovan, D., … Balmaceda, C. (2001). Reduction of paclitaxel-induced peripheral neuropathy with glutamine. *Clinical Cancer Research, 7,* 1192–1197. Retrieved from http://clincancerres.aacrjournals.org/content/7/5/1192.long

37. Wang, W.-S., Lin, J.-K., Lin, T.-C., Chen, W.-S., Jiang, J.-K., Wang, H.-S., … Chen, P.-M. (2007). Oral glutamine is effective for preventing oxaliplatin-induced neuropathy in colorectal cancer patients. *Oncologist, 12,* 312–319. doi:10.1634/theoncologist.12-3-312

38. Cascinu, S., Catalano, V., Cordella, L., Labiance, R., Giordani, P., Baldelli, A.M., … Catalano, G. (2002). Neuroprotective effect of reduced glutathi-one on oxaliplatin-based chemotherapy in advanced colorectal cancer: A randomized, double-blind, placebo-controlled trial. *Journal of Clinical Oncology, 20,* 3478–3483. doi:10.1200/JCO.2002.07.061

39. Cascinu, S., Cordella, L., Del Ferro, E., Fronzoni, M., & Catalana, G. (1995). Neuroprotective effect of reduced glutathione on cisplatin-based chemotherapy in advanced gastric cancer: A randomized double-blind placebo-controlled trial. *Journal of Clinical Oncology, 13,* 26–32. Retrieved from http://jco.ascopubs.org/content/13/1/26.abstract

40. Smyth, J.F., Bowman, A., Perren, T., Wilkinson, P., Prescott, R.J., Quinn, K.J., & Tedeschi, M. (1997). Glutathione reduces the toxicity and improves quality of life of women diagnosed with ovarian cancer treated with cisplatin: Results of a double-blind, randomized trial. *Annals of Oncology, 8,* 569–573. doi:10.1023/A:1008211226339

41. Weinstein, S.M., Abernethy, A.P., Spruill, S.E., Pike, I.M., Kelly, A.T., & Jett, L.G. (2012). A spicamycin derivative (KRN5500) provides neuropathic pain relief in patients with advanced cancer: A placebo-controlled, proof-of-concept trial. *Journal of Pain and Symptom Management, 43,* 679–693. doi:10.1016/j.jpainsymman.2011.05.003

42. Mishra, S., Bhatnagar, S., Goyal, G.N., Rana, S.P.S., & Upadhya, S.P. (2012). A comparative efficacy of amitriptyline, gabapentin, and pregabalin in neuropathic cancer pain: A prospective randomized double-blind place-bo-controlled study. *American Journal of Hospice and Palliative Care, 29,* 177–182. doi:10.1177/1049909111412539

43. Saif, M.W., Syrigos, K., Kaley, K., & Isufi, I. (2010). Role of pregabalin in treatment of oxaliplatin-induced sensory neuropathy. *Anticancer Research, 30,* 2927–2933. Retrieved from http://ar.iiarjournals.org/content/30/7/2927 .long

44. Vondracek, P., Oslejskova, H., Kepak, T., Mazanek, P., Sterba, J., Rysava, M., & Gal, P. (2009). Efficacy of pregabalin in neuropathic pain in paedi-atric oncological patients. *European Journal of Paediatric Neurology, 13,* 332–336. doi:10.1016/j.ejpn.2008.06.011

45. Kautio, A.L., Haanpaa, M., Leminen, A., Kalso, E., Kautiainen, H., & Saarto, T. (2009). Amitriptyline in the prevention of chemotherapy-induced neuropathic symptoms. *Anticancer Research, 29,* 2601–2606. Retrieved from http://ar.iiarjournals.org/content/29/7/2601.long

46. Hammack, J.E., Michalak, J.C., Loprinzi, C.L., Sloan, J.A., Novotny, P.J., Soori, G.S., … Johnson, J.A. (2002). Phase III evaluation of nortriptyline for alleviation of symptoms of cis-platinum–induced peripheral neuropathy. *Pain, 98,* 195–203. doi:10.1016/S0304-3959(02)00047-7

47. Durand, J.P., Deplanque, G., Montheil, V., Gornet, J.M., Scotte, F., Mir, O., … Goldwasser, F. (2012). Efficacy of venlafaxine for the prevention and relief of oxaliplatin-induced acute neurotoxicity: Results of EFFOX, a randomized, double-blind, placebo-controlled phase III trial. *Annals of Oncology, 23,* 200–205. doi:10.1093/annonc/mdr045

48. Donald, G.K., Tobin, I., & Stringer, J. (2011). Evaluation of acupuncture in the management of chemotherapy-induced peripheral neuropathy. *Acupuncture in Medicine, 29,* 230–233. doi:10.1136/acupmed.2011.010025

49. Yoon, J., Jeon, J.-H., Lee, Y.-W., Cho, C.-K., Kwon, K.-R., Shin, J.-E., ... Yoo, H.-S. (2012). Sweet bee venom pharmacopuncture for chemotherapy-induced peripheral neuropathy. *Journal of Acupuncture and Meridian Studies, 5,* 156–165. doi:10.1016/j.jams.2012.05.003

50. Ashton, J.C., & Milligan, E.D. (2008). Cannabinoids for the treatment of neuropathic pain: Clinical evidence. *Current Opinion in Investigational Drugs, 9,* 65–75.

51. Smith, T.J., Coyne, P.J., Parker, G.L., Dodson, P., & Ramakrishnan, V. (2010). Pilot trial of a patient-specific cutaneous electrostimulation device (MC5-A Calmare) for chemotherapy-induced peripheral neuropathy. *Journal of Pain and Symptom Management, 40,* 883–891. doi:10.1016/j.jpainsymman.2010.03.022

52. Nishioka, M., Shimada, M., Kurita, N., Iwata, T., Morimoto, S., Yoshikawa, K., ... Kono, T. (2011). The Kampo medicine, Goshajinkigan, prevents neuropathy in patients treated by FOLFOX regimen. *International Journal of Clinical Oncology, 16,* 322–327. doi:10.1007/s10147-010-0183-1

53. Ghoreishi, Z., Esfahani, A., Djazayeri, A., Djalali, M., Golestan, B., Ayromlou, H., ... Darabi, M. (2012). Omega-3 fatty acids are protective against paclitaxel-induced peripheral neuropathy: A randomized double-blind placebo controlled trial. *BMC Cancer, 12,* 355. doi:10.1186/1471-2407-12-355

54. Truini, A., Biasiotta, A., Di Stefano, G., La Cesa, S., Leone, C., Cartoni, C., ... Cruccu, G. (2011). Palmitoylethanolamide restores myelinated-fibre function in patients with chemotherapy-induced painful neuropathy. *CNS and Neurological Disorders—Drug Targets, 10,* 916–920. doi:10.2174/187152711799219307

55. Argyriou, A.A., Chroni, E., Koutras, A., Ellul, J., Papapetropoulos, S., Katsoulas, G., ... Kalofonos, H.P. (2005). Vitamin E for prophylaxis against chemotherapy-induced neuropathy: A randomized controlled trial. *Neurology, 64,* 26–31. doi:10.1212/01.WNL.0000148609.35718.7D

56. Bove, L., Picardo, M., Maresca, V., Jaredolo, B., & Pace, A. (2001). A pilot study on the relation between cisplatin neuropathy and vitamin E. *Journal of Experimental and Clinical Cancer Research, 20,* 277–280.

57. Kottschade, L.A., Sloan, J.A., Mazurczak, M.A., Johnson, D.B., Murphy, B.P., Rowland, K.M., ... Loprinzi, C.L. (2011). The use of vitamin E for the prevention of chemotherapy-induced peripheral neuropathy: Results of a randomized phase III clinical trial. *Supportive Care in Cancer, 19,* 1769–1777. doi:10.1007/s00520-010-1018-3

58. Pace, A., Giannarelli, D., Galiè, E., Savarese, A., Carpano, S., Della Giulia, M., ... Cognetti, F. (2010). Vitamin E neuroprotection for cisplatin neuropathy: A randomized, placebo-controlled trial. *Neurology, 74,* 762–766. doi:10.1212/WNL.0b013e3181d5279e

59. Pace, A., Savarese, A., Picardo, M., Maresca, V., Pacetti, U., Del Monte, G., ... Bove, L. (2003). Neuroprotective effect of vitamin E supplementation in patients treated with cisplatin chemotherapy. *Journal of Clinical Oncology, 21,* 927–931. doi:10.1200/JCO.2003.05.139

60. von Delius, S., Eckel, F., Wagenpfeil, S., Mayr, M., Stock, K., Kullmann, F., ... Lersch, C. (2007). Carbamazepine for prevention of oxaliplatin-related neurotoxicity in patients with advanced colorectal cancer: Final results of a randomized, controlled, multicenter phase II study. *Investigational New Drugs, 25,* 173–180. doi:10.1007/s10637-006-9010-y

61. Rao, R.D., Flynn, P.J., Sloan, J.A., Wong, G.Y., Novotny, P., Johnson, D.B., ... Loprinzi, C.L. (2008). Efficacy of lamotrigine in the management of chemotherapy-induced peripheral neuropathy. *Cancer, 112,* 2802–2808. doi:10.1002/cncr.23482

62. Bianchi, G., Vitali, G., Caraceni, A., Ravaglia, S., Capri, G., Cundari, S., ... Gianni, L. (2005). Symptomatic and neurophysiological responses of

paclitaxel or cisplatin induced neuropathy to oral acetyl-L-carnitine. *European Journal of Cancer, 41,* 1746–1750. doi:10.1016/j.ejca.2005.04.028

63. Maestri, A., De Pasquale Ceratti, A., Cundari, S., Zanna, C., Cortesi, E., & Crino, L. (2005). A pilot study on the effect of acetyl-L-carnitine in paclitaxel- and cisplatin-induced peripheral neuropathy. *Tumori, 91,* 135–138.

64. Campone, M., Berton-Rigaud, D., Joly-Lobbedez, F., Baurain, J.-F., Rolland, F., Stenzl, A., ... Pautier, P. (2013). A double-blind, randomized phase II study to evaluate the safety and efficacy of acetyl-L-carnitine in the prevention of sagopilone-induced peripheral neuropathy. *Oncologist, 18,* 1190–1191. doi:10.1634/theoncologist.2013-0061

65. Hershman, D.L., Unger, J.M., Crew, K.D., Minasian, L.M., Awad, D., Moinpour, C.M., ... Albain, K.S. (2013). Randomized double-blind placebo-controlled trial of acetyl-L-carnitine for the prevention of taxane-induced neuropathy in women undergoing adjuvant breast cancer therapy. *Journal of Clinical Oncology, 31,* 2627–2633. doi:10.1200/JCO.2012.44.8738

66. Davis, I.D., Kiers, L., MacGregor, L., Quinn, M., Arezo, J., Green, M., ... Daly, M. (2005). A randomized, double-blinded, placebo-controlled phase II trial of recombinant human leukemia inhibitory factor (rhuLIF, emfilermin, AM424) to prevent chemotherapy-induced peripheral neuropathy. *Clinical Cancer Research, 11,* 1890–1898. doi:10.1158/1078-0432.CCR-04-1655

67. Armstrong, T., Almadrones, L., & Gilbert, M.R. (2005). Chemotherapy-induced peripheral neuropathy. *Oncology Nursing Forum, 32,* 305–311. doi:10.1188/05.ONF.305-311

68. Smith, E.M.L. (2013). Current methods for the assessment and management of taxane-related neuropathy. *Clinical Journal of Oncology Nursing, 17*(Suppl.), 22–34. doi:10.1188/13.CJON.S1.22-34

69. Wickham, R. (2007). Chemotherapy-induced peripheral neuropathy: A review and implications for oncology nursing practice. *Clinical Journal of Oncology Nursing, 11,* 361–376. doi:10.1188/07.CJON.361-376

70. Stubblefield, M.D., Burstein, H.J., Burton, A.W., Custodio, C.M., Deng, G.E., Ho, M., ... Von Roenn, J.H. (2009). NCCN task force report: Management of neuropathy in cancer. *Journal of the National Comprehensive Cancer Network, 7*(Suppl. 5), S1–S26.

71. Stubblefield, M.D., McNeely, M.L., Alfano, C.M., & Mayer, D.K. (2012). A prospective surveillance model for physical rehabilitation of women with breast cancer: Chemotherapy-induced peripheral neuropathy. *Cancer, 118*(Suppl. 8), 2250–2260. doi:10.1002/cncr.27463

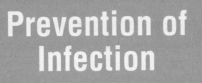

17

Prevention of Infection

Laura J. Zitella, MS, RN, ACNP-BC, AOCN®,
Colleen H. Erb, MSN, ACNP-BC, AOCNP®,
Marilyn J. Hammer, PhD, DC, RN,
Mary E. Peterson, MS, RN, ANP-BC, AOCNP®,
and Barbara J. Wilson, MS, RN, ACNS-BC, AOCN®

Problem and Incidence

Cancer- and treatment-induced immunosuppression leaves patients at great risk for bacterial, fungal, and viral infections.[1-4] Infection is a major cause of morbidity and mortality. Infections find portals of entry primarily through chemotherapy-induced degradation of epithelial mucosal barriers or via indwelling catheters.[5,6] The incidence of infections varies by tumor type and treatment, with more infections occurring in patients with hematologic malignancies. Febrile neutropenia (FN) is one of the most concerning complications of treatments, occurring in about 50% of patients with solid tumors and in 80% or more of patients with hematologic malignancies, often without an identified microorganism. Approximately two-thirds of hospitalized patients with both solid tumor cancers and hematologic malignancies who are neutropenic acquire an infection.[7] Bacteremias account for 20%–30% of infections in patients with FN.[8-11] Patients receiving hematopoietic cell transplantation (HCT) are at high risk for infections because they often have a completely ablated immune system.[12] Pediatric patients with cancer are also at high risk for infections because of aggressive immunosuppressing treatments often used in this population.[13] This material includes prevention of FN but does not include its treatment.

Risk Factors and Assessment

Factors[14,15] that create high risk include
- Anticipated absolute neutrophil count (ANC) of 100/mm^3 or less for seven or more days
- Cancer that is advanced or refractory to treatment
- Hematologic malignancy undergoing induction or consolidation
- Myelodysplastic syndrome
- HCT, with higher risk in allogeneic transplantation; specific risks vary per engraftment phase and continue for more than 100 days post-transplantation.[16]
- Significant comorbid conditions
- Age older than 65
- Chemotherapy including alemtuzumab, high-dose cyclophosphamide, doxorubicin, and docetaxel
- FN or infection with previous therapy
- Immunosuppressive medications (e.g., steroids).

Assessment includes determination of risk for FN with each treatment cycle. The Multinational Association of Supportive Care in Cancer (MASCC) risk index[17] is a tool to estimate risk of infection and treatment approach in patients with FN.

What interventions are effective in preventing febrile neutropenia and infection in people with cancer?

Evidence retrieved through June 31, 2013

Recommended for Practice

Adherence to general published infection control recommendations is crucial for all patients with cancer because of immunodeficiency associated with cancer and its treatment. Comprehensive recommendations for both inpatient and outpatient settings have been published.[16,18-23] The Centers for

Disease Control and Prevention[24] provides basic guidelines for outpatient settings. Key recommendations include the following.

- **Hand hygiene with soap and water or alcohol-based hand rubs** is the most effective means of preventing the transmission of infection.[20,25]
- **Contact precautions for patients with resistant organism colonization** to prevent transmission of multidrug-resistant organisms have been shown to be effective.[26-29]
- **Environmental interventions** for infection control and for disinfection and sterilization of surfaces, medical equipment, and play areas for children are available.[18-23]
  - Water provides potential mold exposure, emphasizing the importance of clean ice machines and water handling.[16,30]
  - For HCT recipients, additional environmental recommendations include high-efficiency particulate air filtration, positive air pressure in patient rooms, self-closing doors, closed windows, sealed electrical outlets, and more than 12 air exchanges per hour in rooms.

Antibiotic prophylaxis for at-risk patients is recommended for patients anticipated to have prolonged severe neutropenia.[9,14,16,31-33] Studies showed reduced fever and infections; however, findings are mixed regarding effect on infection-related and all-cause mortality.[34-41]

- Fluoroquinolones are recommended; levofloxacin and ciprofloxacin have been evaluated the most. Routine prophylaxis needs to be balanced with the potential for growth of fluoroquinolone-resistant organisms in a given setting.
- There is limited evidence for fluoroquinolone use in children.[40,42,43]

Antifungal prophylaxis in at-risk patients is recommended for primary prevention in adults and children anticipated to have prolonged severe neutropenia,[9,14,44-47] in transplantation survivors on chronic steroids,[33] and for secondary prevention in patients with prior fungal infections.[14,48]

- Antifungal prophylaxis with various agents (posaconazole, caspofungin, voriconazole, micafungin, fluconazole, itraconazole, ketoconazole, amphotericin B) reduced fungal infections.[47-66]
- Prophylaxis was effective in children, but evidence is limited.[9,59,60,67]

Antiviral prophylaxis for select at-risk patients, such as those who are seropositive for herpes simplex virus and at risk for infection or reactivation during neutropenia, is recommended.[9,14,16,31-33] Various antivirals have been effective.[68,69] In HCT recipients, prophylaxis is recommended for up to six months or when the patient has been off all immunosuppressive agents for three months. Consider antiviral prophylaxis with

• Induction or consolidation for a hematologic malignancy
• Purine analogs or alemtuzumab
• Allogeneic HCT
• Active acute or chronic graft-versus-host disease (GVHD)
• Expected prolonged ANC reduction.

Central venous catheter care bundles of interventions, including site selection, barriers during insertion, skin prep, dressing regimens, and procedures for catheter hub, cap, and tubing care, are recommended.[20] This bundled care approach reduced central line–associated bloodstream infection (CLABSI) rates in adults and children.[70-72]

Colony-stimulating factors (CSFs) are effective and recommended by professional groups for primary and secondary prophylaxis in patients who are at risk for FN.[9,14,73-78] Research studies[15,39,79-90] and systematic reviews[86,91-98] showed prevention of FN and associated outcomes.

• Studies in children have established the safety and efficacy of CSF prophylaxis.[99-103]
• Various CSF agents appear to have similar safety and effectiveness profiles.[80,85,87,94,101,103-107] The most common adverse effect is bone pain.
• CSF administration 24–72 hours after completion of chemotherapy is recommended.[14,76,84,108,109] One study[90] showed that granulocyte-CSF administered every other day was as effective as every day. Another study[100] showed no benefit to doubling the dose from 5 mcg/kg to 10 mcg/kg.
• Secondary prophylaxis with CSF is recommended for patients who have previously had FN,[14,73,76] who need IV antibiotics during chemotherapy,[83] who have the potential for life-threatening infections in the next treatment cycle, or who need dose reductions below the threshold.[74] Secondary CSF prophylaxis was associated with lower risk of mortality.[82]

Education/counseling of HCT recipients and caregivers to avoid opportunistic infections[9,16,31,32,110] includes

- Performing hand hygiene before patient contact and by patients after contact with animals
- Avoiding patient exposure to individuals with respiratory, varicella, pneumocystis, or other known infections
- Following safe food handling procedures. See the U.S. Department of Agriculture food safety fact sheets.[111]
- Using condoms during sexual intercourse and avoiding mucosal contact with saliva, semen, or vaginal secretions
- Avoiding sharing cups or eating utensils
- Avoiding contact with soil and human feces and use of outhouses (for allogeneic HCT recipients)
- Maintaining good oral hygiene and regular professional dental care.[112]

Influenza vaccination reduces the risk of respiratory infections and hospitalizations.[113,114] Annual vaccination is recommended for all cancer and HCT patients, close contacts, and individuals providing care to these patients.[9,14,16,31-33] No clear consensus exists on the optimal timing of vaccination.[9,14,114]

Pneumococcal and meningococcal vaccination is recommended for patients who are anatomically or functionally asplenic due to irradiation of the spleen.[14,115]

Pneumocystis jiroveci **(formerly *Pneumocystis carinii*) prophylaxis for at-risk patients** is recommended for patients undergoing treatment for acute lymphocytic leukemia, receiving alemtuzumab, receiving T-cell–depleting agents, undergoing prolonged treatment with corticosteroids, receiving temozolomide with radiation therapy, undergoing allogeneic HCT, or with chronic GVHD.[9,14,16,31,33] Trimethoprim-sulfamethoxazole (TMP-SMX) is the preferred treatment. Atovaquone, dapsone, and aerosolized pentamidine are suggested in the case of TMP-SMX intolerance.[14]

Likely to Be Effective

Antibiotic abdominal lavage in colorectal surgery with a clindamycin-gentamicin solution was compared to normal saline lavage. Wound infection and abdominal abscess rates were reduced in patients undergoing surgery for colorectal cancer.[116]

Antimicrobial-coated central venous catheters for short-term use in adults, with coatings such as chlorhexidine and silver sulfadiazine, decreased the incidence of CLABSI.[14,20,22,117,118]

Chlorhexidine-impregnated washcloths/chlorhexidine baths reduced incidence of bloodstream infections and resistant organism acquisition in general cancer and HCT patients[119,120] and has been suggested in guidelines.[20]

Vaccinations in HCT that are recommended include diphtheria, pertussis, *Haemophilus influenzae* type B, inactivated polio vaccine (in children), and the measles, mumps, and rubella (MMR) combination vaccine.[9,14,16,31-33]
- Vaccination is administered 24 months after transplantation in patients without evidence of GVHD or on immunosuppressive drugs.
- Vaccination decisions are individualized based on patients' age and status. General guidelines for childhood immunizations are applicable.
- Hepatitis A and yellow fever immunization may be of benefit in areas where these are endemic.

Benefits Balanced With Harms

IV immunoglobulin may reduce the risk of infection in patients with profound hypogammaglobulinemia or patients with chronic lymphocytic leukemia with low immunoglobulin and recurrent infections, but this has significant adverse effects.[14,121]

Effectiveness Not Established

A number of interventions have been examined that showed mixed results or inconclusive findings because of study limitations.

- **Antibiotic IV catheter lock solutions**[122,123]—These are not recommended because of bacterial resistance concerns.[14,16]
- **Antimicrobial-coated central venous catheters for short-term use in HCT and pediatric patients**[124]—A systematic review concluded the evidence is insufficient for use in children.[72]
- **Antimicrobial-coated sutures**[125,126]
- **Berbamine**, a plant extract[127]
- **Chlorhexidine sponge dressings**[128]—Guidelines suggest use in situations where all other standard interventions have failed.[20]
- **Cranberry juice** to prevent urinary tract infections[129]
- **Electroacupuncture**[130]
- **Granulocyte transfusions** for patients with invasive fungal infections or gram-negative infections and unresponsive to antibiotic treatment[14,131]—One small study examined use in children.[132]
- **Ionic silver surgical dressings**[133]
- **IV port protectors** impregnated with alcohol[134]
- **Laminar air flow**[30,31,135]
- **Mistletoe extract**[136]
- **Protective isolation/protective equipment**[137-140]—Use of gowns, gloves, and masks for reverse isolation is not recommended for routine care.[9] There is no evidence of the need for or effect of filter masks worn by HCT recipients.[30]
- **Staff training**[141]
- **Taurolidine IV catheter lock solution**[142]
- **Tetanus toxoid immunization for HCT recipients**[16,143]
- **Urokinase IV catheter flush**[144]
- **Varicella vaccination for HCT recipients**[30,113]—Only inactivated vaccine has been tested, evidence is limited, and only patients with full immune system recovery should be considered for use.[16,143]

Effectiveness Unlikely

Extended postoperative antibiotics increased surgical site infection rates in a large multisite randomized controlled trial.[145]

Not Recommended for Practice

Dietary restriction of uncooked fresh fruits and vegetables did not reduce the risk of infection in individual studies.[146-149] In one study of HCT recipients, dietary restriction of uncooked fresh fruits and vegetables was associated with higher infection rates and more drug-resistant infections.[150] A systematic review concluded there is no evidence of effectiveness.[151] Guidelines suggest that well-cleaned fruits and vegetables are acceptable.[9,16]

Implantable gentamicin sponge was tested in 602 patients undergoing laparoscopic colorectal surgery. Surgical infections and superficial site infections occurred more frequently in the sponge group.[152]

Live attenuated vaccines should not be used in patients with cancer for at least three months after discontinuation of therapy.[14] Examples of live attenuated vaccines include intranasal influenza vaccine, varicella (chicken pox) vaccine, oral polio vaccine, and MMR.

Routine polio vaccine in adults after HCT is not recommended.[16]

Topical antifungal drugs for oral candidiasis prevention such as nystatin are not supported by evidence.[135,153]

Expert Opinion

Numerous recommendations are identified in published guidelines for HCT recipients and other severely immunosuppressed patients.[9,16,31,154] Some examples are outlined below. Original references should be consulted for a full listing of recommendations.
- Strictly enforce policies restricting contact with visitors or other people who have infections.
- Restrict dried or fresh flowers or plants in patient rooms.
- Follow animal safety guidelines, avoiding contact with animal feces, and minimize contact with ill and exotic animals.

- Avoid use of rectal stimulation by thermometers, enemas, or rectal exams.
- Avoid some foods, such as uncooked or undercooked meat, fish, poultry, seafood, tofu, grain products, or baker's yeast.
- Avoid herbal and nutrient supplement preparations.

Application to Practice

Nurses can provide evidence-based interventions for prevention of infection in the following ways.

- Developing catheter care bundles for the institution—This may include standard orders and policies/procedures directing the insertion, care, and discontinuation of central lines, implementation of uniform standards for central line care, and monitoring for adherence. The Joint Commission has a CLABSI toolkit[155] that may be useful for this work.
- Screening for vaccine administration for patients who are able to receive the vaccines—Caregivers and close contacts should be educated about their need for immunizations and vaccinations.
- Adhering to general infection prevention measures
  - Diligent hand hygiene with soap and water before and after patient contact, between patients, and after contact with objects in the environment or use of alcohol gel when appropriate.
  - Contact precautions for resistant organisms
  - Early removal of urinary catheters
- Educating patients about ways to prevent infection— Patients should be given written materials in the appropriate language and reading levels as well as verbal education. Patients' learning needs should be assessed prior to providing education so the nurse is able to educate the patient most effectively. Topics to cover with patients and families should include
  - Avoidance of opportunistic infections
  - Appropriate hygiene
  - Compliance with prophylactic medications
  - Appropriate nutrition and food handling

– Self-monitoring for fever and signs of infection in patients at risk and when to contact healthcare providers.
• Assessing patients' current medications and associated risk for infections—Ensure that patients at risk are taking preventive medications when appropriate such as antibiotics, antifungals, antivirals, and/or growth factors.

Prevention of Infection Resource Contributors

Topic leader: Barbara J. Wilson, MS, RN, ACNS-BC, AOCN®
Falak Ahmed, RN, BScN, Courtney E. Crannell, RN-BC, MSN, OCN®, Wendy Crego, RN, OCN®, Colleen H. Erb, MSN, ACNP-BC, AOCNP®, Jacqueline Foster, RN, OCN®, MPH, Marilyn J. Hammer, PhD, DC, RN, Huma Moez, RN, BScN, Kathryn Orth, RN, OCN®, Mary E. Peterson, MS, RN, ANP-BC, AOCNP®, Gail Smith, MSN, RN, OCN®, Carrie Williams, RN, MSN/Ed, OCN®, and Laura J. Zitella, MS, RN, ACNP-BC, AOCN®

References

1. Aisenberg, G., Rolston, K.V., & Safdar, A. (2004). Bacteremia caused by *Achromobacter* and *Alcaligenes* species in 46 patients with cancer (1989–2003). *Cancer, 101,* 2134–2140. doi:10.1002/cncr.20604
2. Akinosoglou, K.S., Karkoulias, K., & Marangos, M. (2013). Infectious complications in patients with lung cancer. *European Review for Medical and Pharmacological Sciences, 17,* 8–18. Retrieved from http://www.europeanreview.org/article/2852
3. Derr, R.L., Hsiao, V.C., & Saudek, C.D. (2008). Antecedent hyperglycemia is associated with an increased risk of neutropenic infections during bone marrow transplantation. *Diabetes Care, 31,* 1972–1977. doi:10.2337/dc08-0574
4. Nichols, W.G. (2003). Management of infectious complications in the hematopoietic stem cell transplant recipient. *Journal of Intensive Care Medicine, 18,* 295–312. doi:10.1177/0885066603258009
5. Ghanem, G.A., Boktour, M., Warneke, C., Pham-Williams, T., Kassis, C., Bahna, P., ... Raad, I. (2007). Catheter-related *Staphylococcus aureus* bacteremia in cancer patients: High rate of complications with therapeutic implications. *Medicine, 86,* 54–60. doi:10.1097/MD.0b013e318030d344
6. Xian, C.J. (2003). Roles of growth factors in chemotherapy-induced intestinal mucosal damage repair. *Current Pharmaceutical Biotechnology, 4,* 260–269. doi:10.2174/1389201033489793
7. Caggiano, V., Weiss, R.V., Rickert, T.S., & Linde-Zwirble, W.T. (2005). Incidence, cost, and mortality of neutropenia hospitalization associated with chemotherapy. *Cancer, 103,* 1916–1924. doi:10.1002/cncr.20983
8. Feld, R. (2008). Bloodstream infections in cancer patients with febrile neutropenia. *International Journal of Antimicrobial Agents, 32*(Suppl. 1), S30–S33. doi:10.1016/j.ijantimicag.2008.06.017
9. Freifeld, A.G., Bow, E.J., Sepkowitz, K.A., Boeckh, M.J., Ito, J.I., Mullen, C.A., ... Wingard, J.R. (2011). Clinical practice guideline for the use of antimicrobial agents in neutropenic patients with cancer: 2010 update by the Infectious Diseases Society of America. *Clinical Infectious Diseases, 52*(4), e56–e93. doi:10.1093/cid/cir073

10. Klastersky, J., Ameye, L., Maertens, J., Georgala, A., Muanza, F., Aoun, M., ... Paesmans, M. (2007). Bacteraemia in febrile neutropenic cancer patients. *International Journal of Antimicrobial Agents, 30*(Suppl. 1), S51–S59. doi:10.1016/j.ijantimicag.2007.06.012

11. Nørgaard, M., Larsson, H., Pedersen, G., Schønheyder, H.C., & Sørensen, H.T. (2006). Risk of bacteraemia and mortality in patients with haematological malignancies. *Clinical Microbiology and Infection, 12,* 217–223. doi:10.1111/j.1469-0691.2005.01298.x

12. Junghanss, C., & Marr, K.A. (2002). Infectious risks and outcomes after stem cell transplantation: Are nonmyeloablative transplants changing the picture? *Current Opinion in Infectious Diseases, 15,* 347–353. doi:10.1097/00001432-200208000-00001

13. Dobrasz, G., Hatfield, M., Jones, L.M., Berdis, J.J., Miller, E.E., & Entrekin, M.S. (2013). Nurse-driven protocols for febrile pediatric oncology patients. *Journal of Emergency Nursing, 39,* 289–295. doi:10.1016/j.jen.2013.01.014

14. National Comprehensive Cancer Network. (2013). *NCCN Clinical Practice Guidelines in Oncology: Prevention and treatment of cancer-related infections* [v.1.2013]. Retrieved from http://www.nccn.org/professionals/physician_gls/pdf/infections.pdf

15. Rajan, S.S., Lyman, G.H., Stearns, S.C., & Carpenter, W.R. (2011). Effect of primary prophylactic granulocyte-colony stimulating factor use on incidence of neutropenia hospitalizations for elderly early-stage breast cancer patients receiving chemotherapy. *Medical Care, 49,* 649–657. doi:10.1097/MLR.0b013e318215c42e

16. Tomblyn, M., Chiller, T., Einsele, H., Gress, R., Sepkowitz, K., Storek, J., ... Boeckh, M.J. (2009). Guidelines for preventing infectious complications among hematopoietic cell transplant recipients: A global perspective. *Biology of Blood and Marrow Transplantation, 15,* 1143–1238. doi:10.1016/j.bbmt.2009.06.019

17. QxMD. (n.d.). Febrile neutropenia/MASCC. Retrieved from http://www.qxmd.com/calculate-online/hematology/febrile-neutropenia-mascc

18. Centers for Disease Control and Prevention National Center for Emerging and Zoonotic Infectious Diseases Division of Healthcare Quality Promotion. (2011). *Basic infection control and prevention plan for outpatient oncology settings.* Retrieved from http://www.cdc.gov/hai/pdfs/guidelines/basic-infection-control-prevention-plan-2011.pdf

19. Centers for Disease Control and Prevention National Center for Emerging and Zoonotic Infectious Diseases Division of Healthcare Quality Promotion. (2011, May 2). *Guide to infection prevention for outpatient settings: Minimum expectations for safe care.* Retrieved from http://www.cdc.gov/HAI/settings/outpatient/outpatient-care-guidelines.html

20. O'Grady, N.P., Alexander, M., Burns, L.A., Dellinger, E.P., Garland, J., Heard, S.O., ... Healthcare Infection Control Practices Advisory Committee. (2011). *Guidelines for the prevention of intravascular catheter related infections, 2011.* Retrieved from http://www.cdc.gov/hicpac/pdf/guidelines/bsi-guidelines-2011.pdf

21. Sehulster, L., & Chin, R.Y.W. (2003, June 6). Guidelines for the environmental infection control in health-care facilities: Recommendations of CDC and the Healthcare Infection Control Practices Advisory Committee (HICPAC). *MMWR: Recommendations and Reports, 52*(RR10), 1–42. Retrieved from http://www.cdc.gov/mmwr/preview/mmwrhtml/rr5210a1.htm

22. Wolf, H.H., Leithäuser, M., Maschmeyer, G., Salwender, H., Klein, U., Chaberny, I., ... Mousset, S. (2008). Central venous catheter-related infections in hematology and oncology: Guidelines of the Infectious Diseases Working Party (AGIHO) of the German Society of Hematology and Oncology (DGHO). *Annals of Hematology, 87,* 863–876. doi:10.1007/s00277-008-0509-5

23. Yokoe, D., Casper, C., Dubberke, E., Lee, G., Muñoz, P., Palmore, T., ... Donnelly, J.P. (2009). Infection prevention and control in health-care facilities

in which hematopoietic cell transplant recipients are treated. *Bone Marrow Transplantation, 44,* 495–507. doi:10.1038/bmt.2009.261

24. Centers for Disease Control and Prevention. (2014, January 27). Healthcare-associated infections (HAIs). Retrieved from http://www.cdc.gov/HAI/prevent/prevent_pubs.html

25. Boyce, J.M., & Pittet, D. (2002). Guideline for hand hygiene in health-care settings: Recommendations of the Healthcare Infection Control Practices Advisory Committee and the HICPAC/SHEA/APIC/IDSA Hand Hygiene Task Force. *Infection Control and Hospital Epidemiology, 23*(Suppl. 12), S3–S40. doi:10.1086/503164

26. Montecalvo, M.A., Jarvis, W.R., Uman, J., Shay, D.K., Petrullo, C., Rodney, K., ... Wormser, G.P. (1999). Infection-control measures to reduce transmission of vancomycin-resistant enterococci in an endemic setting. *Annals of Internal Medicine, 131,* 269–272. doi:10.7326/0003-4819-131-4-199908170-00006

27. Shaikh, Z.H.A., Osting, C.A., Hanna, H.A., Arbuckle, R.B., Tarr, J.J., & Raad, I.I. (2002). Effectiveness of a multi-faceted infection control policy in reducing vancomycin usage and vancomycin-resistant enterococci in a tertiary care cancer center. *Journal of Hospital Infection, 51,* 52–58. doi:10.1053/jhin.2002.1161

28. Siegel, J.D., Rhinehart, E., Jackson, M., Chiarello, L., & Healthcare Infection Control Practices Advisory Committee. (2006). *Management of multidrug-resistant organisms in healthcare settings, 2006.* Retrieved from http://www.cdc.gov/hicpac/pdf/MDRO/MDROGuideline2006.pdf

29. Srinivasan, A., Song, X., Ross, T., Merz, W., Brower, R., & Perl, T.M. (2002). A prospective study to determine whether cover gowns in addition to gloves decrease nosocomial transmission of vancomycin-resistant enterococci in an intensive care unit. *Infection Control and Hospital Epidemiology, 23,* 424–428. doi:10.1086/502079

30. Dykewicz, C.A., Kaplan, J.E., Jarvis, W.R., Edlin, B.R., Chen, R.T., Hibbs, B., ... Sullivan, K.M. (2000, October 20). Guidelines for preventing opportunistic infections among hematopoietic stem cell transplant recipients. *MMWR: Recommendations and Reports, 49*(RR10), 1–128. Retrieved from http://www.cdc.gov/mmwr/preview/mmwrhtml/rr4910a1.htm

31. Krüger, W.H., Bohlius, J., Cornely, O.A., Einsele, H., Hebart, H., Massenkeil, G., ... Wolf, H.-H. (2005). Antimicrobial prophylaxis in allogeneic bone marrow transplantation. Guidelines of the Infectious Diseases Working Party (AGIHO) of the German Society of Haematology and Oncology. *Annals of Oncology, 16,* 1381–1390. doi:10.1093/annonc/mdi238

32. Ljungman, P., Engelhard, D., de la Cámara, H., Einsele, H., Locasciulli, A., Martino, R., ... Cordonnier, C. (2005). Vaccination of stem cell transplant recipients: Recommendations of the Infectious Diseases Working Party of the EBMT. *Bone Marrow Transplantation, 35,* 737–746. doi:10.1038/sj.bmt.1704870

33. Rizzo, J.D., Wingard, J.R., Tichelli, A., Lee, S.J., Van Lint, M.T., Burns, L.J., ... Socié, G. (2006). Recommended screening and preventive practices for long-term survivors after hematopoietic cell transplantation: Joint recommendations of the European Group for Blood and Marrow Transplantation, the Center for International Blood and Marrow Transplant Research, and the American Society of Blood and Marrow Transplantation. *Biology of Blood and Marrow Transplantation, 12,* 138–151. doi:10.1016/j.bbmt.2005.09.012

34. Bucaneve, G., Micozzi, A., Menichetti, F., Martino, F., Dionisi, M.S., Martinelli, G., ... Del Favero, A. (2005). Levofloxacin to prevent bacterial infection in patients with cancer and neutropenia. *New England Journal of Medicine, 353,* 977–987. doi:10.1056/NEJMoa044097

35. Cullen, M., Steven, N., Billingham, L., Gaunt, C., Hastings, M., Simmonds, P., ... Stanley, A. (2005). Antibacterial prophylaxis after chemotherapy for solid tumors and lymphoma. *New England Journal of Medicine, 353,* 988–998. doi:10.1056/NEJMoa050078

36. Eleutherakis-Papaiakovou, E., Kostis, E., Migkou, M., Christoulas, D., Terpos, E., Gavriatopoulou, M., ... Papadimitriou, C.A. (2010). Prophylactic antibiotics for the prevention of neutropenic fever in patients undergoing autologous stem-cell transplantation: Results of a single institution, randomized phase 2 trial. *American Journal of Hematology, 85,* 863–867. doi:10.1002/ajh.21855

37. Gafter-Gvili, A., Fraser, A., Paul, M., Vidal, L., Lawrie, T.A., van de Wetering, M.D., ... Leibovici, L. (2012). Antibiotic prophylaxis for bacterial infections in afebrile neutropenic patients following chemotherapy. *Cochrane Database of Systematic Reviews, 2012*(1). doi:10.1002/14651858.CD004386.pub3

38. Imran, H., Tleyjeh, I.M., Arndt, C.A.S., Baddour, L.M., Erwin, P.J., Tsigrelis, C., ... Montori, V.M. (2008). Fluoroquinolone prophylaxis in patients with neutropenia: A meta-analysis of randomized placebo-controlled trials. *European Journal of Clinical Microbiology and Infectious Diseases, 27,* 53–63. doi:10.1007/s10096-007-0397-y

39. Lalami, Y., Paesmans, M., Aoun, M., Munoz-Bermeo, R., Reuss, K., Cherifi, S., & Klastersky, J. (2004). A prospective randomised evaluation of G-CSF or G-CSF plus oral antibiotics in chemotherapy-treated patients at high risk of developing febrile neutropenia. *Supportive Care in Cancer, 12,* 725–730. doi:10.1007/s00520-004-0658-6

40. Laoprasopwattana, K., Khwanna, T., Suwankeeree, P., Sujjanunt, T., Tunyapanit, W., & Chelae, S. (2013). Ciprofloxacin reduces occurrence of fever in children with acute leukemia who develop neutropenia during chemotherapy. *Pediatric Infectious Disease Journal, 32,* e94–e98. doi:10.1097/INF.0b013e3182793610

41. Rahman, M.M., & Khan, M.A. (2009). Levofloxacin prophylaxis to prevent bacterial infection in chemotherapy-induced neutropenia in acute leukemia. *Bangladesh Medical Research Council Bulletin, 35,* 91–94. doi:10.3329/bmrcb.v35i3.4130

42. Barone, A. (2011). Antibacterial prophylaxis in neutropenic children with cancer. *Pediatric Reports, 3*(E3), 9–10. doi:10.4081/pr.2011.e3

43. Bradloy, J.S., & Jackson, M.A. (2011). The use of systemic and topical fluoroquinolones. *Pediatrics, 128,* E1034–E1045. doi:10.1542/peds.2011-1496

44. Cornely, O.A., Böhme, A., Buchheidt, D., Einsele, H., Hoinz, W.J., Karthaus, M., ... Ullmann, A.J. (2009). Primary prophylaxis of invasive fungal infections in patients with hematologic malignancies: Recommendations of the Infectious Diseases Working Party of the German Society for Haematology and Oncology. *Haematologica, 94,* 113–122. doi:10.3324/haematol.11665

45. Maschmeyer, G., Beinert, T., Buchheidt, D., Cornely, O.A., Einsele, H., Heinz, W., ... Mattiuzzi, G. (2009). Diagnosis and antimicrobial therapy of lung infiltrates in febrile neutropenic patients: Guidelines of the Infectious Diseases Working Party of the German Society of Haematology and Oncology. *European Journal of Cancer, 45,* 2462–2472. doi:10.1016/j.ejca.2009.05.001

46. Styczynski, J., & Gil, L. (2008). Prevention of infectious complications in pediatric HCT. *Bone Marrow Transplantation, 42*(Suppl. 2), S77–S81. doi:10.1038/bmt.2008.289

47. Ziakas, P.D., Kourbeti, I.S., Voulgarelis, M., & Mylonakis, E. (2010). Effectiveness of systemic antifungal prophylaxis in patients with neutropenia after chemotherapy: A meta-analysis of randomized controlled trials. *Clinical Therapeutics, 32,* 2316–2336. doi:10.1016/j.clinthera.2011.01.009

48. Song, A., Yang, D.-L., Huang, Y., Jiang, E.-L., Yan, Z.-S., Wei, J.-L., ... Han, M.-Z. (2010). Secondary antifungal prophylaxis in hematological malignancies in a tertiary medical center. *International Journal of Hematology, 92,* 725–731. doi:10.1007/s12185-010-0723-5

49. Bow, E.J., Laverdière, M., Lussier, N., Rotstein, C., Cheang, M.S., & Ioannou, N. (2002). Antifungal prophylaxis for severely neutropenic chemotherapy recipients: A meta-analysis of randomized-controlled clinical trials. *Cancer, 94,* 3230–3246. doi:10.1002/cncr.10610

50. Chaftari, A.-M., Hachem, R.Y., Ramos, E., Kassis, C., Campo, M., Jiang, Y., ... Raad, I.I. (2012). Comparison of posaconazole versus weekly am-

photericin B lipid complex for the prevention of invasive fungal infections in hematopoietic stem-cell transplantation. *Transplantation, 94,* 302–308. doi:10.1097/TP.0b013e3182577485

51. Cordonnier, C., Rovira, M., Maertens, J., Olavarria, E., Faucher, C., Bilger, K., ... Einsele, H. (2010). Voriconazole for secondary prophylaxis of invasive fungal infections in allogeneic stem cell transplant recipients: Results of the VOSIFI study. *Haematologica, 95,* 1762–1768. doi:10.3324/haematol.2009.020073

52. Döring, M., Müller, C., Johann, P.-D., Erbacher, A., Kimmig, A., Schwarze, C.-P., ... Müller, I. (2012). Analysis of posaconazole oral antifungal prophylaxis in pediatric patients under 12 years of age following allogeneic stem cell transplantation. *BMC Infectious Diseases, 12,* 263. doi:10.1186/1471-2334-12-263

53. Egerer, G., & Geist, M.J.P. (2011). Posaconazole prophylaxis in patients with acute myelogenous leukaemia—Results from an observational study. *Mycoses, 54*(Suppl. 1), 7–11. doi:10.1111/j.1439-0507.2010.01979.x

54. Ethier, M.C., Science, M., Beyene, J., Briel, M., Lehrnbecher, T., & Sung, L. (2012). Mould-active compared with fluconazole prophylaxis to prevent invasive fungal diseases in cancer patients receiving chemotherapy or haematopoietic stem-cell transplantation: A systematic review and meta-analysis of randomised controlled trials. *British Journal of Cancer, 106,* 1626–1637. doi:10.1038/bjc.2012.147

55. Glasmacher, A., Prentice, A., Gorschluter, M., Engelhart, S., Hahn, C., Djulbegovic, B., & Schmidt-Wolf, I.G. (2003). Itraconazole prevents invasive fungal infections in neutropenic patients treated for hematologic malignancies: Evidence from a meta-analysis of 3,597 patients. *Journal of Clinical Oncology, 21,* 4615–4626. doi:10.1200/JCO.2003.04.052

56. Gøtzsche, P.C., & Johansen, H.K. (2002). Routine versus selective antifungal administration for control of fungal infections in patients with cancer. *Cochrane Database of Systematic Reviews, 2002*(2). doi:10.1002/14651858.CD000026

57. Hiramatsu, Y., Maeda, Y., Fujii, N., Saito, T., Nawa, Y., Hara, M., ... Tanimoto, M. (2008). Use of micafungin versus fluconazole for antifungal prophylaxis in neutropenic patients receiving hematopoietic stem cell transplantation. *International Journal of Hematology, 88,* 588–595. doi:10.1007/s12185-008-0196-y

58. Kanda, Y., Yamamoto, R., Chizuka, A., Hamaki, T., Suguro, M., Arai, C., ... Togawa, A. (2000). Prophylactic action of oral fluconazole against fungal infection in neutropenic patients: A meta-analysis of 16 randomized, controlled trials. *Cancer, 89,* 1611–1625. doi:10.1002/1097-0142(20001001)89:7<1611::AID-CNCR27>3.0.CO;2-B

59. Kusuki, S., Hashii, Y., Yoshida, H., Takizawa, S., Sato, E., Tokimasa, S., ... Ozono, K. (2009). Antifungal prophylaxis with micafungin in patients treated for childhood cancer. *Pediatric Blood and Cancer, 53,* 605–609. doi:10.1002/pbc.22140

60. Mandhaniya, S., Swaroop, C., Thulkar, S., Vishnubhatla, S., Kabra, S.K., Xess, I., & Bakhshi, S. (2011). Oral voriconazole versus intravenous low dose amphotericin B for primary antifungal prophylaxis in pediatric acute leukemia induction: A prospective, randomized, clinical study. *Journal of Pediatric Hematology/Oncology, 33,* e333–e341. doi:10.1097/MPH.0b013e3182331bc7

61. Oren, I., Rowe, J.M., Sprecher, H., Tamir, A., Benyamini, N., Akria, L., ... Dann, E.J. (2006). A prospective randomized trial of itraconazole vs. fluconazole for the prevention of fungal infections in patients with acute leukemia and hematopoietic stem cell transplant recipients. *Bone Marrow Transplantation, 38,* 127–134. doi:10.1038/sj.bmt.1705418

62. Robenshtok, E., Gafter-Gvili, A., Goldberg, E., Weinberger, M., Yeshurun, M., Leibovici, L., & Paul, M. (2007). Antifungal prophylaxis in cancer patients after chemotherapy or hematopoietic stem-cell transplantation: Systematic

review and meta-analysis. *Journal of Clinical Oncology, 25,* 5471–5489. doi:10.1200/JCO.2007.12.3851

63. Vardakas, K.Z., Michalopoulos, A., & Falagas, M.E. (2005). Fluconazole versus itraconazole for antifungal prophylaxis in neutropenic patients with haematological malignancies: A meta-analysis of randomised-controlled trials. *British Journal of Haematology, 131,* 22–28. doi:10.1111/j.1365 -2141.2005.05727.x

64. Vehreschild, J.J., Sieniawski, M., Reuter, S., Arenz, D., Reichert, D., Maertens, J., ... Cornely, O.A. (2009). Efficacy of caspofungin and itraconazole as secondary antifungal prophylaxis: Analysis of data from a multinational case registry. *International Journal of Antimicrobial Agents, 34,* 446–450. doi:10.1016/j.ijantimicag.2009.06.025

65. Wang, J., Zhan, P., Zhou, R., Xu, J., Shao, X., Yang, Y., & Ouyang, J. (2010). Prophylaxis with itraconazole is more effective than prophylaxis with fluconazole in neutropenic patients with hematological malignancies: A meta-analysis of randomized-controlled trials. *Medical Oncology, 27,* 1082–1088. doi:10.1007/s12032-009-9339-0

66. Wingard, J.R., Carter, S.L., Walsh, T.J., Kurtzberg, J., Small, T.N., Baden, L.R., ... Marr, K.A. (2010). Randomized, double-blind trial of fluconazole versus voriconazole for prevention of invasive fungal infection after allogeneic hematopoietic cell transplantation. *Blood, 116,* 5111–5118. doi:10.1182/blood-2010-02-268151

67. Gramatges, M.M., & Winter, S.S. (2011). Recommendations for broader coverage antifungal prophylaxis in childhood acute myeloid leukemia: ASH evidence-based review 2011. *American Society of Hematology Education Program Book, 2011,* 374–376. doi:10.1182/asheducation-2011.1.374

68. Glenny, A.-M., Mauleffinch, L.M.F., Pavitt, S., & Walsh, T. (2009). Interventions for the prevention and treatment of herpes simplex virus in patients being treated for cancer. *Cochrane Database of Systematic Reviews, 2009*(1). doi:10.1002/14651858.CD006706.pub2

69. Oshima, K., Takahashi, T., Mori, T., Matsuyama, T., Usuki, K., Asano-Mori, Y., ... Kanda, Y. (2010). One-year low-dose valacyclovir as prophylaxis for varicella zoster virus disease after allogeneic hematopoietic stem cell transplantation. A prospective study of the Japan Hematology and Oncology Clinical Study Group. *Transplant Infectious Disease, 12,* 421–427. doi:10.1111/j.1399-3062.2010.00541.x

70. Choi, S.W., Chang, L., Hanauer, D.A., Shaffer-Hartman, J., Teitelbaum, D., Lewis, I., ... Niedner, M.F. (2013). Rapid reduction of central line infections in hospitalized pediatric oncology patients through simple quality improvement methods. *Pediatric Blood and Cancer, 60,* 262–269. doi:10.1002/pbc.24187

71. Rinke, M.L., Chen, A.R., Bundy, D.G., Colantuoni, E., Fratino, L., Drucis, K.M., ... Miller, M.R. (2012). Implementation of a central line maintenance care bundle in hospitalized pediatric oncology patients. *Pediatrics, 130,* e996–e1004. doi:10.1542/peds.2012-0295

72. Secola, R., Lewis, M.A., Pike, N., Needleman, J., & Doering, L. (2012). "Targeting to zero" in pediatric oncology: A review of central venous catheter-related bloodstream infections. *Journal of Pediatric Oncology Nursing, 29,* 14–27. doi:10.1177/1043454211432752

73. Aapro, M.S., Bohlius, J., Cameron, D.A., Dal Lago, L., Donnelly, J.P., Kearney, N., ... Zielinski, C. (2011). 2010 update of EORTC guidelines for the use of granulocyte-colony stimulating factor to reduce the incidence of chemotherapy-induced febrile neutropenia in adult patients with lymphoproliferative disorders and solid tumours. *European Journal of Cancer, 47,* 8–32. doi:10.1016/j.ejca.2010.10.013

74. Crawford, J., Caserta, C., & Roila, F. (2010). Hematopoietic growth factors: ESMO clinical practice guidelines for the applications. *Annals of Oncology, 21*(Suppl. 5), v248–v251. doi:10.1093/annonc/mdq195

75. Muñoz Langa, J., Gascón, P., & de Castro, J. (2012). SEOM clinical guidelines for myeloid growth factors. *Clinical and Translational Oncology, 14,* 491–498. doi:10.1007/s12094-012-0830-2

76. National Comprehensive Cancer Network. (2013). *NCCN Clinical Practice Guidelines in Oncology: Myeloid growth factors* [v.2.2013]. Retrieved from http://www.nccn.org/professionals/physician_gls/pdf/myeloid_growth.pdf

77. O'Shaughnessy, J.A. (2007). Management of febrile neutropenia and cardiac toxicity in the adjuvant treatment of breast cancer. *Clinical Breast Cancer, 8*(Suppl. 1), S11–S21. doi:10.3816/CBC.2007.s.008

78. Phillips, R., Hancock, B., Graham, J., Bromham, N., Jin, H., & Berendse, S. (2012). Prevention and management of neutropenic sepsis in patients with cancer: Summary of NICE guidance. *BMJ, 345*, e5368. doi:10.1136/bmj.e5368

79. Balducci, L., Al-Halawani, H., Charu, V., Tam, J., Shahin, S., Dreiling, L., & Ershler, W.B. (2007). Elderly cancer patients receiving chemotherapy benefit from first-cycle pegfilgrastim. *Oncologist, 12*, 1416–1424. doi:10.1634/theoncologist.12-12-1416

80. Engert, A., Griskevicius, L., Zyuzgin, Y., Lubenau, H., & del Giglio, A. (2009). XM02, the first granulocyte colony–stimulating factor biosimilar, is safe and effective in reducing the duration of severe neutropenia and incidence of febrile neutropenia in patients with non-Hodgkin lymphoma receiving chemotherapy. *Leukemia and Lymphoma, 50*, 374–379. doi:10.1080/10428190902756081

81. Flores, I.Q., & Ershler, W. (2010). Managing neutropenia in older patients with cancer receiving chemotherapy in a community setting. *Clinical Journal of Oncology Nursing, 14*, 81–86. doi:10.1188/10.CJON.81-86

82. Gruschkus, S.K., Lairson, D., Dunn, J.K., Risser, J., & Du, X.L. (2010). Comparative effectiveness of white blood cell growth factors on neutropenia, infection, and survival in older people with non-Hodgkin's lymphoma treated with chemotherapy. *Journal of the American Geriatrics Society, 58*, 1885–1895. doi:10.1111/j.1532-5415.2010.03081.x

83. Gupta, S., Singh, P.K., Bhatt, M.L.B., Pant, M.C., Gupta, R., & Negi, M.P. (2010). Efficacy of granulocyte colony stimulating factor as a secondary prophylaxis along with full-dose chemotherapy following a prior cycle of febrile neutropenia. *Bioscience Trends, 4*, 273–278. Retrieved from http://www.biosciencetrends.com/action/downloaddoc.php?docid=354

84. Hecht, J.R., Pillai, M., Gollard, R., Heim, W., Swan, F., Patel, R., ... Malik, I. (2010). A randomized, placebo-controlled phase II study evaluating the reduction of neutropenia and febrile neutropenia in patients with colorectal cancer receiving pegfilgrastim with every-2-week chemotherapy. *Clinical Colorectal Cancer, 9*, 95–101. doi:10.3816/CCC.2010.n.013

85. Holmes, F.A., Jones, S.E., O'Shaughnessy, J., Vukelja, S., George, T., Savin, M., ... Liang, B.C. (2002). Comparable efficacy and safety profiles of once-per-cycle pegfilgrastim and daily injection filgrastim in chemotherapy-induced neutropenia: A multicenter dose-finding study in women with breast cancer. *Annals of Oncology, 13*, 903–909. doi:10.1093/annonc/mdf130

86. Lyman, G.H., Kuderer, N.M., & Djulbegovic, B. (2002). Prophylactic granulocyte colony-stimulating factor in patients receiving dose-intensive cancer chemotherapy: A meta-analysis. *American Journal of Medicine, 112*, 406–411. doi:10.1016/S0002-9343(02)01036-7

87. Minuk, L.A., Monkman, K., Chin-Yee, I.H., Lazo-Langner, A., Bhagirath, V., Chin-Yee, B.H., & Mangel, J.E. (2012). Treatment of Hodgkin lymphoma with adriamycin, bleomycin, vinblastine and dacarbazine without routine granulocyte-colony stimulating factor support does not increase the risk of febrile neutropenia: A prospective cohort study. *Leukemia and Lymphoma, 53*, 57–63. doi:10.3109/10428194.2011.602771

88. Timmer-Bonte, J.N.H., Punt, C.J.A., vd Heijden, H.F.M., van Die, C.E., Bussink, J., Beijnen, J.H., ... Tjan-Heijnen, V.C. (2008). Prophylactic G-CSF and antibiotics enable a significant dose-escalation of triplet-chemotherapy in non-small cell lung cancer. *Lung Cancer, 60*, 222–230. doi:10.1016/j.lungcan.2007.10.001

89. Weycker, D., Malin, J., Barron, R., Edelsberg, J., Kartashov, A., & Oster, G. (2012). Comparative effectiveness of filgrastim, pegfilgrastim, and

sargramostim as prophylaxis against hospitalization for neutropenic complications in patients with cancer receiving chemotherapy. *American Journal of Clinical Oncology, 35,* 267–274. doi:10.1097/COC.0b013e31820dc075

90. Yakushijin, Y., Shikata, H., Takaoka, I., Horikawa, T., Takeuchi, K., Yamanouchi, J., … Yasukawa, M. (2011). Usage of granulocyte colony-stimulating factor every 2 days is clinically useful and cost-effective for febrile neutropenia during early courses of chemotherapy. *International Journal of Clinical Oncology, 16,* 118–124. doi:10.1007/s10147-010-0134-x

91. Bhana, N. (2007). Granulocyte colony–stimulating factors in the management of chemotherapy-induced neutropenia: Evidence-based review. *Current Opinion in Oncology, 19,* 328–335. doi:10.1097/01.cco.0000275309 .58868.11

92. Bohlius, J., Herbst, C., Reiser, M., Schwarzer, G., & Engert, A. (2008). Granulopoiesis-stimulating factors to prevent adverse effects in the treatment of malignant lymphoma. *Cochrane Database of Systematic Reviews, 2008*(4). doi:10.1002/14651858.CD003189.pub4

93. Gurion, R., Belnik-Plitman, Y., Gafter-Gvili, A., Paul, M., Vidal, L., Ben-Bassat, I., … Raanani, P. (2011). Colony-stimulating factors for prevention and treatment of infectious complications in patients with acute myelogenous leukemia. *Cochrane Database of Systematic Reviews, 2011*(9). doi:10.1002/14651858.CD008238.pub2

94. Herbst, C., Naumann, F., Kruse, E.B., Monsef, I., Bohlius, J., Schulz, H., & Engert, A. (2009). Prophylactic antibiotics or G-CSF for the prevention of infections and improvement of survival in cancer patients undergoing chemotherapy. *Cochrane Database of Systematic Reviews, 2009*(1). doi:10.1002/14651858.CD007107.pub2

95. Kuderer, N.M. (2011). Meta-analysis of randomized controlled trials of granulocyte colony-stimulating factor prophylaxis in adult cancer patients receiving chemotherapy. *Cancer Treatment and Research, 157,* 127–143. doi:10.1007/978-1-4419-7073-2_8

96. Renner, P., Milazzo, S., Liu, J.P., Zwahlen, M., Birkmann, J., & Horneber, M. (2012). Primary prophylactic colony-stimulating factors for the prevention of chemotherapy-induced febrile neutropenia in breast cancer patients. *Cochrane Database of Systematic Reviews, 2012*(10). doi:10.1002/14651858.CD007913.pub2

97. Sung, L., Nathan, P.C., Lange, B., Beyene, J., & Buchanan, G.R. (2004). Prophylactic granulocyte colony-stimulating factor and granulocyte-macrophage colony-stimulating factor decrease febrile neutropenia after chemotherapy in children with cancer: A meta-analysis of randomized controlled trials. *Journal of Clinical Oncology, 22,* 3350–3356. doi:10.1200/JCO.2004.09.106

98. Von Minckwitz, G., Schwenkglenks, M., Skacel, T., Lyman, G.H., Pousa, A.L., Bacon, P., … Aapro, M.S. (2009). Febrile neutropenia and related complications in breast cancer patients receiving pegfilgrastim primary prophylaxis versus current practice neutropaenia management: Results from an integrated analysis. *European Journal of Cancer, 45,* 608–617. doi:10.1016/j.ejca.2008.11.021

99. Borinstein, S.C., Pollard, J., Winter, L., & Hawkins, D.S. (2009). Pegfilgrastim for prevention of chemotherapy-associated neutropenia in pediatric patients with solid tumors. *Pediatric Blood and Cancer, 53,* 375–378. doi:10.1002/pbc.22086

100. Inaba, H., Cao, X., Pounds, S., Pui, C.-H., Rubnitz, J.E., Ribeiro, R.C., & Razzouk, B.I. (2011). Randomized trial of 2 dosages of prophylactic granulocyte-colony-stimulating factor after induction chemotherapy in pediatric acute myeloid leukemia. *Cancer, 117,* 1313–1320. doi:10.1002/cncr.25536

101. Milano-Bausset, E., Gaudart, J., Rome, A., Coze, C., Gentet, J.C., Padovani, L., … André, N. (2009). Retrospective comparison of neutropenia in children with Ewing sarcoma treated with chemotherapy and granulocyte colony-stimulating factor (G-CSF) or pegylated G-CSF. *Clinical Therapeutics, 31,* 2388–2395. doi:10.1016/j.clinthera.2009.11.013

102. Paksu, M.S., Paksu, S., Akbalik, M., Ozyurek, E., Duru, F., Albayrak, D., & Fisgin, T. (2012). Comparison of the approaches to non-febrile neutropenia developing in children with acute lymphoblastic leukemia. *Fundamental and Clinical Pharmacology, 26,* 418–423. doi:10.1111/j.1472-8206.2011.00938.x

103. Spunt, S.L., Irving, H., Frost, J., Sender, L., Guo, M., Yang, B.-B., ... Santana, V.M. (2010). Phase II, randomized, open-label study of pegfilgrastim-supported VDC/IE chemotherapy in pediatric sarcoma patients. *Journal of Clinical Oncology, 28,* 1329–1336. doi:10.1200/JCO.2009.24.8872

104. Chan, A., Leng, X.Z., Chiang, J.Y.L., Tao, M., Quek, R., Tay, K., & Lim, S.T. (2011). Comparison of daily filgrastim and pegfilgrastim to prevent febrile neutropenia in Asian lymphoma patients. *Asia-Pacific Journal of Clinical Oncology, 7,* 75–81. doi:10.1111/j.1743-7563.2010.01355.x

105. Green, M.D., Koelbl, H., Baselga, J., Galid, A., Guillem, V., Gascon, P., ... Piccart, M.J. (2003). A randomized double-blind multicenter phase III study of fixed-dose single-administration pegfilgrastim versus daily filgrastim in patients receiving myelosuppressive chemotherapy. *Annals of Oncology, 14,* 29–35. doi:10.1093/annonc/mdg019

106. Sveikata, A., Liutkauskienė, S., Juozaitytė, E., Characiejus, D., Tamošaitytė, L., & Šeštakauskas, K. (2011). An open-label multicenter safety, tolerability, and efficacy study of recombinant granulocyte colony-stimulating factor in the prevention of neutropenic complications in breast cancer patients. *Medicina, 47,* 428–433. Retrieved from http://medicina.kmu.lt/1108/11111806.pdf

107. Waller, C.F., Semiglazov, V.F., Tjulandin, S., Bentsion, D., Chan, S., & Challand, R. (2010). A phase III randomized equivalence study of biosimilar filgrastim versus Amgen filgrastim in patients receiving myelosuppressive chemotherapy for breast cancer. *Onkologie, 33,* 504–511. doi:10.1159/000319693

108. Burris, H.A., III, Belani, C.P., Kaufman, P.A., Gordon, A.N., Schwartzberg, L.S., Paroly, W.S., ... Saven, A. (2010). Pegfilgrastim on the same day versus next day of chemotherapy in patients with breast cancer, non-small-cell lung cancer, ovarian cancer, and non-Hodgkin lymphoma: Results of four multicenter, double-blind, randomized phase II studies. *Journal of Oncology Practice, 6,* 133–140. doi:10.1200/JOP.091094

109. Loibl, S., Mueller, V., von Minckwitz, G., Conrad, B., Koehne, C.-H., Kremers, S., ... Moebus, V. (2011). Comparison of pegfilgrastim on day 2 vs. day 4 as primary prophylaxis of intense dose-dense chemotherapy in patients with node-positive primary breast cancer within the prospective, multicenter GAIN study: (GBG 33). *Supportive Care in Cancer, 19,* 1789–1795. doi:10.1007/s00520-010-1020-9

110. Majhail, N.S., Rizzo, J.D., Lee, S.J., Aljurf, M., Atsuta, Y., Bonfim, C., ... Tichelli, A. (2012). Recommended screening and preventive practices for long-term survivors after hematopoietic cell transplantation. *Biology of Blood and Marrow Transplantation, 18,* 348–371. doi:10.1016/j.bbmt.2011.12.519

111. U.S. Department of Agriculture Food Safety and Inspection Service. (2013, August 28). Basics for handling food safely. Retrieved from http://www.fsis.usda.gov/wps/portal/fsis/topics/food-safety-education/get-answers/food-safety-fact-sheets/safe-food-handling/basics-for-handling-food-safely/CT_Index

112. Kashiwazaki, H., Matsushita, T., Sugita, J., Shigematsu, A., Kasashi, K., Yamazaki, Y., ... Inoue, N. (2012). Professional oral health care reduces oral mucositis and febrile neutropenia in patients treated with allogeneic bone marrow transplantation. *Supportive Care in Cancer, 20,* 367–373. doi:10.1007/s00520-011-1116-x

113. Cheuk, D.K.L., Chiang, A.K.S., Lee, T.L., Chan, G.C.F., & Ha, S.Y. (2011). Vaccines for prophylaxis of viral infections in patients with hematological malignancies. *Cochrane Database of Systematic Reviews, 2011*(3). doi:10.1002/14651858.CD006505.pub2

114. Pollyea, D.A., Brown, J.M.Y., & Horning, S.J. (2010). Utility of influenza vaccination for oncology patients. *Journal of Clinical Oncology, 28,* 2481–2490. doi:10.1200/JCO.2009.26.6908

115. Kroger, A.T., Sumaya, C.V., Pickering, L.K., & Atkinson, W.L. (2011, January 28). General recommendations on immunization: Recommendations of the Advisory Committee on Immunization Practices (ACIP). *MMWR: Recommendations and Reports, 60*(RR02), 1–61. Retrieved from http://www.cdc.gov/mmwr/preview/mmwrhtml/rr6002a1.htm?s_cid=rr6002a1_e

116. Ruiz-Tovar, J., Santos, J., Arroyo, A., Llavero, C., Armañanzas, L., López-Delgado, A., … Calpena, R. (2012). Effect of peritoneal lavage with clindamycin-gentamicin solution on infections after elective colorectal cancer surgery. *Journal of the American College of Surgeons, 214,* 202–207. doi:10.1016/j.jamcollsurg.2011.10.014

117. Chemaly, R.F., Sharma, P.S., Youssef, S., Gerber, D., Hwu, P., Hanmod, S.S., … Raad, I.I. (2010). The efficacy of catheters coated with minocycline and rifampin in the prevention of catheter-related bacteremia in cancer patients receiving high-dose interleukin-2. *International Journal of Infectious Diseases, 14,* e548–e552. doi:10.1016/j.ijid.2009.08.007

118. Schierholz, J.M., Nagelschmidt, K., Nagelschmidt, M., Lefering, R., Yücel, N., & Beuth, J. (2010). Antimicrobial central venous catheters in oncology: Efficacy of a rifampicin-miconazole-releasing catheter. *Anticancer Research, 30,* 1353–1358. Retrieved from http://ar.iiarjournals.org/content/30/4/1353.long

119. Bass, P., Karki, S., Rhodes, D., Gonelli, S., Land, G., Watson, K., … Cheng, A.C. (2013). Impact of chlorhexidine-impregnated washcloths on reducing incidence of vancomycin-resistant enterococci colonization in hematology-oncology patients. *American Journal of Infection Control, 41,* 345–348. doi:10.1016/j.ajic.2012.04.324

120. Climo, M.W., Yokoe, D.S., Warren, D.K., Perl, T.M., Bolon, M., Herwaldt, L.A., … Wong, E.S. (2013). Effect of daily chlorhexidine bathing on hospital-acquired infection. *New England Journal of Medicine, 368,* 533–542. doi:10.1056/NEJMoa1113849

121. Raanani, P., Gafter-Gvili, A., Paul, M., Ben-Bassat, I., Leibovici, L., & Shpilberg, O. (2009). Immunoglobulin prophylaxis in chronic lymphocytic leukemia and multiple myeloma: Systematic review and meta-analysis. *Leukemia and Lymphoma, 50,* 764–772. doi:10.1080/10428190902856824

122. Ferreira Chacon, J.M., Hato de Almeida, E., de Lourdes Simões, R., Ozório, V.L.C., Alves, B.C., Mello de Andréa, M.L., … Biernat, J.C. (2011). Randomized study of minocycline and edetic acid as a locking solution for central line (Port-A-Cath) in children with cancer. *Chemotherapy, 57,* 285–291. doi:10.1159/000328976

123. Snaterse, M., Rüger, W., Scholte op Reimer, W.J.M., & Lucas, C. (2010). Antibiotic-based catheter lock solutions for prevention of catheter-related bloodstream infection: A systematic review of randomised controlled trials. *Journal of Hospital Infection, 75,* 1–11. doi:10.1016/j.jhin.2009.12.017

124. Vokurka, S., Kabatova-Maxova, K., Skardova, J., & Bystricka, E. (2009). Antimicrobial chlorhexidine/silver sulfadiazine-coated central venous catheters versus those uncoated in patients undergoing allogeneic stem cell transplantation. *Supportive Care in Cancer, 17,* 145–151. doi:10.1007/s00520-008-0454-9

125. Chen, S.Y., Chen, T.M., Dai, N.T., Fu, J.P., Chang, S.C., Deng, S.C., & Chen, S.G. (2011). Do antibacterial-coated sutures reduce wound infection in head and neck cancer reconstruction? *European Journal of Surgical Oncology, 37,* 300–304. doi:10.1016/j.ejso.2011.01.015

126. Williams, N., Sweetland, H., Goyal, S., Ivins, N., & Leaper, D.J. (2011). Randomized trial of antimicrobial-coated sutures to prevent surgical site infection after breast cancer surgery. *Surgical Infections, 12,* 469–474. doi:10.1089/sur.2011.045

127. Zhao, Y., Tan, Y., Wu, G., Liu, L., Wang, Y., Luo, Y., … Huang, H. (2011). Berbamine overcomes imatinib-induced neutropenia and permits cytoge-

netic responses in Chinese patients with chronic-phase chronic myeloid leukemia. *International Journal of Hematology, 94,* 156–162. doi:10.1007/s12185-011-0887-7

128. Chambers, S.T., Sanders, J., Patton, W.N., Ganly, P., Birch, M., Crump, J.A., & Spearing, R.L. (2005). Reduction of exit-site infections of tunneled intravascular catheters among neutropenic patients by sustained-release chlorhexidine dressings: Results from a prospective randomized controlled trial. *Journal of Hospital Infection, 61,* 53–61. doi:10.1016/j.jhin.2005.01.023

129. Cowan, C.C., Hutchison, C., Cole, T., Barry, S.J.E., Paul, J., Reed, N.S., & Russell, J.M. (2011). A randomised double-blind placebo-controlled trial to determine the effect of cranberry juice on decreasing the incidence of urinary symptoms and urinary tract infections in patients undergoing radiotherapy for cancer of the bladder or cervix. *Clinical Oncology, 24,* e31–e38. doi:10.1016/j.clon.2011.05.009

130. Lu, W., Matulonis, U.A., Doherty-Gilman, A., Lee, H., Dean-Clower, E., Rosulek, A., … Penson, R.T. (2009). Acupuncture for chemotherapy-induced neutropenia in patients with gynecologic malignancies: A pilot randomized, sham-controlled clinical trial. *Journal of Alternative and Complementary Medicine, 15,* 745–753. doi:10.1089/acm.2008.0589.

131. Mousset, S., Hermann, S., Klein, S.A., Bialleck, H., Duchscherer, M., Bomke, B., … Martin, H. (2005). Prophylactic and interventional granulocyte transfusions in patients with haematological malignancies and life-threatening infections during neutropenia. *Annals of Hematology, 84,* 734–741. doi:10.1007/s00277-005-1055-z

132. Pham, H.P., Rogoza, K., Stotler, B., Duffy, D., Parker-Jones, S., Ginzburg, Y., … Schwartz, J. (2012). Granulocyte transfusion therapy in pediatric patients after hematopoietic stem cell transplantation: A 5-year single tertiary care center experience. *Journal of Pediatric Hematology/Oncology, 34,* e332–e336. doi:10.1097/MPH.0b013e3182580d40

133. Biffi, R., Fattori, L., Bertani, E., Radice, D., Rotmensz, N., Misitano, P., … Nespoli, A. (2012). Surgical site infections following colorectal cancer surgery: A randomized prospective trial comparing common and advanced antimicrobial dressing containing ionic silver. *World Journal of Surgical Oncology, 10,* 94. doi:10.1186/1477-7819-10-94

134. Sweet, M.A., Cumpston, A., Briggs, F., Craig, M., & Hamadani, M. (2012). Impact of alcohol-impregnated port protectors and needleless neutral pressure connectors on central line–associated bloodstream infections and contamination of blood cultures in an inpatient oncology unit. *American Journal of Infection Control, 40,* 931–934. doi:10.1016/j.ajic.2012.01.025

135. Zitella, L., Gobel, B.H., O'Leary, C., Friese, C.R., Woolery, M., Hauser, J., & Andrews, F. (2009). ONS PEP resource: Prevention of infection. In L.H. Eaton & J.M. Tipton (Eds.), *Putting evidence into practice: Improving oncology patient outcomes* (pp. 273–283). Pittsburgh, PA: Oncology Nursing Society.

136. Tröger, W., Jezdić, S., Ždrale, Z., Tišma, N., Hamre, H.J., & Matijašević, M. (2009). Quality of life and neutropenia in patients with early stage breast cancer: A randomized pilot study comparing additional treatment with mistletoe extract to chemotherapy alone. *Breast Cancer: Basic and Clinical Research, 3,* 35–45. Retrieved from http://www.la-press.com/quality-of-life-and-neutropenia-in-patients-with-early-stage-breast-ca-article-a1532-abstract

137. Mank, A., & van der Lelie, H. (2003). Is there still an indication for nursing patients with prolonged neutropenia in protective isolation? An evidence-based nursing and medical study of 4 years experience for nursing patients with neutropenia without isolation. *European Journal of Oncology Nursing, 71,* 17–23. doi:10.1054/ejon.2002.0216

138. Nauseef, W.M., & Maki, D.G. (1981). A study of the value of simple protective isolation in patients with granulocytopenia. *New England Journal of Medicine, 304,* 448–453. doi:10.1056/NEJM198102193040802

139. Schlesinger, A., Paul, M., Gafter-Gvili, A., Rubinovitch, B., & Leibovici, L. (2009). Infection-control interventions for cancer patients after chemother-

apy: A systematic review and meta-analysis. *Lancet Infectious Diseases, 9*, 97–107. doi:10.1016/S1473-3099(08)70284-6

140. Stoll, P., Silla, L.M., Cola, C.M., Splitt, B.I., & Moreira, L.B. (2013). Effectiveness of a Protective Environment implementation for cancer patients with chemotherapy-induced neutropenia on fever and mortality incidence. *American Journal of Infection Control, 41*, 357–359. doi:10.1016/j.ajic.2012.05.018

141. Chaberny, I.F., Ruseva, E., Sohr, D., Buchholz, S., Ganser, A., Mattner, F., & Gastmeier, P. (2009). Surveillance with successful reduction of central line-associated bloodstream infections among neutropenic patients with hematologic or oncologic malignancies. *Annals of Hematology, 88*, 907–912. doi:10.1007/s00277-008-0687-1

142. Handrup, M.M., Møller, J.K., & Schrøder, H. (2013). Central venous catheters and catheter locks in children with cancer: A prospective randomized trial of taurolidine versus heparin. *Pediatric Blood and Cancer, 60*, 1292–1298. doi:10.1002/pbc.24482

143. Ljungman, P., Cordonnier, C., Einsele, H., Englund, J., Machada, C.M., Storek, J., & Small, T. (2009). Vaccination of hematopoietic cell transplant recipients. *Bone Marrow Transplantation, 44*, 521–526. doi:10.1038/bmt.2009.263

144. Arora, R.S., Roberts, R., Eden, T.O.B., & Pizer, B. (2010). Interventions other than anticoagulants and systemic antibiotics for prevention of central venous catheter–related infections in children with cancer. *Cochrane Database of Systematic Reviews, 2010*(12). doi:10.1002/14651858.CD007785.pub2

145. Imamura, H., Kurokawa, Y., Tsujinaka, T., Inoue, K., Kimura, Y., Iijima, S., … Furukawa, H. (2012). Intraoperative versus extended antimicrobial prophylaxis after gastric cancer surgery: A phase 3, open-label, randomised controlled, non-inferiority trial. *Lancet Infectious Diseases, 12*, 381–387. doi:10.1016/S1473-3099(11)70370-X

146. DeMille, D., Deming, P., Lupinacci, P., & Jacobs, L. (2006). The effect of the neutropenic diet in the outpatient setting: A pilot study. *Oncology Nursing Forum, 33*, 337–343. doi:10.1188/ONF.06.337-343

147. Gardner, A., Mattiuzzi, G., Faderl, S., Borthakur, G., Garcia-Manero, G., Pierce, S., … Estey, E. (2008). Randomized comparison of cooked and noncooked diets in patients undergoing remission induction therapy for acute myeloid leukemia. *Journal of Clinical Oncology, 26*, 5684–5688. doi:10.1200/JCO.2008.16.4681

148. Moody, K., Finlay, J., Mancuso, C., & Charlson, M. (2006). Feasibility and safety of a pilot randomized trial of infection rate: Neutropenic diet versus standard food safety guidelines. *Journal of Pediatric Hematology/Oncology, 28*, 126–133. doi:10.1097/01.mph.0000210412.33630.fb

149. van Tiel, F.H., Harbers, M.M., Terporten, P.H.W., van Boxtel, R.T.C., Kessels, A.G., Voss, G.B.W.E., & Schouten, H.C. (2007). Normal hospital and low-bacterial diet in patients with cytopenia after intensive chemotherapy for hematologic malignancy: A study of safety. *Annals of Oncology, 18*, 1080–1084. doi:10.1093/annonc/mdm082

150. Trifilio, S., Helenowoki, I., Giel, M., Gobel, B., Pi, J., Greenberg, D., & Mehta, J. (2012). Questioning the role of a neutropenic diet following hematopoietic stem cell transplantation. *Biology of Blood and Marrow Transplantation, 18*, 1385–1390. doi:10.1016/j.bbmt.2012.02.015

151. van Dalen, E.C., Mank, A., Leclercq, E., Mulder, R.L., Davies, M., Kersten, M.J., & van de Wetering, M.D. (2012). Low bacterial diet versus control diet to prevent infection in cancer patients treated with chemotherapy causing episodes of neutropenia. *Cochrane Database of Systematic Reviews, 2012*(9). doi:10.1002/14651858.CD006247.pub2

152. Bennett-Guerrero, E., Pappas, T.N., Koltun, W.A., Fleshman, J.W., Lin, M., Garg, J., … SWIPE 2 Trial Group. (2010). Gentamicin-collagen sponge for infection prophylaxis in colorectal surgery. *New England Journal of Medicine, 363*, 1038–1049. doi:10.1056/NEJMoa1000837

153. Clarkson, J.E., Worthington, H.V., & Eden, T.O.B. (2007). Interventions for pre-venting oral candidiasis for patients with cancer receiving treatment. *Cochrane Database of Systematic Reviews, 2007*(1). doi:10.1002/14651858.CD003807.pub3

154. Irwin, M., Erb, C., Williams, C., Wilson, B.J., & Zitella, L.J. (2013). *Putting evidence into practice: Improving oncology patient outcomes: Prevention of infection.* Pittsburgh, PA: Oncology Nursing Society.

155. Joint Commission. (n.d.). CLABSI toolkit and monograph. Retrieved from http://www.jointcommission.org/Topics/Clabsi_toolkit.aspx

18

Radiodermatitis

Tracy K. Gosselin, PhD, RN, MSN, AOCN®,
Marilyn Omabegho, RN, MSN, OCN®, NE-BC,
and Margaret Irwin, PhD, RN, MN

Problem and Incidence

Radiodermatitis often occurs within the first two to four weeks of radiation therapy and is characterized by a progression of skin changes from dry skin to mild erythema to moist desquamation. Depending upon the site of radiation therapy and severity of radiodermatitis, the patient may have pain and pruritus that affect quality of life, body image, and sleep.[1] The incidence of radiodermatitis can be as high as 95% depending upon the population of patients receiving treatment.[2,3] Studies documenting incidence have primarily occurred in women receiving treatment for breast cancer.

Risk Factors and Assessment

Patients are at greater risk with
- Higher total dose, larger field size, and presence of overlapping fields
- Obesity and skin folds within the treatment field
- Concurrent chemotherapy (especially with paclitaxel, docetaxel, or cetuximab)
- Smoking
- Poor nutritional status
- Concurrent ultraviolet light exposure
- Certain comorbid conditions (e.g., diabetes, autoimmune diseases).

Assessment tools include
- Radiation Therapy Oncology Group (RTOG) Acute Radiation Morbidity Screening Criteria

- National Cancer Institute Cancer Therapy Evaluation Program *Common Terminology Criteria for Adverse Events* (CTCAE) (open access)[4]
- RTOG and European Organisation for Research and Treatment of Cancer Toxicity Criteria
- Oncology Nursing Society *Radiation Therapy Patient Care Record*, using the CTCAE.

What interventions are effective in preventing and managing radiodermatitis in people with cancer?

Evidence retrieved through June 30, 2013

Recommended for Practice

Intensity-modulated radiation therapy was associated with less severe radiodermatitis than conventional radiation therapy.[5-8]

Skin hygiene and usual care practices, including washing the skin[9-14] and use of deodorant,[15] are beneficial.

Likely to Be Effective

Calendula officinalis reduced the severity of radiodermatitis in one large randomized controlled trial[16] and a systematic review.[17] Calendula has been recommended in professional guidelines.[9]

Silver sulfadiazine was associated with lower severity of radiodermatitis in 102 women receiving therapy for breast cancer.[18]

Effectiveness Not Established

Multiple topical agents, dressings, and systemic interventions have been tested. Evidence is generally limited by small sample sizes, few studies, and study design limitations.

- **Topical agents**
  - **Anionic polar phospholipid cream**[19]
  - **Ascorbic acid topical solution**[20]
  - **Barrier ointment, semi-occlusive (Aquaphor®)**[2]
  - **Chamomile cream and almond ointment**[21]
  - **Glutathione and anthocyanin (RayGel®)**[22]
  - **Herbal medicine** administered as a topical mixture[23]
  - **Hyaluronic acid (sodium hyaluronate)**[24-26]—A meta-analysis showed evidence supporting hyaluronic acid.[17] One underpowered study showed worse outcomes with topical hyaluronic acid.[27] Lotion containing both hyaluronic acid and urea was associated with lower severity of radiodermatitis.[28]
  - **Light-emitting diode photomodulation to irradiated skin**[29]—A systematic review suggested it might be beneficial.[8]
  - **Lipiderm**[30]
  - **MAS065D (Xclair®)**[31]
  - **Sodium sucrose octasulfate**[32]
  - **Sucralfate lotion**[33]
  - **Theta cream**[34]
  - **Topical steroids**[35-38]—Systematic reviews suggest that topical corticosteroids might be beneficial.[8,17]
  - **Urea lotion**[39]
  - **Wheatgrass extract**[40]
- **Dressings**
  - **Granulocyte macrophage colony–stimulating factor impregnated gauze**[41]
  - **Hydrocolloid dressing**[42-46]
  - **Hydrophyllic foam**[47,48]
  - **No-sting barrier film (Cavilon™)**[49]—A systematic review showed some evidence in support of barrier films.[17]
  - **Silver leaf dressing**[50-52]—This type of dressing was suggested as potentially beneficial by a systematic review of evidence.[8]
- **Systemic treatments**
  - **Dietary supplements** of resveratrol, lycopene, vitamin C, and anthocyanins[53]

- **Sucralfate** given orally[8,17,54]
- **Wobe-Mugos**, a proteolytic enzyme mixture[55]
- **Zinc supplements**[56]

Effectiveness Unlikely

Aloe vera resulted in no benefit in several studies and systematic reviews.[8,19,57-60] Aloe vera was associated with higher toxicity in one meta-analysis.[17]

Trolamine (Biafine®) was not beneficial in several studies[2,16,30,61-63] and one systematic review.[17]

Expert Opinion

Topical unscented moisturizers can be used in the absence of infection,[64,65] and the use of any moisturizing agent is likely to be better than no treatment.[17] Additional expert opinion recommendations include the following.[65,66]
- Do not use baby powder or cornstarch on the skin.
- Protect skin from sun exposure during and following treatment. Use sunscreen with a protection factor of at least 30 after completion of treatment, and cover irradiated skin during treatment.
- Avoid use of tapes and adhesives to prevent mechanical skin injury.
- Do not use ice or heating pads on skin in the treatment field.
- Avoid swimming and using hot tubs or saunas.
- Wear loose-fitting clothing.
- If receiving radiation to the perineal or rectal area, use sitz baths daily.

Application to Practice

Reliable and valid assessment for radiodermatitis needs to be incorporated into routine nursing practice.

Patients should continue to wash the area being treated with mild soap, and deodorant can be used on intact skin. Good skin hygiene is beneficial.

Patient education materials should outline self-care practices that can be performed, including use of topical agents to maintain moisture that have the highest levels of supportive evidence and expert opinion recommendations to avoid skin trauma and behaviors that may increase risk. Agents that are associated with negative results should be avoided.

Encouragement and treatment to assist patients to stop smoking should be employed.

Radiodermatitis Resource Contributors

Topic leaders: Maurene McQuestion, RN, BScN, CON(C), MSc, and Tracy K. Gosselin, PhD, RN, MSN, AOCN®
Laura Beamer, DNP, CNP, CNS, APNG, AOCNP®, AOCNS®, Deb Feight, RN, MSN, CNS, AOCN®, Christine Merritt, MSN, RN, Marilyn Omabegho, RN, MSN, OCN®, NE-BC, and Anne Shaftic, MSN, RN, NP-C, AOCNP®

References

1. Schnur, J.B., Zivin, J.G., Mattson, D.M.K., Jr., Green, S., Jandorf, L.H., Wenicke, A.G., & Montgomery, G.H. (2012). Acute skin toxicity-related, out-of-pocket expenses in patients with breast cancer treated with external beam radiotherapy: A descriptive, exploratory study. *Supportive Care in Cancer, 20,* 3105–3113. doi:10.1007/s00520-012-1435-6
2. Gosselin, T.K., Schneider, S.M., Plambeck, M.A., & Rowe, K. (2010). A prospective randomized, placebo-controlled skin care study in women diagnosed with breast cancer undergoing radiation therapy. *Oncology Nursing Forum, 37,* 619–626. doi:10.1188/10.ONF.619-626
3. McQuestion, M. (2011). Evidence-based skin care management in radiation therapy: Clinical update. *Seminars in Oncology Nursing, 27,* e1–e17. doi:10.1016/j.soncn.2011.02.009
4. National Cancer Institute Cancer Therapy Evaluation Program. (2010, June 14). *Common terminology criteria for adverse events* [v.4.03]. Retrieved from http://evs.nci.nih.gov/ftp1/CTCAE/CTCAE_4.03_2010-06-14 _QuickReference_5x7.pdf
5. Freedman, G.M., Anderson, P.R., Li, J., Jinsheng, L., Eisenberg, D.F., Hanlon, A.L., ... Nicolaou, N. (2006). Intensity modulated radiation therapy (IMRT) decreases acute skin toxicity for women receiving radiation for breast cancer. *American Journal of Clinical Oncology, 29,* 66–70. doi:10.1097/01 .coc.0000197661.09628.03
6. Freedman, G.M., Li, T., Nicolaou, N., Chen, Y., Ma, C.C.-M., & Anderson, P.R. (2009). Breast intensity-modulated radiation therapy reduces time

spent with acute dermatitis for women of all breast sizes during radiation. *International Journal of Radiation Oncology, Biology, Physics, 74*, 689–694. doi:10.1016/j.ijrobp.2008.08.071

7. Pignol, J.-P., Olivotto, I., Rakovitch, E., Gardner, S., Sixel, K., Beckham, W., … Paszat, L. (2008). A multicenter randomized trial of breast intensity-modulated radiation therapy to reduce acute radiation dermatitis. *Journal of Clinical Oncology, 26*, 2085–2092. doi:10.1200/JCO.2007.15.2488

8. Salvo, N., Barnes, E., van Draanen, J., Stacey, E., Mitera, G., Breen, D., … De Angelis, C. (2010). Prophylaxis and management of acute radiation-induced skin reactions: A systematic review of the literature. *Current Oncology, 17*, 94–112. Retrieved from http://www.ncbi.nlm.nih.gov/pmc/articles/PMC2913836

9. Bolderston, A., Lloyd, N.S., Wong, R.K.S., Holden, L., & Robb-Blenderman, L. (2005, February 21). *The prevention and management of acute skin reactions related to radiation therapy.* Retrieved from https://www.cancercare.on.ca/common/pages/UserFile.aspx?fileId=34406

10. Campbell, I.R., & Illingworth, M.H. (1992). Can patients wash during radiotherapy to the breast or chest wall? A randomized controlled trial. *Clinical Oncology, 4*, 78–82. doi:10.1016/S0936-6555(05)80971-9

11. Koukourakis, G.V., Kelekis, N., Kouvaris, J., Beli, I.K., & Kouloulias, V.E. (2010). Therapeutics interventions with anti-inflammatory creams in post radiation acute skin reactions: A systematic review of most important clinical trials. *Recent Patents on Inflammation and Allergy Drug Discovery, 4*, 149–158. doi:10.2174/187221310791163099

12. Meegan, M.A., & Haycocks, T.R. (1997). An investigation into the management of acute skin reactions from tangential breast irradiation. *Canadian Journal of Medical Radiation, 28*, 169–173.

13. Roy, I., Fortin, A., & Larochelle, M. (2001). The impact of skin washing with water and soap during breast irradiation: A randomized study. *Radiotherapy and Oncology, 58*, 333–339. doi:10.1016/S0167-8140(00)00322-4

14. Westbury, C., Hines, F., Hawkes, E., Ashley, S., & Brada, M. (2000). Advice on hair and scalp care during cranial radiotherapy: A prospective randomized trial. *Radiotherapy and Oncology, 54*, 109–116. doi:10.1016/S0167-8140(99)00146-2

15. Théberge, V., Harel, F., & Dagnault, A. (2009). Use of axillary deodorant and effect on acute skin toxicity during radiotherapy for breast cancer: A prospective randomized noninferiority trial. *International Journal of Radiation Oncology, Biology, Physics, 75*, 1048–1052. doi:10.1016/j.ijrobp.2008.12.046

16. Pommier, P., Gomez, F., Sunyach, M.P., D'Hombres, A., Carrie, C., & Montbarbon, X. (2004). Phase III randomized trial of *Calendula officinalis* compared with trolamine for the prevention of acute dermatitis during irradiation for breast cancer. *Journal of Clinical Oncology, 22*, 1447–1453. doi:10.1200/JCO.2004.07.063

17. Kumar, S., Juresic, E., Barton, M., & Shafiq, J. (2010). Management of skin toxicity during radiation therapy: A review of the evidence. *Journal of Medical Imaging and Radiation Oncology, 54*, 264–279. doi:10.1111/j.1754-9485.2010.02170.x

18. Hemati, S., Asnaashari, O., Sarvizadeh, M., Motlagh, B.N., Akbari, M., Tajvidi, M., & Gookizadeh, A. (2012). Topical silver sulfadiazine for the prevention of acute dermatitis during irradiation for breast cancer. *Supportive Care in Cancer, 20*, 1613–1618. doi:10.1007/s00520-011-1250-5

19. Merchant, T.E., Bosley, C., Smith, J., Baratti, P., Pritchard, D., David, T., … Xiong, X. (2007). A phase III trial comparing an anionic phospholipid-based cream and aloe vera-based gel in the prevention of radiation dermatitis in pediatric patients. *Radiation Oncology, 2*, 45. doi:10.1186/1748-717X-2-45

20. Halperin, E.D., Gaspar, L., George, S., Darr, D., & Pinnell, S. (1993). A double-blind, randomized, prospective trial to evaluate topical vitamin C solution for the prevention of radiation dermatitis. *International Journal of Radiation Oncology, Biology, Physics, 26*, 413–416. doi:10.1016/0360-3016(93)90958-X

21. Maiche, A.G., Gröhn, P., & Mäki-Hokkonen, H. (1991). Effect of chamomile cream and almond ointment on acute radiation skin reaction. *Acta Oncologica, 30,* 395–396.

22. Enomoto, T.M., Johnston, T., Peterson, N., Homer, L., Walts, D., & Johnson, N. (2005). Combination glutathione and anthocyanins as an alternative for skin care during external-beam radiation. *American Journal of Surgery, 189,* 627–631. doi:10.1016/j.amjsurg.2005.02.001

23. Rizza, L., D'Agostino, A., Girlando, A., & Puglia, C. (2010). Evaluation of the effect of topical agents on radiation-induced skin disease by reflectance spectrophotometry. *Journal of Pharmacy and Pharmacology, 62,* 779–785. doi:10.1211/jpp.62.06.0015

24. Kirova, Y.M., Fromantin, I., De Rycke, Y., Fourquet, A., Morvan, E., Padiglione, S., … Bollet, M.A. (2011). Can we decrease the skin reaction in breast cancer patients using hyaluronic acid during radiation therapy? Results of phase III randomised trial. *Radiotherapy and Oncology, 100,* 205–209. doi:10.1016/j.radonc.2011.05.014

25. Liguori, V., Guillemin, C., Pesce, G.F., Mirimanoff, R.O., & Bernier, J. (1997). Double-blind, randomized clinical study comparing hyaluronic acid cream to placebo in patients treated with radiotherapy. *Radiotherapy and Oncology, 42,* 155–161. doi:10.1016/S0167-8140(96)01882-8

26. Ravo, V., Calvanese, M.G., Di Franco, R., Crisci, V., Murino, P., Manzo, R., … Muto, P. (2011). Prevention of cutaneous damages induced by radiotherapy in breast cancer: An institutional experience. *Tumori, 97,* 732–736. doi:10.1700/1018.11089

27. Pinnix, C., Perkins, G.H., Strom, E.A., Tereffe, W., Woodward, W., Oh, J.L., … Yu, T. (2012). Topical hyaluronic acid vs. standard of care for the prevention of radiation dermatitis after adjuvant radiotherapy for breast cancer: Single-blind randomized phase III clinical trial. *International Journal of Radiation Oncology, Biology, Physics, 83,* 1089–1094. doi:10.1016/j.ijrobp.2011.09.021

28. Pardo Masferrer, J., Murcia Mejía, M., Vidal Fernández, M., Alvarado Astudillo, A., Hernandez Armenteros, M.L., Macias Hernández, V., … Mirada Ferre, A. (2010). Prophylaxis with a cream containing urea reduces the incidence and severity of radio-induced dermatitis. *Clinical and Translational Oncology, 12,* 43–48. doi:10.1007/s12094-010-0465-0

29. Fife, D., Rayhan, D.J., Behnam, S., Ortiz, A., Elkeeb, L., Aquino, L., … Kelly, K.M. (2010). A randomized, controlled, double-blind study of light emitting diode photomodulation for the prevention of radiation dermatitis in patients with breast cancer. *Dermatologic Surgery, 36,* 1921–1927. doi:10.1111/j.1524-4725.2010.01801.x

30. Fenig, E., Brenner, B., Katz, A., Sulkes, J., Lapidot, M., Schachter, J., … Gutman, H. (2001). Topical Biafine and Lipiderm for the prevention of radiation dermatitis: A randomized prospective trial. *Oncology Reports, 8,* 305–309. doi:10.3892/or.8.2.305

31. Leonardi, M.C., Gariboldi, S., Ivaldi, G.B., Ferrari, A., Serafini, F., Didier, F., … Orecchia, R. (2008). A double-blind, randomized, vehicle-controlled clinical study to evaluate the efficacy of MAS065D in limiting the effects of radiation on the skin: Interim analysis. *European Journal of Dermatology, 18,* 317–321. doi:10.1684/ejd.2008.0396

32. Evensen, J.F., Bjordal, K., Jacobsen, A.-B., Løkkevic, E., & Tausjø, J.E. (2001). Effects of Na-sucrose octasulfate on skin and mucosa reactions during radiotherapy of head and neck cancers. *Acta Oncologica, 40,* 751–755. doi:10.1080/02841860152619188

33. Falkowski, S., Trouillas, P., Duroux, J.-L., Bonnetblanc, J.-M., & Clavère, P. (2011). Radiodermatitis prevention with sucralfate in breast cancer: Fundamental and clinical studies. *Supportive Care in Cancer, 19,* 57–65. doi:10.1007/s00520-009-0788-y

34. Röper, N., Kaisig, D., Auer, F., Mergen, E., & Molls, M. (2004). Theta-cream versus bepanthol lotion in breast cancer patients under radiotherapy. *Strahlentherapie und Onkologie, 180,* 315–322. doi:10.1007/s00066-004-1174-9

35. Boström, A., Lindman, H., Swartling, C., Berne, B., & Bergh, J. (2001). Potent corticosteroid cream (mometasone furoate) significantly reduces acute radiation dermatitis: Results from a double-blind, randomized study. *Radiotherapy and Oncology, 59,* 257–265. doi:10.1016/S0167-8140(01)00327-9

36. Miller, R.C., Schwartz, D.J., Sloan, J.A., Griffin, P.C., Deming, R.L., Anders, J.C., … Martenson, J.A. (2011). Mometasone furoate effect on acute skin toxicity in breast cancer patients receiving radiotherapy: A phase III double-blind, randomized trial from the North Central Cancer Treatment Group N06C4. *International Journal of Radiation Oncology, Biology, Physics, 79,* 1460–1466. doi:10.1016/j.ijrobp.2010.01.031

37. Omidvari, S., Saboori, H., Mohammadianpanah, M., Mosalaei, A., Ahmadloo, N., Mosleh-Shirazi, M.A., … Namaz, S. (2007). Topical betamethasone for prevention of radiation dermatitis. *Indian Journal of Dermatology, Venerology, and Leprology, 73,* 209–214. doi:10.4103/0378-6323.32755

38. Shukla, P.N., Gairola, M., Mohanti, B.K., & Rath, G.K. (2006). Prophylactic beclomethasone spray to the skin during postoperative radiotherapy of carcinoma breast: A prospective randomized study. *Indian Journal of Cancer, 43,* 180–184. doi:10.4103/0019-509X.29424

39. Momm, F., Weissenberger, C., Bartelt, S., & Henke, M. (2003). Moist skin care can diminish acute radiation-induced skin toxicity. *Strahlentherapie und Onkologie, 179,* 708–712. doi:10.1007/s00066-003-1142-9

40. Wheat, J., Currie, G., & Coulter, K. (2007). Management of acute radiation skin toxicity with wheatgrass extract in breast radiation therapy: A pilot study. *Australian Journal of Medical Herbalism, 19,* 77–80.

41. Kouvaris, J.R., Kouloulias, V.E., Plataniotis, G.A., Balafouta, E.J., & Vlahos, L.J. (2001). Dermatitis during radiation for vulvar carcinoma: Prevention and treatment with granulocyte-macrophage colony-stimulating factor impregnated gauze. *Wound Repair and Regeneration, 9,* 187–193. doi:10.1046/j.1524-475x.2001.00187.x

42. Gollins, S., Gaffney, C., Slade, S., & Swindell, R. (2008). RCT on gentian violet versus a hydrogel dressing for radiotherapy-induced moist skin desquamation. *Journal of Wound Care, 17,* 268–275. Retrieved from http://www.internurse.com/cgi-bin/go.pl/library/article.cgi?uid=29589;article=JWC_17_6_268_275

43. Kedge, E.M. (2009). A systematic review to investigate the effectiveness and acceptability of interventions for moist desquamation in radiotherapy patients. *Radiography, 15,* 247–257. doi:10.1016/j.radi.2008.08.002

44. Macmillan, M.S., Wells, M., MacBridge, S., Raab, G.M., Munro, A., & MacDougall, H. (2007). Randomized comparison of dry dressings versus hydrogel in management of radiation-induced moist desquamation. *International Journal of Radiation Oncology, Biology, Physics, 68,* 864–872. doi:10.1016/j.ijrobp.2006.12.049

45. Mak, S.S., Molassiotis, A., Wan, W.-M., Lee, I.Y.M., & Chan, E.S.J. (2000). The effects of hydrocolloid dressing and gentian violet on radiation-induced moist desquamation wound healing. *Cancer Nursing, 23,* 220–229. doi:10.1097/00002820-200006000-00010

46. Mak, S.S., Zee, C.Y., Molassiotis, A., Chan, S.J., Leung, S.F., Mo, K.F., & Johnson, P.J. (2005). A comparison of wound treatments in nasopharyngeal cancer patients receiving radiation therapy. *Cancer Nursing, 28,* 436–445. doi:10.1097/00002820-200511000-00005

47. Diggelmann, K.V., Zytkovicz, A.E., Tuaine, J.M., Bennett, N.C., Kelly, L.E., & Herst, P.M. (2010). Mepilex Lite dressings for the management of radiation-induced erythema: A systematic inpatient controlled clinical trial. *British Journal of Radiology, 83,* 971–978. doi:10.1259/bjr/62011713

48. Perez, Y.L., Medina, J.A., Perez, I.L., & Garcia, C.M. (2011). Prevention and treatment of radiodermatitis using a non-adhesive foam dressing. *Journal of Wound Care, 20,* 130–135.

49. Graham, P., Browne, L., Capp, A., Fox, C., Graham, J., Hollis, J., & Nasser, E. (2004). Randomized, paired comparison of no-sting barrier film versus sorbolene cream (10% glycerine) skin care during post-mastectomy irra-

diation. *International Journal of Radiation Oncology, Biology, Physics, 58,* 241–246. doi:10.1016/S0360-3016(03)01431-7

50. Aquino-Parsons, C., Lomas, S., Smith, K., Hayes, J., Lew, S., Bates, A.T., & Macdonald, A.G. (2010). Phase III study of silver leaf nylon dressing vs. standard care for reduction of inframammary moist desquamation in patients undergoing adjuvant whole breast radiation therapy. *Journal of Medical Imaging and Radiation Sciences, 41,* 215–221. doi:10.1016/j.jmir.2010.08.005

51. Niazi, T.M., Vuong, T., Azoulay, L., Marijnen, C., Bujko, K., Nasr, E., … Cummings, B. (2012). Silver clear nylon dressing is effective in preventing radiation-induced dermatitis in patients with lower gastrointestinal cancer: Results from a phase III study. *International Journal of Radiation Oncology, Biology, Physics, 84,* e305–e310. doi:10.1016/j.ijrobp.2012.03.062

52. Vavassis, P., Gelinas, M., Chabot Tr, J., & Nguyen-Tân, P.F. (2008). Phase 2 study of silver leaf dressing for treatment of radiation-induced dermatitis in patients receiving radiotherapy to the head and neck. *Journal of Otolaryngology-Head and Neck Surgery, 37,* 124–129.

53. DiFranco, R., Calvanese, M., Murino, P., Manzo, R., Guida, C., Di Gennaro, D., … Ravo, V. (2012). Skin toxicity from external beam radiation therapy in breast cancer patients: Protective effects of resveratrol, lycopene, vitamin C and anthocianin (Ixor®). *Radiation Oncology, 7,* 12. doi:10.1186/1748717X-7-12

54. Lievens, Y., Haustermans, K., Van der Weyngaert, D., Van den Bogaert, W., Scalliet, P., Hutsebaut, L., … Lambin, P. (1998). Does sucralfate reduce the acute side-effects in head and neck cancer treated with radiotherapy? A double-blind randomized trial. *Radiation and Oncology, 47,* 149–153. doi:10.1016/S0167-8140(97)00231-4

55. Gujral, M.S., Patnaik, P.M., Kayl, R., Parikh, H.K., Conradt, C., Tamhankar, C.P., & Daftary, G.V. (2001). Efficacy of hydrolytic enzymes in preventing radiation therapy-induced side effects in patients with head and neck cancers. *Cancer Chemotherapy and Pharmacology, 47*(Suppl.), S23–S28. doi:10.1007/s002800170005

56. Lin, L. C., Que, J., Lin, L.-K., & Lin, F.-C. (2006). Zinc supplementation to improve mucositis and dermatitis in patients after radiotherapy for head-and-neck cancers: A double-blind, randomized study. *International Journal of Radiation Oncology, Biology, Physics, 65,* 745–750. doi:10.1016/j.ijrobp.2006.01.015

57. Heggie, S., Bryant, G.P., Tripcony, L., Keller, J., Rose, P., Glendenning, M., & Heath, J. (2002). A phase III study on the efficacy of topical aloe vera gel on irradiated breast tissue. *Cancer Nursing, 25,* 442–451. doi:10.1097/00002820-200212000-00007

58. Olsen, D.L., Raub, W., Jr., Bradley, C., Johnson, M., Macias, J.L., Love, V., & Markoe, A. (2001). The effect of aloe vera gel/mild soap versus mild soap alone in preventing skin reactions in patients undergoing radiation therapy. *Oncology Nursing Forum, 28,* 543–547.

59. Vogler, B.K., & Ernst, E. (1999). Aloe vera: A systematic review of its clinical effectiveness. *British Journal of General Practice, 49,* 823–828. Retrieved from http://www.ncbi.nlm.nih.gov/pmc/articles/PMC1313538

60. Williams, M.S., Burk, M., Loprinzi, C.L., Hill, M., Schomberg, P.J., Near-hood, K., … Eggleston, W.D. (1996). Phase III double-blind evaluation of an aloe vera gel as a prophylactic agent for radiation-induced skin toxicity. *International Journal of Radiation Oncology, Biology, Physics, 36,* 345–349. doi:10.1016/S0360-3016(96)00320-3

61. Elliott, E.A., Wright, J.R., Swann, R.S., Nguyen-Tân, F., Takita, C., Bucci, M.K., … Berk, L. (2006). Phase III trial of an emulsion containing trolamine for the prevention of radiation dermatitis in patients with advanced squamous cell carcinoma of the head and neck: Results of Radiation Therapy Oncology Group Trial 99-13. *Journal of Clinical Oncology, 24,* 2092–2096. doi:10.1200/JCO.2005.04.9148

62. Fisher, J., Scott, C., Stevens, R., Marconi, B., Champion, L., Freedman, G.M., … Wong, G. (2000). Randomized phase III study comparing best

supportive care to Biafine as a prophylactic agent for radiation-induced skin toxicity for women undergoing breast irradiation: Radiation Therapy Oncology Group (ROTG) 97-13. *International Journal of Radiation Oncology, Biology, Physics, 48,* 1307–1310. doi:10.1016/S0360-3016(00)00782-3

63. Szumacher, E., Wighton, A., Franssen, E., Chow, E., Tsao, M., Ackerman, I., ... Hayter, C. (2001). Phase II study assessing the effectiveness of Biafine cream as a prophylactic agent for radiation-induced acute skin toxicity to the breast in women undergoing radiotherapy with concominant CMF chemotherapy. *International Journal of Radiation Oncology, Biology, Physics, 51,* 81–86. doi:10.1016/S0360-3016(01)01576-0

64. Bernier, J., Bonner, J., Vermorken, J.B., Bensadoun, R.-J., Dummer, R., Giralt, J., ... Ang, K.K. (2008). Consensus guidelines for the management of radiation dermatitis and coexisting acne-like rash in patients receiving radiotherapy plus EGFR inhibitors for the treatment of squamous cell carcinoma of the head and neck. *Annals of Oncology, 19,* 142–149. doi:10.1093/annonc/mdm400

65. McQuestion, M. (2010). Radiation-induced skin reactions. In M.L. Haas & G.J. Moore-Higgs (Eds.), *Principles of skin care and the oncology patient* (pp. 115–140). Pittsburgh, PA: Oncology Nursing Society.

66. British Columbia Cancer Agency. (2006). *Care of radiation skin reactions.* Retrieved from http://www.bccancer.bc.ca/NR/rdonlyres/6065FF4A-7A08 -4DA2-9C13-293890A7ABB2/16217/RadiationSkinReactions2006web.pdf

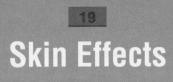

19

Skin Effects

Lee Ann Johnson, PhD(c), RN

Problem and Incidence

Adverse skin reactions are a significant problem for many patients[1] and are caused by multiple chemotherapy and biotherapy agents. Reactions range from mild to severe and negatively affect quality of life, physical abilities, and psychosocial well-being.[1-4] Increased use of targeted therapies, especially epidermal growth factor receptor inhibitors (EGFRIs), has led to an overall increase in reported skin reactions[5] with 49%–100% of patients on these therapies reporting some type of toxicity.[6] Many types of skin reactions are associated with cancer treatment; this resource focuses on rash, palmar-plantar erythrodysesthesia (PPE), xerosis, pruritus, and paronychia.

Clinical presentations of skin reactions vary according to the agent used. Carboplatin may cause allergic reactions that manifest as rash, urticaria, erythema, and pruritus.[7] Interleukin-2 may cause erythematous rash, pruritus, and dry, peeling skin.[8] Interferon alfa causes diffuse skin reactions.[9]

Rash is the most commonly reported skin reaction.[10] Rash occurs in 80%–95% of patients receiving monoclonal antibodies,[11] 67%–75% of patients receiving erlotinib,[12] and 50%–100% of patients receiving high-dose cytarabine as part of a regimen.[13] Multiple other chemotherapeutic agents have been associated with development of skin rash.[14] Among patients receiving EGFRIs, 80% of physicians reported that patients had rash, and 32% had to prescribe medications for associated pain.[2] Rash can have a significant effect on body image and quality of life.

PPE, also known as hand-foot syndrome, is the most severe cutaneous reaction.[1] It begins as mild redness and discomfort on the palms and soles and progresses to intense burning pain and tenderness, swelling, desquamation, severe crusting, ulceration, and epidermal necrosis.[10,15,16] It is associated with capecitabine, continuous-infusion fluorouracil (5-FU), pegylated liposomal doxorubicin (PLD), and docetaxel. The overall incidence of PPE associated with capecitabine is 45%–65% and is 42%–82% with 5-FU.[17-19]

Xerosis is abnormally dry, flaky, dull skin[10,15] and is associated with chemotherapy and EGFRIs. It occurs in 4%–100% of patients.[6] Dry skin can result in painful fissures on fingers or feet.

Pruritus is intense itching often associated with rash and xerosis.[10,15,20] Pruritus has been reported in approximately 15% of patients.[6]

Paronychia, painful inflammation of tissue around the fingernails and toenails,[15] is reported in approximately 12%–58% of patients.[6] All patients receiving EGFRIs are at risk for nail changes, which can lead to significant pain and functional limitation.[21]

Risk Factors and Assessment

Several factors have been associated with increased risk of skin reactions, including
- EGFRI therapy
- Treatment with certain chemotherapy agents (e.g., capecitabine, continuous-infusion 5-FU, PLD, docetaxel)
- Fair skin
- Older age
- Exposure to ultraviolet light (rash).

Assessment of dermatologic adverse effects includes determination of the severity of skin reactions and the patient's subjective response and associated symptoms. Patients need to be monitored for development of skin reactions for detection and initiation of treatment as early as possible. Review of patient medications should be done to determine other potential causes of skin rash, such as hypersensitivity reactions to other drugs.

Paronychia has the potential to become superinfected. Bacterial, viral, and fungal cultures of the skin are generally recommended.[2,21,22]

Patients can benefit from referral to dermatology specialists for further assessment and management of treatment-related skin effects.

Assessment tools include
- National Cancer Institute Cancer Therapy Evaluation Program *Common Terminology Criteria for Adverse Events* (open access)[10]—Papulopustular eruption, PPE, nail changes, erythema, pruritus, xerosis
- Skindex-16
- The Dermatology Life Quality Index.[23]

What interventions are effective in preventing and managing skin effects (rash, PPE, pruritus, xerosis, and paronychia) from systemic treatment in people with cancer?

Evidence retrieved through June 30, 2013

Likely to Be Effective

Chemotherapy dose interruption or modification reduces adverse skin reactions.[2,22,24,25] Drug manufacturers provide recommended dosage modification schemas.

Effectiveness Not Established

A number of topical, local, and systemic interventions for prevention and treatment of skin effects from cancer treatment have been suggested, but little research evidence exists to support interventions. Most evidence in this area is anecdotal, from case series, or consensus-based guidelines, and guideline recommendations are not consistent for all interventions.

- **Regional cooling with ice packs** during administration of PLD was associated with lower incidence of PPE in a retrospective review.[26-28]
- **Topical interventions**
  - **Benzoyl peroxide**[3,21]—Professional guidelines do not recommend use of benzoyl peroxide.[25,29]
  - **Colloidal oatmeal lotion** for general prevention[30]—Topical agents containing colloidal oatmeal have been recommended in guidelines for general skin care and prevention.[21]
  - **Emollients and moisturizers** for general prevention[31]—Use of emollients and moisturizers has been recommended in consensus guidelines for xerosis and general prophylactic skin care.[21,32,33]
  - **Petroleum-based topical agents**[34-36]—These topical agents have been recommended in guidelines for xerosis.[21]
  - **Pimecrolimus**[37]—Not recommended for rash in guidelines[21]
  - **Sunscreen** for prevention of rash[22,38]—Sunscreens with sun protection factor of at least 30 and protection from both ultraviolet A and B rays have been recommended.[22,25,32,33]
  - **Tazarotene** in combination with systemic minocycline for prevention of skin lesions[39]
  - **Topical antibiotics**, including clindamycin, erythromycin, metronidazole, and nadifloxacin[2,3,6,25,40]
  - **Topical steroids** for treatment of paronychia and rash[2,21,22,32,33]
- **Systemic interventions**
  - **Antibiotics**, including tetracycline, minocycline, doxycycline, amoxicillin, and gentamycin for prophylaxis or empiric treatment[2,6,21,22,25,29,32,33,38,41-43]—Antibiotic administration is recommended for culture-proven infections. Empiric use without cultures is not recommended in guidelines.[21]
  - **Antihistamines** for pruritus[21]
  - **Corticosteroids** for treatment of rash[2,21,22,24,26,44-46]
  - **Cyclooxygenase-2 inhibitors** for prevention of PPE in patients receiving capecitabine[47,48]

- **Low-dose aspirin** for prevention of skin effects with gefitinib[49]
- **Multicomponent intervention (Skin Toxicity Evaluation Protocol with Panitumumab, or STEPP)**, including prophylactic use of skin moisturizer, use of sunscreen, topical corticosteroid, and systemic doxycycline, followed by standardized treatment for skin reactions according to severity grading[50]
- **Retinoids** for cases of severe effects or conditions unresponsive to other treatment are recommended in some guidelines[2,25] and specifically not recommended by others.[21]

Effectiveness Unlikely

Urea-based topical treatment was ineffective in a large study of patients treated with capecitabine.[51] One small study showed some benefit,[31] and some experts recommend use of urea-based skin care products.[22,32]

Not Recommended for Practice

Pyridoxine has been suggested for prevention of PPE.[48,52,53] Clinical trials do not support its use.[54-56]

Expert Opinion

Multiple professional groups have identified consensus-based recommendations of behaviors that patients can employ to potentially reduce skin effects from treatments.[2,6,21,32] These include

- Clipping or removing nails
- Soaking nails in diluted white vinegar or bleach for management of paronychia
- Maintaining skin moisture with emollients and avoidance of activities and agents that dry the skin, including
  - Avoiding frequent hand washing, showers, and baths
  - Using mild bath or shower oils rather than soap
  - Avoiding use of lotions containing alcohol or perfumes

- Cleansing with daily antiseptic baths for paronychia
- Avoiding trauma to the skin and skin contact with irritants such as solvents or disinfectants
  - Wear well-fitting protective footwear.
  - Wear gloves while cleaning.
- Using medical-grade cyanoacrylate glue for skin fissures
- Avoiding skin exposure to ultraviolet rays.

Application to Practice

Nurses can educate patients on the potential skin effects of treatment and counsel patients to inform healthcare providers of any skin or nail changes for immediate management. Nurses can directly assess skin condition and impact on the patient using objective assessment tools and ensure that these effects are addressed.

Nurses can educate patients regarding behaviors from expert opinion that may be helpful to prevent or reduce skin reactions, such as

- Avoiding temperature extremes to the skin
- Minimizing sun exposure by keeping skin covered and using sunscreens that protect against both ultraviolet A and B rays
- Using hypoallergenic skin care products that do not contain alcohol
- Using nonocclusive makeup.

Nurses can educate patients on appropriate interventions to be done at home to protect nails, including

- Keeping nails short
- Moisturizing hands and feet regularly
- Avoiding products with harmful chemicals
- Wearing shoes that do not push on the nail fold. It has been suggested that nail trauma is not likely to cause paronychia but will exacerbate it and can cause discomfort.

Nurses can educate patients in treatments for specific skin reactions suggested by expert opinion and advocate or implement those interventions that have the highest strength of evidence.

Referral to dermatology specialists can be beneficial.

Skin Effects Resource Contributors

Topic leader: Lori Williams, PhD, RN, AOCN®, OCN®
Julie Carlson, RN, MSN, APN, AOCNS®, Ann Fuhrman, RN, BSN,
OCN®, Jeanene Robison, RN, MSN, AOCN®, and Gary Shelton,
MSN, NP, ANP-BC, AOCNP®

References

1. Bensadoun, R.-J., Humbert, P., Krutman, J., Luger, T., Triller, R., Rougier, A., ... Dreno, B. (2013). Daily baseline skin care in the prevention, treatment, and supportive care of skin toxicity in oncology patients: Recommendations from a multinational expert panel. *Cancer Management and Research, 5,* 401–408. doi:10.2147/CMAR.S52256

2. Burtness, B., Anadkat, M., Basti, S., Hughes, M., Lacouture, M.E., McClure, J.S., ... Spencer, S. (2009). NCCN Task Force report: Management of dermatologic and other toxicities associated with EGFR inhibition in patients with cancer. *Journal of the National Comprehensive Cancer Network, 7*(Suppl. 1), S5–S21. Retrieved from http://www.jnccn.org/content/7/Suppl_1/S-5.full.pdf+html

3. de Noronha e Menezes, N.M., Lima, R., Moreira, A., Varela, P., Barroso, A., Baptista, A., & Parente, B. (2009). Description and management of cutaneous side effects during erlotinib and cetuximab treatment in lung and colorectal cancer patients: A prospective and descriptive study of 19 patients. *European Journal of Dermatology, 19,* 248–251. doi:10.1684/ejd.2009.0650

4. Lynch, T.J., Jr., Kim, E.S., Eaby, B., Garey, J., West, D.P., & Lacouture, M.E. (2007). Epidermal growth factor receptor–associated cutaneous toxicities: An evolving paradigm in clinical management. *Oncologist, 12,* 610–621. doi:10.1634/theoncologist.12-5-610

5. Lacouture, M.E., Basti, S., Patel, J., & Benson, A., III. (2006). The SERIES clinic: An interdisciplinary approach to the management of toxicities of EGFR inhibitors. *Journal of Supportive Oncology, 4,* 236–238.

6. Potthoff, K., Hofheinz, R., Hassel, J.C., Volkenandt, M., Lordick, F., Hartmann, J.T., ... Wollenberg, A. (2011). Interdisciplinary management of EGFR-inhibitor–induced skin reactions: A German expert opinion. *Annals of Oncology, 22,* 524–535. doi:10.1093/annonc/mdq387

7. Wilkes, G.M., & Barton-Burke, M. (2010). *Oncology nursing drug handbook.* Burlington, MA: Jones and Bartlett.

8. Schwartzentruber, D.J. (2000). Interleukin-2: Clinical applications: Principles of administration and management of side effects. In S.A. Rosenberg (Ed.), *Principles and practice of the biologic therapy of cancer* (3rd ed., pp. 32–50). Philadelphia, PA: Lippincott Williams & Wilkins.

9. Esper, P., Gale, D., & Muehlbauer, P. (2007). What kind of rash is it? Deciphering the dermatologic toxicities of biologic and targeted therapies. *Clinical Journal of Oncology Nursing, 11,* 659–666. doi:10.1188/07.CJON.659-666

10. National Cancer Institute Cancer Therapy Evaluation Program. (2010, June 14). *Common terminology criteria for adverse events* [v.4.03]. Re-

trieved from http://evs.nci.nih.gov/ftp1/CTCAE/CTCAE_4.03_2010-06-14_QuickReference_5x7.pdf

11. Fakih, M., & Vincent, M. (2010). Adverse events associated with anti-EGFR therapies for the treatment of metastatic colorectal cancer. *Current Oncology, 17*(Suppl. 1), S18–S30. doi:10.3747/co.v17iS1.615

12. Boone, S.L., Rademaker, A., Liu, D., Pfeiffer, C., Mauro, D.J., & Lacouture, M.E. (2007). Impact and management of skin toxicity associated with anti-epidermal growth factor receptor therapy: Survey results. *Oncology, 72*, 152–159. doi:10.1159/000112795

13. Wright, L.G. (2006). Maculopapular skin rashes associated with high-dose chemotherapy: Prevalence and risk factors. *Oncology Nursing Forum, 33*, 1095–1103. doi:10.1188/06.ONF.1095-1103

14. Robison, J. (Ed.). (2011). Skin reactions: Rash, palmar-plantar erythrodysesthesia, xerosis, paronychia, photosensitivity, and pruritus. In L.H. Eaton, J.M. Tipton, & M. Irwin (Eds.), *Putting evidence into practice: Improving oncology patient outcomes, volume 2* (pp. 77–121). Pittsburgh, PA: Oncology Nursing Society.

15. Polovich, M., Whitford, J.M., & Olsen, M. (Eds.). (2009). *Chemotherapy and biotherapy guidelines and recommendations for practice* (3rd ed.). Pittsburgh, PA: Oncology Nursing Society.

16. Rossi, D., Alessandroni, P., Catalano, V., Giordani, P., Fedeli, S.L., Fedeli, A., ... Catalano, G. (2007). Safety profile and activity of lower capecitabine dose in patients with metastatic breast cancer. *Clinical Breast Cancer, 7*, 857–860. doi:10.3816/CBC.2007.n.050

17. Heo, Y.S., Chang, H.M., Kim, T.W., Ryu, M., Ahn, J., Kim, S.B., ... Kang, Y. (2004). Hand-foot syndrome in patients treated with capecitabine-containing combination chemotherapy. *Journal of Clinical Pharmacology, 44*, 1166–1172. doi:10.1177/0091270004268321

18. Brant, J.M., Wilkes, G.M., & Doyle, D. (2005). Palmar-plantar erythrodysesthesia. *Clinical Journal of Oncology Nursing, 9*, 103–106. doi:10.1188/05.CJON.103-106

19. Fabian, C.J., Molina, R., Slavik, M., Dahlberg, S., Giri, S., & Stephens, R. (1990). Pyridoxine therapy for palmar-plantar erythrodysesthesia associated with continuous 5-fluorouracil infusion. *Investigational New Drugs, 8*, 57–63. doi:10.1007/BF00216925

20. Dest, V.M. (2010). Systematic therapy–induced skin reactions. In M.L. Haas & G.J. Moore-Higgs (Eds.), *Principles of skin care and the oncology patient* (pp. 141–166). Pittsburgh, PA: Oncology Nursing Society.

21. Lacouture, M.E., Anadkat, M.J., Bensadoun, R.-J., Bryce, J., Chan, A., Epstein, J.B., ... Murphy, B.A. (2011). Clinical practice guidelines for the prevention and treatment of EGFR inhibitor-associated dermatologic toxicities. *Supportive Care in Cancer, 19*, 1079–1095. doi:10.1007/s00520-011-1197-6

22. Balagula, Y., Garbe, C., Myskowski, P.L., Hauschild, A., Rapoport, B.L., Boers-Doets, C.B., & Lacouture, M.E. (2011). Clinical presentation and management of dermatological toxicities of epidermal growth factor receptor inhibitors. *International Journal of Dermatology, 50*, 129–146. doi:10.1111/j.1365-4632.2010.04791.x

23. Finlay, A.Y., & Khan, G.K. (1992). Dermatology Life Quality Index (DLQI). Retrieved from http://www.drugcoverage.org/Enbrel/pdf/2E3E5EDF13964842A597E02005C3FE9A_AMEE_5288E_DLQI_TP_v01_230708_ENGLISH.pdf

24. Grunwald, V., Kalanovic, D., & Merseburger, A.S. (2010). Management of sunitinib-related adverse events: An evidence- and expert-based consensus approach. *World Journal of Urology, 28*, 343–351. doi:10.1007/s00345-010-0565-z

25. Pinto, C., Barone, C.A., Girolomoni, G., Russi, E.G., Merlano, M.C., Ferrari, D., & Maiello, E. (2011). Management of skin toxicity associated with cetuximab treatment in combination with chemotherapy or radiotherapy. *Oncologist, 16*, 228–238. doi:10.1634/theoncologist.2010-0298

26. Mangili, G., Petrone, M., Gentile, C., De Marzi, P., Viganò, R., & Rabaiotti, E. (2008). Prevention strategies in palmar-plantar erythrodysesthesia onset: The role of regional cooling. *Gynecologic Oncology, 108,* 332–335. doi:10.1016/j.ygyno.2007.10.021

27. Molpus, K.L., Anderson, L.B., Craig, C.L., & Pulee, J.G. (2004). The effect of regional cooling on toxicity associated with intravenous infusion of pegylated liposomal doxorubicin in recurrent ovarian carcinoma. *Gynecologic Oncology, 93,* 513–516. doi:10.1016/j.ygyno.2004.02.019

28. Tanyi, J.L., Smith, J.A., Ramos, L., Parker, C.L., Munsel, M.F., & Wolf, J.K. (2009). Predisposing risk factors for palmar-plantar erythrodysesthesia when using liposomal doxorubicin to treat recurrent ovarian cancer. *Gynecologic Oncology, 114,* 219–224. doi:10.1016/j.ygyno.2009.04.007

29. Molinari, E., De Quatrebarbes, J., André, T., & Aractingi, S. (2005). Cetuximab-induced acne. *Dermatology, 211,* 330–333. doi:10.1159/000088502

30. Alexandrescu, D.T., Vaillant, J.G., & Dasanu, C.A. (2006). Effect of treatment with a colloidal oatmeal lotion on the acneform eruption induced by epidermal growth factor receptor and multiple tyrosine-kinase inhibitors. *Clinical and Experimental Dermatology, 32,* 71–74. doi:10.1111/j.1365-2230.2006.02285.x

31. Ocvirk, J., & Rebersek, M. (2008). Managing cutaneous side effects with K1 vitamine creme reduces cutaneous toxicities induced by cetuximab [Abstract]. *Journal of Clinical Oncology, 26*(Suppl. 15), 20750.

32. Gutzmer, R., Becker, J.C., Enk, A., Garbe, C., Hauschild, A., Leverkus, M., ... Homey, B. (2011). Management of cutaneous side effects of EGFR inhibitors: Recommendations from a German expert panel for the primary treating physician. *Journal of the German Society of Dermatology, 9,* 195–203. doi:10.1111/j.1610-0387.2010.07561.x

33. Reguiai, Z., Bachet, J.B., Bachmeyer, C., Peuvrel, L., Beylot-Barry, M., Bezier, M., ... Bouché, O. (2012). Management of cutaneous adverse events induced by anti-EGFR (epidermal growth factor receptor): A French interdisciplinary therapeutic algorithm. *Supportive Care in Cancer, 20,* 1395–1404. doi:10.1007/s00520-012-1451-6

34. Fluhr, J.W., Miteva, M., Primavera, G., Ziemer, M., Elsner, P., & Borardosca, E. (2007). Functional assessment of a skin care system in patients on chemotherapy. *Skin Pharmacology and Physiology, 20,* 253–259. doi:10.1159/000104423

35. Ocvirk, J., & Cencelj, S. (2009). Management of cutaneous side-effects of cetuximab therapy in patients with metastatic colorectal cancer. *Journal of the European Academy of Dermatology and Venereology, 24,* 453–459. doi:10.1111/j.1468-3083.2009.03446.x

36. Racca, P., Fanchini, L., Caliendo, V., Ritorto, G., Evangelista, W., Volpatto, R., ... Ciuffreda, L. (2008). Efficacy and skin toxicity management with cetuximab in metastatic colorectal cancer: Outcomes from an oncologic/dermatologic cooperation. *Clinical Colorectal Cancer, 7,* 48–54. doi:10.3816/CCC.2008.n.007

37. Scope, A., Lieb, J.A., Dusza, S.W., Phelan, D.L., Myskowski, P.L., Saltz, L., & Halpern, A.C. (2009). A prospective randomized trial of topical pimecrolimus for cetuximab-associated acne-like eruption. *Journal of the American Academy of Dermatology, 61,* 614–620. doi:10.1016/j.jaad.2009.03.046

38. Jatoi, A., Thrower, A., Sloan, J.A., Flynn, P.J., Wentworth-Hartung, N.L., Dakhil, S.R., ... Loprinzi, C.L. (2010). Does sunscreen prevent epidermal growth factor receptor (EGFR) inhibitor-induced rash? Results of a placebo-controlled trial from the North Central Cancer Treatment Group (N05C4). *Oncologist, 15,* 1016–1022. doi:10.1634/theoncologist.2010-0082

39. Scope, A., Agero, A.L., Dusza, S.W., Myskowski, P.L., Lieb, J.A., Saltz, L., ... Halpern, A.C. (2007). Randomized double-blind trial of prophylactic oral minocycline and topical tazarotene for cetuximab-associated acne-like eruption. *Journal of Clinical Oncology, 25,* 5390–5396. doi:10.1200/JCO.2007.12.6987

40. Katzer, K., Tietze, J., Klein, E., Heinemann, V., Ruzicka, T., & Wollenberg, A. (2010). Topical therapy with nadifloxacin cream and prednicarbate cream

improves acneform eruptions caused by the EGFR-inhibitor cetuximab—A report of 29 patients. *European Journal of Dermatology, 20*, 82–84. doi:10.1684/ejd.2010.0806

41. Baas, J.M., Krens, L.L., Guchelaar, H.-J., Ouwerkerk, J., de Jong, F.A., Lavrijsen, A.P., & Gelderblom, H. (2012). Recommendations on management of EGFR inhibitor-induced skin toxicity: A systematic review. *Cancer Treatment Reviews, 38*, 505–514. doi:10.1016/j.ctrv.2011.09.004

42. Jatoi, A., Dakhil, S.R., Sloan, J.A., Kugler, J.W., Rowland, K.M., Jr., Schaefer, P.L., ... Loprinzi, C.L. (2011). Prophylactic tetracycline does not diminish the severity of epidermal growth factor receptor (EGFR) inhibitor-induced rash: Results from the North Central Cancer Treatment Group (Supplementary N03CB). *Supportive Care in Cancer, 19*, 1601–1607. doi:10.1007/s00520-010-0988-5

43. Jatoi, A., Rowland, K., Sloan, J.A., Gross, H.M., Fishkin, P.A., Kahanic, S.P., ... Loprinzi, C.L. (2008). Tetracycline to prevent epidermal growth factor receptor inhibitor-induced skin rashes: Results of a placebo-controlled trial from the North Central Cancer Treatment Group (N03CB). *Cancer, 113*, 847–853. doi:10.1002/cncr.23621

44. Drake, R.D., Lin, W.M., King, M., Farrar, D., Miller, D.S., & Coleman, R.L. (2004). Oral dexamethasone attenuates Doxil®-induced palmar-plantar erythrodysesthesias in patients with recurrent gynecologic malignancies. *Gynecologic Oncology, 94*, 320–324. doi:10.1016/j.ygyno.2004.05.027

45. Janusch, M., Fischer, M., Marsch, W., Holzhausen, H.J., Kegel, T., & Helmbold, P. (2006). The hand-foot syndrome—A frequent secondary manifestation in antineoplastic chemotherapy. *European Journal of Dermatology, 16*, 494–499.

46. Kollmannsberger, C., Schittenhelm, M., Honecker, F., Tillner, J., Weber, D., Oechsle, K., ... Bokemeyer, C. (2006). A phase I study of the humanized monoclonal anti-epidermal growth factor receptor (EGFR) antibody EMD 72000 (matuzumab) in combination with paclitaxel in patients with EGFR-positive advanced non-small-cell lung cancer (NSCLC). *Annals of Oncology, 17*, 1007–1013. doi:10.1093/annonc/mdl042

47. Zhang, R.-X., Wu, X.-J., Lu, S.-X., Pan, Z.-Z., Wan, D.-S., & Chen, G. (2011). The effect of COX-2 inhibitor on capecitabine-induced hand-foot syndrome in patients with stage II/III colorectal cancer: A phase II randomized prospective study. *Journal of Cancer Research and Clinical Oncology, 137*, 953–957. doi:10.1007/s00432-010-0958-9

48. Zhang, R.-X., Wu, X.-J., Wan, D.-S., Lu, Z.-H., Kong, L.-H., Pan, Z.-Z., & Chen, G. (2012). Celecoxib can prevent capecitabine-related hand-foot syndrome in stage II and III colorectal cancer patients: Result of a single-center, prospective randomized phase III trial. *Annals of Oncology, 23*, 1348–1353. doi:10.1093/annonc/mdr400

49. Kanazawa, S., Yamaguchi, K., Kinoshita, Y., Muramatsu, M., Komiyama, Y., & Nomura, S. (2006). Aspirin reduces adverse effects of gefitinib. *Anti-Cancer Drugs, 17*, 423–427. doi:10.1097/01.cad.0000203385.45163.76

50. Lacouture, M.E., Mitchell, E.P., Piperdi, B., Pillai, M.V., Shearer, H., Iannotti, N., ... Yassine, M. (2010). Skin Toxicity Evaluation Protocol with Panitumumab (STEPP), a phase II, open-label, randomized trial evaluating the impact of a pre-emptive skin treatment regimen on skin toxicities and quality of life in patients with metastatic colorectal cancer. *Journal of Clinical Oncology, 28*, 1351–1357. doi:10.1200/JCO.2008.21.7828

51. Wolf, S.L., Qin, R., Menon, S.P., Rowland, K.M., Jr., Thomas, S., Delaune, R., ... Loprinzi, C.L. (2010). Placebo-controlled trial to determine the effectiveness of a urea/lactic acid-based topical keratolytic agent for prevention of capecitabine-induced hand-foot syndrome: North Central Cancer Treatment Group Study N05C5. *Journal of Clinical Oncology, 28*, 5182–5187. doi:10.1200/JCO.2010.31.1431

52. Edwards, S.J. (2003). Prevention and treatment of adverse effects related to chemotherapy for recurrent ovarian cancer. *Seminars in Oncology Nursing, 19*(3, Suppl. 1), 19–39. doi:10.1016/S0749-2081(03)00059-7

53. Saif, M.W., & Elfiky, A.A. (2007). Identifying and treating fluoropyrimidine-associated hand-and-foot syndrome in White and non-White patients. *Journal of Supportive Oncology, 5,* 337–343. Retrieved from http://www.oncologypractice.com/jso/journal/articles/0507337.pdf

54. Kang, Y.-K., Lee, S.S., Yoon, D.H., Lee, S.Y., Chun, Y.J., Kim, M.S., ... Kim, T.W. (2010). Pyridoxine is not effective to prevent hand-foot syndrome associated with capecitabine therapy: Results of a randomized, double-blind, placebo-controlled study. *Journal of Clinical Oncology, 28,* 3824–3829. doi:10.1200/JCO.2010.29.1807

55. von Gruenigen, V., Frasure, H., Fusco, N., DeBernardo, R., Eldermire, E., Eaton, S., & Waggoner, S. (2010). A double-blind, randomized trial of pyridoxine versus placebo for the prevention of pegylated liposomal doxorubicin-related hand-foot syndrome in gynecologic oncology patients. *Cancer, 116,* 4735–4743. doi:10.1002/cncr.25262

56. Yoshimoto, N., Yamashita, T., Fujita, T., Hayashi, H., Tsunoda, N., Kimura, M., ... Iwata, H. (2010). Impact of prophylactic pyridoxine on occurrence of hand-foot syndrome in patients receiving capecitabine for advanced or metastatic breast cancer. *Breast Cancer, 17,* 298–302. doi:10.1007/s12282-009-0171-3

Sleep-Wake Disturbances

Ann M. Berger, PhD, APRN, AOCNS®, FAAN,
Genevieve Desaulniers, MS, CPNP-PC, RN,
Ellyn E. Matthews, PhD, RN, AOCN®, CBSM,
Julie L. Otte, PhD, RN, OCN®,
and Margaretta S. Page, MS, RN

Problem and Incidence

Sleep-wake disturbances are alterations in nighttime sleep with resultant daytime impairment. Insomnia, sleep-related movement disorders (restless legs syndrome and periodic limb movement disorder), and sleep-related breathing disorders are most common. Insomnia includes difficulty falling asleep, staying asleep, waking too early or inability to fall back to sleep, and feeling that sleep is nonrestorative.[1-5]

Sleep-wake disturbances are reported by 30%–90% of patients with cancer and are present in a variety of cancer diagnoses, affecting adults, children, and caregivers. They can be present before diagnosis, often worsen during treatment, and can persist after treatment is complete. Disturbed sleep may affect daytime sleepiness, functional ability, immune function, and overall quality of life.[1,4,6,7]

Risk Factors and Assessment

Screening patients who are at risk for sleep-wake disturbances enables providers to identify those patients who should receive a full assessment for the problem. Factors that contribute to risk of sleep-wake disturbances may be physiologic, psychosocial, and environmental.[9-13]

Predisposing factors include
- Female gender
- Older age
- Personal/family history of sleep disturbances or disorders
- Personal/family history of mood disorders or mental health problems
- Hyperarousal.

Precipitating factors include
- Side effects of treatment and medications, such as
  - Diarrhea, constipation, nausea
  - Incontinence, nocturia
  - Dyspnea, orthopnea, coughing
  - Hot flashes, night sweats
  - Pain, peripheral neuropathy
  - Immunologic changes, fever
  - Symptom cluster of sleep disturbance, pain, and fatigue
- Psychological distress in response to cancer
- Change in sedating or other sleep-altering medications (e.g., antidepressants)
- Sleep-disruptive environmental issues such as noise or temperature.

Perpetuating factors include maladaptive sleep behaviors and beliefs such as
- Excessive daytime napping or stimulant consumption
- Unrealistic sleep expectations.

Common instruments and methods for assessment include[6,12]
- Polysomnography to rule out underlying sleep disorders
- Actigraphy (using a wristwatch-like device that provides information about an individual's time to fall asleep, awakenings, and total sleep time by using movement sensors to record activity/rest rhythms)
- Subjective patient-reported outcome measures, including
  - Pittsburgh Sleep Quality Index
  - Insomnia Severity Index
  - Daily sleep diary
  - National Institutes of Health PROMIS® Sleep Disturbance Short Form 8a.[14]

What interventions are effective in managing sleep-wake disturbances in people with cancer?

Evidence retrieved through October 31, 2013

Likely to Be Effective

Cognitive behavioral strategies (combinations of restructuring and reducing unhelpful thoughts, stimulus control, sleep scheduling and restriction, relaxation, and sleep hygiene) have been shown to change negative thoughts and behaviors surrounding an individual's sleep and function in a number of studies and systematic reviews.[15-39]

Effectiveness Not Established

Pharmacologic therapies: Medications to induce sleep have not been well studied in patients with cancer. There is no evidence to recommend a specific medication. The National Cancer Institute Sleep Disorders PDQ® lists commonly prescribed medications.[40] The medications studied in cancer are the following.

- **Anticonvulsants:** Pregabalin[41]
- **Antidepressants:** Mirtazapine,[42,43] paroxetine,[44] trazadone,[45] and venlafaxine[46,47]
- **Antipsychotics:** Quetiapine[48]
- **Sedatives/hypnotics:** Zolpidem[47]

Herbal supplements: No studies have shown the efficacy of herbal therapy in patients with cancer.

- **Guarana**[49]
- **Kefir**, a probiotic[50]
- **Valerian**[51]

Nonpharmacologic and complementary therapies: Nonpharmacologic and complementary approaches have shown mixed effects for sleep outcomes or were evaluated in small studies that are inconclusive.

- **Acupressure**[52,53]

- **Acupuncture**[54-58]
- **Cranial stimulation** where low-intensity electrical stimulation to the brain is provided via electrodes attached to the earlobes[59]
- **Electroacupuncture**[53]
- **Electroencephalography neurofeedback**, which provides visual or auditory display of brain activity to the individual to facilitate brain self-regulation through biofeedback[60]
- **Exercise** such as brisk walking, strength training, and aerobics[2,61-74]—Results have been mixed.
- **Expressive writing**[75-78]
- **Haptotherapy**[79]
- **Healing touch**[80]
- **Massage/aromatherapy massage**[81-84]
- **Mind-body-spirit therapy/Qigong**, which involves the combination of gentle exercise, relaxation, and meditation practices[85]
- **Mindfulness-based stress reduction** consisting of a combination of psychoeducation, meditation, and stress-reducing mental exercises[86-93]
- **Progressive muscle relaxation with and without visual or guided imagery**[22,30,31,94,95]
- **Psychoeducation**[30,38,96-100]—Education is recommended in professional guidelines,[12] but research outcomes have been mixed.
- **Relaxation and imagery** using breathing exercises[30,31,101]
- **Stellate ganglion block** to sympathetic nerves in the neck has been studied for effects on hot flashes and associated sleep disruption.[102,103]
- **Support groups**[104]
- **Warm water foot bath**[105]
- **Yoga**[106-112]—Yoga has shown mixed effects on sleep.

Expert Opinion

Sleep hygiene practices to facilitate quality sleep and daytime alertness include the following.[113]
- Avoid stimulant drinks after noon, daytime napping, and eating a full meal prior to bed.
- Initiate a routine one to two hours before bedtime using a preferred relaxation technique, but do not watch television or use a computer screen in the bedroom.

- Maintain a comfortable sleeping environment that is dark, cool, and quiet.
- Go to bed around the same time each night only when sleepy, and get out of bed when unable to fall asleep.
- Rise the same time each day and have exposure to at least 20 minutes of bright natural light, preferably in the morning.

Application to Practice

Patients who demonstrate multiple risk factors for or indicate sleep-wake disturbance should be specifically assessed for this problem. Use of tools such as patient-reported outcome measures can be used to assess the patient and evaluate the effectiveness of interventions.

A sleep assessment for complaints requiring referral to a certified sleep specialist should be the initial step in treatment.[12] Referrals should be made for

- Chronic sleep complaints limiting function and/or moderate to severe subjective measurement of sleep quality
- Symptoms suggestive of sleep disorders (e.g., sleep apnea, restless legs syndrome) that require diagnostic testing.

Cognitive behavioral therapy (CBT) or standard CBT for insomnia (CBT-I) can promote healthy sleep. Nurses can apply these approaches by educating patients to adopt sleep hygiene practices, assisting patients to increase awareness of why sleep is problematic, identifying thoughts and behaviors that disrupt sleep, developing strategies to address these, and adopting behaviors that promote relaxation. Patients may need to be referred to a certified CBT-I therapist.

Other interventions currently lack sufficient evidence for recommendation but may prove beneficial after further study and may be helpful to some patients.

Sleep-Wake Disturbances Resource Contributors

Topic leader: Ann M. Berger, PhD, APRN, AOCNS®, FAAN
Genevieve Desaulniers, MS, CPNP-PC, RN, Ellyn E. Matthews,
PhD, RN, AOCN®, CBSM, Julie L. Otte, PhD, RN, OCN®,
Margaretta S. Page, MS, RN, and Catherine Vena, PhD, RN

Marcia Y. Shade, MSN, BSN, BS, is acknowledged for her assistance in the preparation of this material.

References

1. Palesh, O.G., Roscoe, J.A., Mustian, K.M., Roth, T., Savard, J., Ancoli-Israel, S., ... Morrow, G.R. (2010). Prevalence, demographics, and psychological associations of sleep disruption in patients with cancer: University of Rochester Cancer Center-Community Clinical Oncology Program. *Journal of Clinical Oncology, 28,* 292–298. doi:10.1200/JCO.2009.22.5011

2. Phillips, K.M., Jim, H.S., Donovan, K.A., Pinder-Schenck, M., & Jacobsen, P.B. (2012). Characteristics and correlates of sleep disturbances in cancer patients. *Supportive Care in Cancer, 20,* 357–365. doi:10.1007/s00520-011-1106-z

3. Sanford, S.D., Wagner, L.I., Beaumont, J.L., Butt, Z., Sweet, J.J., & Cella, D. (2013). Longitudinal prospective assessment of sleep quality: Before, during, and after adjuvant chemotherapy for breast cancer. *Supportive Care in Cancer, 21,* 959–967. doi:10.1007/s00520-012-1612-7

4. Savard, J., Villa, J., Ivers, H., Simard, S., & Morin, C.M. (2009). Prevalence, natural course, and risk factors of insomnia comorbid with cancer over a 2-month period. *Journal of Clinical Oncology, 27,* 5233–5239. doi:10.1200/JCO.2008.21.6333

5. Sharma, N., Hansen, C.H., O'Connor, M., Thekkumpurath, P., Walker, J., Kleiboer, A., ... Sharpe, M. (2012). Sleep problems in cancer patients: Prevalence and association with distress and pain. *Psycho-Oncology, 21,* 1003–1009. doi:10.1002/pon.2004

6. Berger, A.M. (2009). Update on the state of the science: Sleep-wake disturbances in adult patients with cancer. *Oncology Nursing Forum, 36,* E165–F177. doi:10.1188/09.ONF.E165 E177

7. Page, M.S., Berger, A.M., & Johnson, L.B. (2006). Putting evidence into practice: Evidence-based interventions for sleep-wake disturbances. *Clinical Journal of Oncology Nursing, 10,* 753–767. doi:10.1188/06.CJON.753-767

8. Savard, J., Ivers, H., Villa, J., Caplette-Gingras, A., & Morin, C.M. (2011). Natural course of insomnia comorbid with cancer: An 18-month longitudinal study. *Journal of Clinical Oncology, 29,* 3580–3586. doi:10.1200/JCO.2010.33.2247

9. Bardwell, W.A., Profant, J., Casden, D.R., Dimsdale, J.E., Ancoli-Isreal, S., Natarajan, L., ... Pierce, J.P. (2008). The relative importance of specific risk factors for insomnia in women treated for early-stage breast cancer. *Psycho-Oncology, 17,* 9–18. doi:10.1002/pon.1192

10. Berger, A.M., Parker, K.P., Young-McCaughan, S., Mallory, G.A., Barsevick, A.M., Beck, S.L., ... Hall, M. (2005). Sleep wake disturbances in people with cancer and their caregivers: State of the science [Online Exclusive]. *Oncology Nursing Forum, 32,* E98–E126. doi:10.1188/05.ONF.E98-E126

11. Davidson, J.R., MacLean, A.W., Brundage, M.D., & Schulze, K. (2002). Sleep disturbance in cancer patients. *Social Science and Medicine, 54,* 1309–1321. doi:10.1016/S0277-9536(01)00043-0

12. Howell, D., Oliver, T.K., Keller-Olaman, S., Davidson, J., Garland, S., Samuels, C., ... Taylor, C. (2013). A Pan-Canadian practice guideline:

Prevention, screening, assessment, and treatment of sleep disturbances in adults with cancer. *Supportive Care in Cancer, 21,* 2695–2706. doi:10.1007/s00520-013-1823-6

13. Spielman, A.J., Caruso, L.S., & Glovinsky, P.B. (1987). A behavioral perspective on insomnia treatment. *Psychiatric Clinics of North America, 10,* 541–553.

14. National Institutes of Health. (n.d.). Measures. Retrieved from http://www.nihpromis.org/measures/measureshome

15. Allison, P.J., Nicolau, B., Edgar, L., Archer, J., Black, M., & Hier, M. (2004). Teaching head and neck cancer patients coping strategies: Results of a feasibility study. *Oral Oncology, 40,* 538–544. doi:10.1016/j.oraloncology.2003.11.008

16. Arving, C., Sjoden, P.O., Bergh, J., Hellbom, M., Johansson, B., Glimelius, B., & Brandberg, Y. (2007). Individual psychosocial support for breast cancer patients: A randomized study of nurse versus psychologist interventions and standard care. *Cancer Nursing, 30,* E10–E19. doi:10.1097/01.NCC.0000270709.64790.05

17. Barsevick, A., Beck, S.L., Dudley, W.N., Wong, B., Berger, A.M., Whitmer, K., ... Stewart, K. (2010). Efficacy of an intervention for fatigue and sleep disturbance during cancer chemotherapy. *Journal of Pain and Symptom Management, 40,* 200–216. doi:10.1016/j.jpainsymman.2009.12.020

18. Berger, A.M., Kuhn, B.R., Farr, L.A., Lynch, J.C., Agrawal, S., Chamberlain, J., & Von Essen, S.G. (2009). Behavioral therapy intervention trial to improve sleep quality and cancer-related fatigue. *Psycho-Oncology, 18,* 634–646. doi:10.1002/pon.1438

19. Berger, A.M., Kuhn, B.R., Farr, L.A., Von Essen, S., Chamberlain, J., Lynch, J.C., & Agrawal, S. (2009). One-year outcomes of a behavioral therapy intervention trial to improve sleep quality and cancer-related fatigue. *Journal of Clinical Oncology, 27,* 6033–6040. doi:10.1200/JCO.2008.20.8306

20. Berger, A.M., VonEssen, S., Kuhn, B.R., Piper, B.F., Farr, L., Agrawal, S., ... Higginbotham, P. (2003). Adherence, sleep, and fatigue outcomes after adjuvant breast cancer chemotherapy: Results of a feasibility intervention study. *Oncology Nursing Forum, 30,* 513–522. doi:10.1188/03.ONF.513-522

21. Berger, A.M., VonEssen, S., Kuhn, B.R., Piper, B.F., Farr, L., Agrawal, S., ... Higginbotham, P. (2002). Feasibility of a sleep intervention during adjuvant breast cancer chemotherapy. *Oncology Nursing Forum, 29,* 1431–1441. doi:10.1188/02.ONF.1431-1441

22. Carpenter, J.S., Neal, J.G., Payne, J., Kimmick, G., & Storniolo, A.M. (2007). Cognitive-behavioral intervention for hot flashes. *Oncology Nursing Forum, 34,* E1–E8. doi:10.1188/07.ONF.E1-E8

23. Cohen, M., & Fried, G. (2007). Comparing relaxation training and cognitive-behavioral group therapy for women with breast cancer. *Research on Social Work Practice, 17,* 313–323. doi:10.1177/1049731506293741

24. Dalton, J.A., Keefe, F.J., Carlson, J., & Youngblood, R. (2004). Tailoring cognitive-behavioral treatment for cancer pain. *Pain Management Nursing, 5,* 3–18. doi:10.1016/S1524-9042(03)00027-4

25. Davidson, J.R., Waisberg, J.L., Brundage, M.D., & MacLean, A.W. (2001). Nonpharmacologic group treatment of insomnia: A preliminary study with cancer survivors. *Psycho-Oncology, 10,* 389–397. doi:10.1002/pon.525

26. Dirksen, S.R., & Epstein, D.R. (2008). Efficacy of an insomnia intervention on fatigue, mood and quality of life in breast cancer survivors. *Journal of Advanced Nursing, 61,* 664–675. doi:10.1111/j.1365-2648.2007.04560.x

27. Epstein, D.R., & Dirksen, S.R. (2007). Randomized trial of a cognitive-behavioral intervention for insomnia in breast cancer survivors. *Oncology Nursing Forum, 34,* E51–E59. doi:10.1188/07.ONF.E51-E59

28. Espie, C.A., Fleming, L., Cassidy, J., Samuel, L., Taylor, L.M., White, C.A., ... Paul, J. (2008). Randomized controlled clinical effectiveness trial of cognitive behavior therapy compared with treatment as usual for persistent insomnia in patients with cancer. *Journal of Clinical Oncology, 26,* 4651–4658. doi:10.1200/JCO.2007.13.9006

29. Fiorentino, L., McQuaid, J.R., Liu, L., Natarajan, L., He, F., Cornejo, M., ... Ancoli-Israel, S. (2009). Individual cognitive behavioral therapy for insomnia in breast cancer survivors: A randomized controlled crossover pilot study. *Nature and Science of Sleep, 2010*(2), 1–8. doi:10.2147/NSS.S8004

30. Kwekkeboom, K.L., Cherwin, C.H., Lee, J.W., & Wanta, B. (2010). Mind-body treatments for the pain-fatigue-sleep disturbance symptom cluster in persons with cancer. *Journal of Pain and Symptom Management, 39*, 126–138. doi:10.1016/j.jpainsymman.2009.05.022

31. Kwekkeboom, K.L., Abbott-Anderson, K., Cherwin, C., Roiland, R., Serlin, R.C., & Ward, S.E. (2012). Pilot randomized controlled trial of a patient-controlled cognitive-behavioral intervention for the pain, fatigue, and sleep disturbance symptom cluster in cancer. *Journal of Pain and Symptom Management, 44*, 810–822. doi:10.1016/j.jpainsymman.2011.12.281

32. Langford, D.J., Lee, K., & Miaskowski, C. (2012). Sleep disturbance interventions in oncology patients and family caregivers: A comprehensive review and meta-analysis. *Sleep Medicine Reviews, 16*, 397–414. doi:10.1016/j.smrv.2011.07.002

33. Quesnel, C., Savard, J., Simard, S., Ivers, H., & Morin, C.M. (2003). Efficacy of cognitive-behavioral therapy for insomnia in women treated for nonmetastatic breast cancer. *Journal of Consulting and Clinical Psychology, 71*, 189–200. doi:10.1037/0022-006X.71.1.189

34. Ritterband, L.M., Bailey, E.T., Thorndike, F.P., Lord, H.R., Farrell-Carnahan, L., & Baum, L.D. (2012). Initial evaluation of an Internet intervention to improve the sleep of cancer survivors with insomnia. *Psycho-Oncology, 21*, 695–705. doi:10.1002/pon.1969

35. Savard, J., Simard, S., Ivers, H., & Morin, C.M. (2005). Randomized study on the efficacy of cognitive-behavioral therapy for insomnia secondary to breast cancer, part I: Sleep and psychological effects. *Journal of Clinical Oncology, 23*, 6083–6096. doi:10.1200/JCO.2005.09.548

36. Savard, J., Simard, S., Giguère, I., Ivers, H., Morin, C.M., Maunsell, E., ... Marceau, D. (2006). Randomized clinical trial on cognitive therapy for depression in women with metastatic breast cancer: Psychological and immunological effects. *Palliative and Supportive Care, 4*, 219–237. doi:10.1017/S1478951506060305

37. Savard, J., Villa, J., Simard, S., Ivers, H., & Morin, C.M. (2011). Feasibility of a self-help treatment for insomnia comorbid with cancer. *Psycho-Oncology, 20*, 1013–1019. doi:10.1002/pon.1818

38. Vilela, L.D., Nicolau, B., Mahmud, S., Edgar, L., Hier, M., Black, M., ... Allison, P.J. (2006). Comparison of psychosocial outcomes in head and neck cancer patients receiving a coping strategies intervention and control subjects receiving no intervention. *Journal of Otolaryngology, 35*, 88–96. doi:10.2310/7070.2005.5002

39. Wanchai, A., Armer, J.M., & Stewart, B.R. (2011). Nonpharmacologic supportive strategies to promote quality of life in patients experiencing cancer-related fatigue: A systematic review. *Clinical Journal of Oncology Nursing, 15*, 203–214. doi:10.1188/11.CJON.203-214

40. National Cancer Institute. (2014, April 23). Sleep disorders (PDQ®) [Health professional version]. Retrieved from http://www.cancer.gov/cancertopics/pdq/supportivecare/sleepdisorders/HealthProfessional

41. Manas, A., Ciria, J.P., Fernandez, M.C., Gonzalvez, M.L., Morillo, V., Perez, M., ... TENOR collaborative study group. (2011). Post hoc analysis of pregabalin vs. non-pregabalin treatment in patients with cancer-related neuropathic pain: Better pain relief, sleep and physical health. *Clinical and Translational Oncology, 13*, 656–663. doi:10.1007/s12094-011-0711-0

42. Cankurtaran, E.S., Ozalp, E., Soygur, H., Akbiyik, D.I., Turhan, L., & Alkis, N. (2008). Mirtazapine improves sleep and lowers anxiety and depression in cancer patients: Superiority over imipramine. *Supportive Care in Cancer, 16*, 1291–1298. doi:10.1007/s00520-008-0425-1

43. Kim, S., Shin, I., Kim, J., Kim, Y., Kim, K., Kim, K., Yang, S., ... Yoon, J. (2008). Effectiveness of mirtazapine for nausea and insomnia in cancer

patients with depression. *Psychiatry and Clinical Neurosciences, 62,* 75–83. doi:10.1111/j.1440-1819.2007.01778.x

44. Palesh, O.G., Mustian, K.M., Peppone, L.J., Janelsins, M., Sprod, L.K., Kesler, S., … Morrow, G.R. (2012). Impact of paroxetine on sleep problems in 426 cancer patients receiving chemotherapy: A trial from the University of Rochester Cancer Center Community Clinical Oncology Program. *Sleep Medicine, 13,* 1184–1190. doi:10.1016/j.sleep.2012.06.001

45. Tanimukai, H., Murai, T., Okazaki, N., Matsuda, Y., Okamoto, Y., Kabeshita, Y., … Tsuneto, S. (2013). An observational study of insomnia and nightmare treated with trazodone in patients with advanced cancer. *American Journal of Hospice and Palliative Care, 30,* 359–362. doi:10.1177/1049909112452334

46. Carpenter, J.S., Storniolo, A.M., Johns, S., Monahan, P.O., Azzouz, F., Elam, J.L., … Shelton, R.C. (2007). Randomized, double-blind, placebo-controlled crossover trials of venlafaxine for hot flashes after breast cancer. *Oncologist, 12,* 124–135. doi:10.1634/theoncologist.12-1-124

47. Joffe, H., Partridge, A., Giobbie-Hurder, A., Li, X., Habin, K., Goss, P., … Garber, J. (2010). Augmentation of venlafaxine and selective serotonin reuptake inhibitors with zolpidem improves sleep and quality of life in breast cancer patients with hot flashes: A randomized, double-blind, placebo-controlled trial. *Menopause, 17,* 908–916. doi:10.1097/gme.0b013e3181dbee1b

48. Pasquini, M., Speca, A., & Biondi, M. (2009). Quetiapine for tamoxifen-induced insomnia in women with breast cancer. *Psychosomatics, 50,* 159–161. doi:10.1176/appi.psy.50.2.159

49. de Oliveira Campos, M.P., Riechelmann, R., Martins, L.C., Hassan, B.J., Casa, F.B., & Del Giglio, A. (2011). Guarana (*Paullinia cupana*) improves fatigue in breast cancer patients undergoing systemic chemotherapy. *Journal of Alternative and Complementary Medicine, 17,* 505–512. doi:10.1089/acm.2010.0571

50. Can, G., Topuz, E., Derin, D., Durna, Z., & Aydiner, A. (2009). Effect of kefir on the quality of life of patients being treated for colorectal cancer. *Oncology Nursing Forum, 36,* E335–E342. doi:10.1188/09.ONF.E335-E342

51. Barton, D.L., Atherton, P.J., Bauer, B.A., Moore, D.F., Jr., Mattar, B.I., Lavasseur, B.I., … Loprinzi, C.L. (2011). The use of *Valeriana officinalis* (valerian) in improving sleep in patients who are undergoing treatment for cancer: A phase III randomized, placebo-controlled, double-blind study (NCCTG Trial, N01C5). *Journal of Supportive Oncology, 9,* 24–31. doi:10.1016/j.suponc.2010.12.008

52. Cerrone, R., Giani, L., Galbiati, B., Messina, G., Casiraghi, M., Proserpio, E., … Gardani, G. (2008). Efficacy of HT 7 point acupressure stimulation in the treatment of insomnia in cancer patients and in patients suffering from disorders other than cancer. *Minerva Medica, 99,* 535–537. Retrieved from http://www.minervamedica.it/en/journals/minerva-medica/article.php?cod=R10Y2008N06A0535

53. Frisk, J., Kallstrom, A.C., Wall, N., Fredrikson, M., & Hammar, M. (2012). Acupuncture improves health-related quality-of-life (HRQoL) and sleep in women with breast cancer and hot flashes. *Supportive Care in Cancer, 20,* 715–724. doi:10.1007/s00520-011-1134-8

54. Beer, T.M., Benavides, M., Emmons, S.L., Hayes, M., Liu, G., Garzotto, M., … Eilers, K. (2010). Acupuncture for hot flashes in patients with prostate cancer. *Urology, 76,* 1182–1188. doi:10.1016/j.urology.2010.03.033

55. de Valois, B.A., Young, T.E., Robinson, N., McCourt, C., & Maher, E.J. (2010). Using traditional acupuncture for breast cancer-related hot flashes and night sweats. *Journal of Alternative and Complementary Medicine, 16,* 1047–1057. doi:10.1089/acm.2009.0472

56. Feng, Y., Wang, X.Y., Li, S.D., Zhang, Y., Wang, H.M., Li, M., … Zhang, Z. (2011). Clinical research of acupuncture on malignant tumor patients for improving depression and sleep quality. *Journal of Traditional Chinese Medicine, 31,* 199–202. doi:10.1016/S0254-6272(11)60042-3

57. Garcia, M.K., McQuade, J., Haddad, R., Patel, S., Lee, R., Yang, P., ... Cohen, L. (2013). Systematic review of acupuncture in cancer care: A synthesis of the evidence. *Journal of Clinical Oncology, 31,* 952–960. doi:10.1200/JCO.2012.43.5818

58. Otte, J.L., Carpenter, J.S., Zhong, X., & Johnstone, P.A. (2011). Feasibility study of acupuncture for reducing sleep disturbances and hot flashes in postmenopausal breast cancer survivors. *Clinical Nurse Specialist, 25,* 228–236. doi:10.1097/NUR.0b013e318229950b

59. Lyon, D.E., Schubert, C., & Taylor, A.G. (2010). Pilot study of cranial stimulation for symptom management in breast cancer. *Oncology Nursing Forum, 37,* 476–483. doi:10.1188/10.ONF.476-483

60. Alvarez, J., Meyer, F.L., Granoff, D.L., & Lundy, A. (2013). The effect of EEG biofeedback on reducing postcancer cognitive impairment. *Integrative Cancer Therapies, 12,* 475–487. doi:10.1177/1534735413477192

61. Cheville, A.L., Kollasch, J., Vandenberg, J., Shen, T., Grothey, A., Gamble, G., & Basford, J.R. (2013). A home-based exercise program to improve function, fatigue, and sleep quality in patients with stage IV lung and colorectal cancer: A randomized controlled trial. *Journal of Pain and Symptom Management, 45,* 811–821. doi:10.1016/j.jpainsymman.2012.05.006

62. Coleman, E.A., Coon, S., Hall-Barrow, J., Richards, K., Gaylor, D., & Stewart, B. (2003). Feasibility of exercise during treatment for multiple myeloma. *Cancer Nursing, 26,* 410–419. doi:10.1097/00002820-200310000-00012

63. Courneya, K.S., Sellar, C.M., Trinh, L., Forbes, C.C., Stevinson, C., McNeely, M.L., ... Reiman, T. (2012). A randomized trial of aerobic exercise and sleep quality in lymphoma patients receiving chemotherapy or no treatments. *Cancer Epidemiology, Biomarkers and Prevention, 21,* 887–894. doi:10.1158/1055-9965.EPI-12-0075

64. Kwiatkowski, F., Mouret-Reynier, M.A., Duclos, M., Leger-Enreille, A., Bridon, F., Hahn, T., ... Bignon, Y.J. (2013). Long term improved quality of life by a 2-week physical and educational intervention shortly after breast cancer chemotherapy completion. Results of the 'Programme of Accompanying women after breast Cancer treatment completion in Thermal resorts' (PACThe) randomised clinical trial of 251 patients. *European Journal of Cancer, 49,* 1530–1538. doi:10.1016/j.ejca.2012.12.021

65. Mishra, S.I., Scherer, R.W., Geigle, P.M., Berlanstein, D.R., Topaloglu, O., Gotay, C.C., & Snyder, C. (2012). Exercise interventions on health-related quality of life for cancer survivors. *Cochrane Database of Systematic Reviews, 2012*(8). doi:10.1002/14651858.CD007566.pub2

66. Mock, V., Dow, K.H., Meares, C.J., Grimm, P.M., Dienemann, J.A., Haisfield-Wolfe, M.E., ... Gage, I. (1997). Effects of exercise on fatigue, physical functioning, and emotional distress during radiation therapy for breast cancer. *Oncology Nursing Forum, 24,* 991–1000.

67. Payne, J.K., Held, J., Thorpe, J., & Shaw, H. (2008). Effect of exercise on biomarkers, fatigue, sleep disturbances, and depressive symptoms in older women with breast cancer receiving hormonal therapy. *Oncology Nursing Forum, 35,* 635–642. doi:10.1188/08.ONF.635-642

68. Rabin, C., Pinto, B., Dunsinger, S., Nash, J., & Trask, P. (2009). Exercise and relaxation intervention for breast cancer survivors: Feasibility, acceptability, and effects. *Psycho-Oncology, 18,* 258–266. doi:10.1002/pon.1341

69. Rajotte, E.J., Yi, J.C., Baker, K.S., Gregerson, L., Leiserowitz, A., & Syrjala, K.L. (2012). Community-based exercise program effectiveness and safety for cancer survivors. *Journal of Cancer Survivorship: Research and Practice, 6,* 219–228. doi:10.1007/s11764-011-0213-7

70. Sprod, L.K., Palesh, O.G., Janelsins, M.C., Peppone, L.J., Heckler, C.E., Adams, M.J., ... Mustian, K.M. (2010). Exercise, sleep quality, and mediators of sleep in breast and prostate cancer patients receiving radiation therapy. *Community Oncology, 7,* 463–471. doi:10.1016/S1548-5315(11)70427-2

71. Tang, M.-F., Liou, T.-H., & Lin, C.-C. (2010). Improving sleep quality for cancer patients: Benefits of a home-based exercise intervention. *Supportive Care in Cancer, 18,* 1329–1339. doi:10.1007/s00520-009-0757-5

72. Wang, Y.J., Boehmke, M., Wu, Y.W., Dickerson, S.S., & Fisher, N. (2011). Effects of a 6-week walking program on Taiwanese women newly diagnosed with early-stage breast cancer. *Cancer Nursing, 34,* E1–E13. doi:10.1097/NCC.0b013e3181e4588d

73. Wenzel, J.A., Griffith, K.A., Shang, J., Thompson, C.B., Hedlin, H., Stewart, K.J., … Mock, V. (2013). Impact of a home-based walking intervention on outcomes of sleep quality, emotional distress, and fatigue in patients undergoing treatment for solid tumors. *Oncologist, 18,* 476–484. doi:10.1634/theoncologist.2012-0278

74. Young-McCaughan, S., Mays, M.Z., Arzola, S.M., Yoder, L.H., Dramiga, S.A., Leclerc, K.M., … Leclerc, K.M. (2003). Research and commentary: Change in exercise tolerance, activity and sleep patterns, and quality of life in patients with cancer participating in a structured exercise program. *Oncology Nursing Forum, 30,* 441–454. doi:10.1188/03.ONF.441-454

75. de Moor, C., Sterner, J., Hall, M., Warneke, C., Gilani, Z., Amato, R., & Cohen, L. (2002). A pilot study of the effects of expressive writing on psychological and behavioral adjustment in patients enrolled in a Phase II trial of vaccine therapy for metastatic renal cell carcinoma. *Health Psychology, 21,* 615–619. doi:10.1037/0278-6133.21.6.615

76. de Moor, J.S., Moyé, L., Low, M.D., Rivera, E., Singletary, S.E., Fouladi, R.T., & Cohen, L. (2008). Expressive writing as a presurgical stress management intervention for breast cancer patients. *Journal of the Society for Integrative Oncology, 6,* 59–66.

77. Low, C.A., Stanton, A.L., Bower, J.E., & Gyllenhammer, L. (2010). A randomized controlled trial of emotionally expressive writing for women with metastatic breast cancer. *Health Psychology, 29,* 460–466. doi:10.1037/a0020153

78. Mosher, C.E., Duhamel, K.N., Lam, J., Dickler, M., Li, Y., Massie, M.J., & Norton, L. (2012). Randomised trial of expressive writing for distressed metastatic breast cancer patients. *Psychology and Health, 27,* 88–100. doi:10.1080/08870446.2010.551212

79. van den Berg, M., Visser, A., Schoolmeesters, A., Edelman, P., & van den Borne, B. (2006). Evaluation of haptotherapy for patients with cancer treated with chemotherapy at a day clinic. *Patient Education and Counseling, 60,* 336–343. doi:10.1016/j.pec.2005.10.012

80. Weze, C., Leathard, H.L., Grange, J., Tiplady, P., & Stevens, G. (2004). Evaluation of healing by gentle touch in 35 clients with cancer. *European Journal of Oncology Nursing, 8,* 40–49. doi:10.1016/j.ejon.2003.10.004

81. Jane, S.W., Chen, S.L., Wilkie, D.J., Lin, Y.C., Foreman, S.W., Beaton, R.D., … Llao, M.N. (2011). Effects of massage on pain, mood status, relaxation, and sleep in Taiwanese patients with metastatic bone pain: A randomized clinical trial. *Pain, 152,* 2432–2442. doi:10.1016/j.pain.2011.06.021

82. Smith, M.C., Kemp, J., Hemphill, L. & Vojir, C.P. (2002). Outcomes of therapeutic massage for hospitalized cancer patients. *Journal of Nursing Scholarship 34,* 257–262. doi:10.1111/j.1547-5069.2002.00257.x

83. Soden, K., Vincent, K., Craske, S., Lucas, C., & Ashley, S. (2004). A randomized controlled trial of aromatherapy massage in a hospice setting. *Palliative Medicine, 18,* 87–92. doi:10.1191/0269216304pm874oa

84. Sturgeon, M., Wetta-Hall, R., Hart, T., Good, M., & Dakhil, S. (2009). Effects of therapeutic massage on the quality of life among patients with breast cancer during treatment. *Journal of Alternative and Complementary Medicine, 15,* 373–380. doi:10.1089/acm.2008.0399

85. Chen, Z., Meng, Z., Milbury, K., Bei, W., Zhang, Y., Thornton, B., … Cohen, L. (2013). Qigong improves quality of life in women undergoing radiotherapy for breast cancer: Results of a randomized controlled trial. *Cancer, 119,* 1690–1698. doi:10.1002/cncr.27904

86. Andersen, S.R., Wurtzen, H., Steding-Jessen, M., Christensen, J., Andersen, K.K., Flyger, H., … Dalton, S.O. (2013). Effect of mindfulness-based stress reduction on sleep quality: Results of a randomized trial among Danish breast cancer patients. *Acta Oncologica, 52,* 336–344. doi:10.3109/0284186X.2012.745948

87. Carlson, L.E., & Garland, S.N. (2005). Impact of mindfulness-based stress reduction (MBSR) on sleep, mood, stress and fatigue symptoms in cancer outpatients. *International Journal of Behavioral Medicine, 12,* 278–285. doi:10.1207/s15327558ijbm1204_9

88. Carlson, L.E., Speca, M., Patel, K.D., & Goodey, E. (2003). Mindfulness-based stress reduction in relation to quality of life, mood, symptoms of stress, and immune parameters in breast and prostate cancer outpatients. *Psychosomatic Medicine, 65,* 571–581. doi:10.1097/01.PSY .0000074003.35911.41

89. Carlson, L.E., Speca, M., Patel, K.D., & Goodey, E. (2004). Mindfulness-based stress reduction in relation to quality of life, mood, symptoms of stress and levels of cortisol, dehydroepiandrosterone sulfate (DHEAS) and melatonin in breast and prostate cancer outpatients. *Psychoneuroendocrinology, 29,* 448–474. doi:10.1016/S0306-4530(03)00054-4

90. Lengacher, C.A., Reich, R.R., Post-White, J., Moscoso, M., Shelton, M.M., Barta, M., … Budhrani, P. (2012). Mindfulness based stress reduction in post-treatment breast cancer patients: An examination of symptoms and symptom clusters. *Journal of Behavioral Medicine, 35,* 86–94. doi:10.1007/ s10865-011-9346-4

91. Nakamura, Y., Lipschitz, D.L., Kuhn, R., Kinney, A.Y., & Donaldson, G.W. (2013). Investigating efficacy of two brief mind-body intervention programs for managing sleep disturbance in cancer survivors: A pilot randomized controlled trial. *Journal of Cancer Survivorship: Research and Practice, 7,* 165–182. doi:10.1007/s11764-012-0252-8

92. Shapiro, S.L., Bootzin, R.R., Figueredo, A.J., Lopez, A.M., & Schwartz, G.E. (2003). The efficacy of mindfulness-based stress reduction in the treatment of sleep disturbance in women with breast cancer: An exploratory study. *Journal of Psychosomatic Research, 54,* 85–91. doi:10.1016/ S0022-3999(02)00546-9

93. Winbush, N.Y., Gross, C.R., & Kreitzer, M.J. (2007). The effects of mindfulness-based stress reduction on sleep disturbance: A systematic review. *Explore, 3,* 585–591. doi:10.1016/j.explore.2007.08.003

94. Cannici, J., Malcolm, R., & Peek, L.A. (1983). Treatment of insomnia in cancer patients using muscle relaxation training. *Journal of Behavioral Therapy and Experimental Psychiatry, 14,* 251–256. doi:1016/0005 -7916(83)90056-3

95. Demiralp, M., Oflaz, F., & Komurcu, S. (2010). Effects of relaxation training on sleep quality and fatigue in patients with breast cancer undergoing adjuvant chemotherapy. *Journal of Clinical Nursing, 19,* 1073–1083. doi:10.1111/j.1365-2702.2009.03037.x

96. Bruera, E., Yennurajalingam, S., Palmer, J.L., Perez-Cruz, P.E., Frisbee-Hume, S., Allo, J.A., … Cohen, M.Z. (2013). Methylphenidate and/ or a nursing telephone intervention for fatigue in patients with advanced cancer: A randomized, placebo-controlled, phase II trial. *Journal of Clinical Oncology, 31,* 2421–2427. doi:10.2100/JCO.2012.45.3696

97. Kim, Y., Roscoe, J.A., & Morrow, G.R. (2002). The effects of information and negative affect on severity of side effects from radiation therapy for prostate cancer. *Supportive Care in Cancer, 10,* 416–421. doi:10.1007/ s00520-002-0359-y

98. Kwekkeboom, K.L., Abbott-Anderson, K., & Wanta, B. (2010). Feasibility of a patient-controlled cognitive-behavioral intervention for pain, fatigue, and sleep disturbance in cancer. *Oncology Nursing Forum, 37,* E151–E159. doi:10.1188/10.ONF.E151-E159

99. Simeit, R., Deck, R., & Conta-Marx, B. (2004). Sleep management training for cancer patients with insomnia. *Supportive Care in Cancer, 12,* 176–183. doi:10.1007/s00520-004-0594-5

100. Williams, S.A., & Schreier, A.M. (2005). The role of education in managing fatigue, anxiety, and sleep disorders in women undergoing chemotherapy for breast cancer. *Applied Nursing Research, 18,* 138–147. doi:10.1016/ j.apnr.2004.08.005

101. Serra, D., Parris, C.R., Carper, E., Homel, P., Fleishman, S.B., Harrison, L.B., & Chadha, M. (2012). Outcomes of guided imagery in patients receiving radiation therapy for breast cancer. *Clinical Journal of Oncology Nursing, 16,* 617–623. doi:10.1188/12.CJON.617-623

102. Haest, K., Kumar, A., Van Calster, B., Leunen, K., Smeets, A., Amant, F., … Neven, P. (2012). Stellate ganglion block for the management of hot flashes and sleep disturbances in breast cancer survivors: An uncontrolled experimental study with 24 weeks of follow-up. *Annals of Oncology, 23,* 1449–1454. doi:10.1093/annonc/mdr478

103. Lipov, E.G., Joshi, J.R., Sanders, S., Wilcox, K., Lipov, S., Xie, H., … Slavin, K. (2008). Effects of stellate-ganglion block on hot flushes and night awakenings in survivors of breast cancer: A pilot study. *Lancet Oncology, 9,* 523–532. doi:10.1016/S1470-2045(08)70131-1

104. Fobair, P., Koopman, C., DiMiceli, S., O'Hanlan, K., Butler, L.D., Classen, C., … Spiegel, D. (2002). Psychosocial intervention for lesbians with primary breast cancer. *Psycho-Oncology, 11,* 427–438. doi:10.1002/pon.624

105. Yang, H.-L., Chen, X.-P., Lee, K.-C., Fang, F.-F., & Chao, Y.-F. (2010). The effects of warm-water footbath on relieving fatigue and insomnia of the gynecologic cancer patients on chemotherapy. *Cancer Nursing, 33,* 454–460. doi:10.1097/NCC.0b013e3181d761c1

106. Bower, J.E., Garet, D., Sternlieb, B., Ganz, P.A., Irwin, M.R., Olmstead, R., & Greendale, G. (2012). Yoga for persistent fatigue in breast cancer survivors: A randomized controlled trial. *Cancer, 118,* 3766–3775. doi:10.1002/cncr.26702

107. Buffart, L.M., van Uffelen, J.G., Riphagen, I.I., van Mechelen, W., Brown, W.J., & Chinapaw, M.J. (2012). Physical and psychosocial benefits of yoga in cancer patients and survivors, a systematic review and meta-analysis of randomized controlled trials. *BMC Cancer, 12,* 559. doi:10.1186/1471-2407-12-559

108. Carson, J.W., Carson, K.M., Porter, L.S., Keefe, F.J., & Seewaldt, V.L. (2009). Yoga of Awareness program for menopausal symptoms in breast cancer survivors: Results from a randomized trial. *Supportive Care in Cancer, 17,* 1301–1309. doi:10.1007/s00520-009-0587-5

109. Cohen, L., Warneke, C., Fouladi, R.T., Rodriguez, M.A., & Chaoul-Reich, A. (2004). Psychological adjustment and sleep quality in a randomized trial of the effects of a Tibetan yoga intervention in patients with lymphoma. *Cancer, 100,* 2253–2260. doi:10.1002/cncr.20236

110. Dhruva, A., Miaskowski, C., Abrams, D., Acree, M., Cooper, B., Goodman, S., & Hecht, F.M. (2012). Yoga breathing for cancer chemotherapy-associated symptoms and quality of life: Results of a pilot randomized controlled trial. *Journal of Alternative and Complementary Medicine, 18,* 473–479. doi:10.1089/acm.2011.0555

111. Mustian, K.M., Sprod, L.K., Janelsins, M., Peppone, L.J., Palesh, O.G., Chandwani, K., … Morrow, G.R. (2013). Multicenter, randomized controlled trial of yoga for sleep quality among cancer survivors. *Journal of Clinical Oncology, 31,* 3233–3241. doi:10.1200/JCO.2012.43.7707.

112. Zhang, J., Yang, K.-H., Tian, J.-H., & Wang, C.-M. (2012). Effects of yoga on psychologic function and quality of life in women with breast cancer: A meta-analysis of randomized controlled trials. *Journal of Alternative and Complementary Medicine, 18,* 994–1002. doi:10.1089/acm.2011.0514

113. National Sleep Foundation. (2013). Sleep hygiene. Retrieved from www.sleepfoundation.org/article/ask-the-expert/sleep-hygiene

Index

The letter f after a page number indicates that relevant content appears in a figure.